Out of Operating Room Anesthesia

Basavana G. Goudra • Preet Mohinder Singh

Editors

Out of Operating Room Anesthesia

A Comprehensive Review

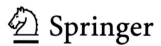 Springer

Editors
Basavana Goudra, MD, FRCA, FCARCSI
Associate Professor of Anesthesiology and
Critical Care Medicine
Perelman School of Medicine
Hospital of the University of Pennsylvania
Philadelphia
PA
USA

Preet Mohinder Singh
All India Inst. Med. Sci. (AIIMS)
New Delhi
Delhi
India

ISBN 978-3-319-39148-9   ISBN 978-3-319-39150-2   (eBook)
DOI 10.1007/978-3-319-39150-2

Library of Congress Control Number: 2016954334

Printed on acid-free paper

This Springer imprint is published by Springer Nature
The registered company is Springer International Publishing AG Switzerland
The registered company address is: Gewerbestrasse 11, 6330 Cham, Switzerland

Foreword

Out of Operating Room Anesthesia: A Comprehensive Review (*OORA*) discusses the delivery of anesthesia care for surgery and invasive diagnostic and therapeutic procedures in areas other than in the standard operating room. Delivery of anesthesia care in these settings is a widely accepted practice that has grown by leaps and bound in recent years, and will certainly continue to grow in the years to come. This growth brings with it new challenges that are unique to this field. In particular, as the delivery of care outside the typical operating room environment has become more commonplace, so has the tendency to undertake more complex surgeries and procedures with increasingly complicated (ASA III-IV, debilitated and elderly) patients. For example, the procedure may only be a colonoscopy. However, in a patient who is 157 cm (5′ 2″) and weighs 118 kg (260 lbs) with a history of sleep apnea and a Mallampati III airway, the risk of a respiratory arrest with minimal sedation is nontrivial. The pressures to care for significant numbers of patients daily in the out of operating room setting while maintaining the same safety and quality standards expected in the operating room create an enormous challenge. Therefore, now is the perfect time to codify in a monograph, practices and principles that can guide the delivery of patient care in this now significant segment of anesthesiology.

OORA provides a much-needed guide to the important specialty of out of operating room anesthesia care. Dr. Goudra has done an outstanding job compiling a comprehensive set of topics and presenting them in a way that is easy for any anesthesia caregiver to readily comprehend, and most importantly, place into practice. The contributing authors are all well-respected practitioners in out of the operating room anesthesia care from the United States and Ireland. The monograph consists of 32 chapters organized in 8 logical parts. Parts 1 and 2 lay out, respectively, general principles and specific patient safety concerns administering anesthesia care to patients outside of the operating room. Much of the core management material is presented in Parts 3–5 in the monograph where the authors discuss anesthesia care for gastroenterology (Part 3), cardiac (Part 4) and neuroradiology (Part 5) procedures. Parts 6 and 7 describe the management of selected special cases, whereas Part 8 outlines the enormous possibilities for anesthesiology research in areas outside of the operating room. Dr. Goudra and colleagues have expanded into a monograph a significant volume of material that typically appears in only a few chapters in a standard anesthesiology textbook.

Dr. Goudra is uniquely qualified to write and edit OORA. He draws upon more than 20 years of experience as an anesthesiologist practicing in India, Ireland, the United Kingdom, and the United States. In addition to being an experienced practitioner in the out of operating room setting, he has devised a number of anesthesia innovations including novel designs for a bite block, airway, and a mask airway. I recently spent time with Dr. Goudra in the operating room at the University of Pennsylvania to learn first-hand his approaches for managing total intravenous anesthesia. It is without question time very well spent!

I strongly support and endorse the work that Dr. Goudra and his colleagues have so nicely assembled in OORA. It is a must read for anesthesiologists, residents, fellows, and nurse anesthetists to gain up-to-date, step-by-step management recommendations for delivering anesthesia care outside the operating room. OORA is an important contribution to maintaining and improving care in this now significant segment of anesthesiology practice.

Sincerely,
Emery N. Brown, MD, PhD
Warren M. Zapol Professor of Anaesthesia
Harvard Medical School
Department of Anesthesia, Critical Care and Pain Medicine
Massachusetts General Hospital
Edward Hood Taplin Professor of Medical Engineering
Institute for Medical Engineering and Science
Professor of Computational Neuroscience
Picower Institute for Learning and Memory
Department of Brain and Cognitive Sciences
Massachusetts Institute of Technology
May 2016

Preface

Out of operating room anesthesia challenges are discussed in almost all anesthesia textbooks. Moreover, there are at least two books dedicated to the area already available. With this in the background, one might wonder the necessity and timeliness of yet another book. The project can only be justified with one or more of the following three criteria and we hope that all three are met in this maiden edition.

The field of out of operating room anesthesia has evolved beyond belief. About two decades ago, most gastrointestinal (GI) endoscopic procedures were diagnostic and performed either awake or after administration of midazolam. Nearly all neuroradiological procedures were diagnostic scans, occasionally requiring sedation or general anesthesia. Electrophysiological procedures were largely restricted to cardioversions and pacemaker insertions. As we fast-forward two decades, the array of procedures performed in all these areas is of epic proportions. Therapeutic GI endoscopic procedures are performed in large numbers on a daily basis. Apart from highly evolved pacemaker insertions and reinsertions, the growth in the area of cardiac ablation is phenomenal. Neuroradiological approaches involving coils and stents have already limited the scope of neurosurgery. Thoracic surgery has seen a major decline as a result of therapeutic bronchoscopy. The ongoing research promises that 10–20 years henceforth, the out of operating procedures will overtake operating room procedures—both in volume and complexity. In all these locations, the presence of anesthesia provider is ubiquitous. Consequently, there is an absolute need for another dedicated book in the out of operating room area.

Another factor is the content. This book is much more practice oriented. Although topics such as organization, layout, and management of the out of operating room practice are important, we have deliberately left them out. Instead, extensive focus is on the various aspects of administration of anesthesia. As editors, we would like to consider all the chapters as outstanding.

The third reason to write a book is to present the subject matter in a unique style. Wherever appropriate, the chapters are bulleted and we believe that this feature would increase the pleasure of reading. A brief abstract is presented for many chapters summarizing the salient features. Additionally, tables and figures are used as applicable.

Although family support is essential during such endeavors and we appreciate their support, more importantly we would like to acknowledge the precise and dependable assistance provided by Wade Grayson, the developmental editor at Springer. We also appreciate the guidance accorded by Joanna Renwick, Clinical Medicine Editor at Springer. It was a pleasure to work with both of them.

Philadelphia, PA, USA   Basavana Goudra, MD FRCA FCARCSI
New Delhi, Delhi, India   Preet Mohinder Singh, MD DNB

Contents

Contributors

Mian Ahmad Drexel University College of Medicine, Hahnemann University Hospital, Philadelphia, PA, USA

Mansoor M. Aman, MD Department of Anesthesiology and Perioperative Medicine, Drexel University College of Medicine/Hahnemann University Hospital, Philadelphia, PA, USA

Jonathan Anson, MD Anesthesiology and Perioperative Medicine, Penn State Milton S. Hershey Medical Center, Hershey, PA, USA

Shubhangi Arora, MBBS, MD Department of Anesthesia, Brigham and Women's Hospital, Boston, MA, USA

Carlos A. Artime, MD Department of Anesthesiology, McGovern Medical School at The University of Texas Health Science Center at Houston, Houston, TX, USA

Radha Arunkumar, MD Department of Anesthesiology and Perioperative Medicine, The University of Texas MD Anderson Cancer Center, Houston, TX, USA

Maimouna Bah, MD Department of Anesthesiology, Hahnemann University Hospital, Philadelphia, PA, USA

Alexander Bailey, MD Department of Anesthesiology, Emory University Hospital, Atlanta, GA, USA

Carolyn Barbieri, MD Department of Anesthesiology and Perioperative Medicine, Penn State Milton S Hershey Medical Center, Hershey, PA, USA

Kara M. Barnett, MD Department of Anesthesiology and Critical Care Medicine, Memorial Sloan Kettering Cancer Center, New York, NY, USA

John Barrett, MD Department of Emergency Medicine, Hospital of the University of Pennsylvania, Philadelphia, PA, USA

Anuradha Borle Department of Anesthesiology, Pain Medicine and Critical Care, All India Institute of Medical Sciences, New Delhi, Delhi, India

Gwendolyn L. Boyd, MD Department of Anesthesiology and Perioperative Medicine, University of Alabama at Birmingham, UAB Callahan Eye Hospital and University of Alabama Hospital, Birmingham, AL, USA

Melissa Ann Brodsky, MD Department of Anesthesiology and Perioperative Medicine, Drexel University College of Medicine, Hahnemann University Hospital, Wayne, PA, USA

Janette Brohan, MB, BCh, BAO Department of Anaesthesia, Cork University Hospital, Cork, Ireland

Arne O. Budde, MD, DEAA Anesthesiology and Perioperative Medicine, Penn State Milton S Hershey Medical Center, Center for Perioperative Services, Hershey, PA, USA

Jean Gabriel Charchaflieh, MD, PhD Department of Anesthesiology, Yale University School of Medicine, New Haven, CT, USA

Rajiv R. Doshi, MD Department of Anesthesia, Critical Care, and Pain Medicine, Beth Israel Deaconess Medical Center, Boston, MA, USA

Elizabeth W. Duggan, MD Department of Anesthesiology, Emory University Hospital, Atlanta, GA, USA

Michael Duggan, MD Division of Cardiothoracic Anesthesiology, Department of Anesthesiology, Emory University Hospital, Atlanta, GA, USA

George A. Dumas, MD Department of Anesthesiology and Perioperative Medicine, University of Alabama at Birmingham, Birmingham, AL, USA

John Fitzgerald, MB, FRCA, FCAI, EDIC Department of Anesthesia, The Rotunda Hospital, Dublin, Ireland

Monica Ganatra, MD, MPH Department of Anesthesiology, Yale New Haven Hospital, New Haven, CT, USA

Shelley Joseph George, MD Department of Anesthesiology, Hahnemann University Hospital, Philadelphia, PA, USA

Basavana Goudra, MD, FRCA, FCARCSI Department of Anesthesiology and Critical Care Medicine, Hospital of the University of Pennsylvania, Philadelphia, PA, USA

Sprague W. Hazard III , MD Anesthesiology and Perioperative Medicine, Penn State Milton S Hershey Medical Center, Hershey, PA, USA

Nikki Higgins, MB, BSc, FCAI, FJFICMI Department of Anesthesia, The Rotunda Hospital, Dublin, Ireland

McKenzie Hollon, MD Department of Anesthesiology, Emory University Hospital, Atlanta, GA, USA

Nicole Jackman, MD, PhD Department of Anesthesia and Perioperative Care, Brain and Spinal Injury Center (BASIC), University of California, San Francisco, San Francisco, CA, USA

Peter John Lee, MB, BCh, BAO, FCARCSI, MD Department of Anaesthesia, Intensive Care and Pain Medicine, Cork University Hospital, Cork, Ireland

John M. Levenick, MD Department of Anesthesiology and Perioperative Medicine, Penn State Milton S. Hershey Medical Center, Hershey, PA, USA

Todd Justin Liu, BA, MD Anesthesiology and Critical Care Medicine, Memorial Sloan Kettering, New York, NY, USA

John P.R. Loughrey, MB, FCAI, FFPMCAI Department of Anesthesia, The Rotunda Hospital, Dublin, Ireland

Amy Catherine Lu, MD MPH Department of Anesthesiology, Perioperative, and Pain Medicine, Stanford University, Stanford, CA, USA

Julie Mani, MD Department of Anesthesiology, Drexel University College of Medicine, Hahnemann University Hospital, Philadelphia, PA, USA

Mary Elizabeth McAlevy, MD Department of Anesthesiology and Perioperative Medicine, Penn State Milton S. Hershey Medical Center, Hershey, PA, USA

Pascal Owusu-Agyemang, MD Department of Anesthesiology and Perioperative Medicine, The University of Texas MD Anderson Cancer Center, Houston, TX, USA

Jonathan Z. Pan, MD, PhD Department of Anesthesia and Perioperative Care, Brain and Spinal Injury Center (BASIC) University of California, San Francisco, San Francisco, CA, USA

Andrea Riphaus, MD, PhD Department of Medicine, KRH Klinikum Agnes Karll Laatzen, Hannover, Germany

Mona Sarkiss, MD, PhD Department of Anesthesiology and Perioperative Medicine, University of Texas MD Anderson Cancer Center, Houston, TX, USA

Kathy L. Schwock, MD Department of Anesthesiology, Emory University, Atlanta, GA, USA

Bunty Shah, MD Anesthesiology and Perioperative Medicine, Penn State Milton S. Hershey Medical Center, Hershey, PA, USA

Preet Mohinder Singh, MD, DNB, MNAMS Department of Anesthesiology, Critical Care and Pain Medicine, All India Institute of Medical Sciences, New Delhi, Delhi, India

Ashish C. Sinha, MD, PhD, MBA Department of Anesthesiology and Perioperative Medicine, Drexel University College of Medicine/Hahnemann University Hospital, Philadelphia, PA, USA

Erin Springer, MD Department of Anesthesiology, Yale New Haven Hospital, New Haven, CT, USA

Michele L. Sumler, MD Department of Anesthesiology, Emory University Hospital, Atlanta, GA, USA

Rayhan Ahmed Tariq, MD Department of Anesthesiology and Perioperative Medicine, Drexel University College of Medicine, Phiadelphia, PA, USA

Christopher J.D. Tems, MD Department of Emergency Medicine, Hospital of the University of Pennsylvania, Philadelphia, PA, USA

Luis E. Tollinche, MD Anesthesia and Critical Care Medicine, Memorial Sloan Kettering Cancer Center, New York, NY, USA

Anjan Trikha, MD, DA, FICA, MNAMS Department of Anesthesiology, Pain Medicine and Critical Care, All India Institute of Medical Sciences, New Delhi, Delhi, India

Mary Ann Vann, MD Department of Anesthesia, Critical Care, and Pain Medicine, Beth Israel Deaconess Medical Center, Boston, MA, USA

Bharathram Vasudevan, MBBS Department of Anesthesiology, Pain Medicine and Critical Care, All India Institute of Medical Sciences, New Delhi, Delhi, India

Nancy Vinca, MD Department of Anesthesiology, Hospital of the University of Pennsylvania, Philadelphia, PA, USA

Till Wehrmann, MD, PhD Department of Gastroenterology, DKD Helios Klinik Wiesbaden, Wiesbaden, Germany

Gregory E.R. Weller, MD, PhD Department of Anesthesiology & Perioperative Medicine, Penn State Hershey Medical Center, Hershey, PA, USA

Meghan Whitley, DO Anesthesiology and Perioperative Medicine, Penn State Milton S. Hershey Medical Center, Hershey, PA, USA

Igor O. Zhukov, MD Division of Cardiothoracic Anesthesiology, Emory University, Atlanta, GA, USA

Yuriy O. Zhukov, MD Department of Cardiothoracic Surgery, University Hospitals Elyria Medical Center, Elyria, OH, USA

About the Editors

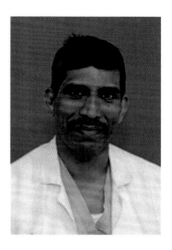

Basavana G. Goudra, MD, FRCA, FCARCSI, is an Associate Professor of Anesthesiology and Critical Care at the University of Pennsylvania's Perelman School of Medicine. He obtained his primary medical education from Bangalore Medical College, Bangalore, India. After training as a junior resident at the prestigious Jawaharlal Institute of Medical Education and Research (JIPMER), Pondicherry, he moved to Ireland for Specialist training. Subsequently, he worked as a fellow in pediatric anesthesia at the Cincinnati Children's Hospital, Cincinnati, Ohio, before moving to the UK to work as a consultant anesthetist at Russells Hall Hospital, NHS, England. His main area of focus is out of operating room anesthesia with an emphasis on anesthesia for endoscopic procedures and total intravenous anesthesia. He has conducted clinical research and published extensively in this area. Additionally, he has invented airway devices "Goudra Bite Block" and "Goudra Mask Airway" that are likely to improve the safety and efficiency of out of operating room anesthesia practice.

Preet M. Singh, MBBS, MD, DNB, is a renowned consultant anesthesiologist working at one of the topmost hospitals in India (All India Institute of Medical Sciences, New Delhi). After obtaining a postgraduate degree in anesthesia in 2010, Dr Singh has been actively contributing and publishing in the field of clinical anesthesia. He has published more than 100 scholarly articles in various well-known international scientific journals. In addition, he has authored multiple chapters on various aspects of anesthesia in many well-known anesthesiology books. His key interest areas include "out of operating room anesthesia," "chronic pain," and "anesthesia for the high risk." His research work in the out of operating room anesthesia field is well recognized and has received numerous citations across the globe.

Part I
General Concepts

Chapter 1
Pharmacology of Sedative Drugs Used in Out of Operating Room Anesthesia

Carlos A. Artime

Abstract Due to the minimally-invasive nature of many out of operating room procedures, patient comfort and appropriate procedural conditions can oftentimes be achieved without general anesthesia. Depending on the nature of the procedure, mild, moderate, or deep sedation may be appropriate. This chapter presents the pharmacology of various drugs used for sedation. Pharmacologic considerations for obese and elderly patients are also presented.

Keywords Sedation • Pharmacology • Midazolam • Fentanyl • Remifentanil • Ketamine • Dexmedetomidine

Introduction

- Due to the minimally-invasive nature of many out of operating room (OOR) procedures, patient comfort and appropriate procedural conditions can oftentimes be achieved without general anesthesia.
- Depending on the nature of the procedure, mild, moderate, or deep sedation may be appropriate.
- This chapter presents the pharmacology of various drugs used for sedation. A summary of the significant features of these drugs is found in Table 1.1.

C.A. Artime, MD
Department of Anesthesiology, McGovern Medical School at The University of Texas Health Science Center at Houston, 6431 Fannin St., MSB 5.020, Houston, TX 77030, USA
e-mail: carlos.artime@uth.tmc.edu

© Springer International Publishing Switzerland 2017   3
B.G. Goudra, P.M. Singh (eds.), *Out of Operating Room Anesthesia*,
DOI 10.1007/978-3-319-39150-2_1

Table 1.1 Summary of the drugs most commonly used for sedation

Drug	Sedative dose	Notes
Midazolam	1–2 mg IV, repeated PRN (0.025–0.1 mg/kg)	Frequently used in combination with fentanyl or for its amnestic properties when other agents are utilized as the primary sedative
Fentanyl	25–100 µg IV, repeated PRN (0.25–1 µg/kg)	Usually used in combination with other agents (e.g., midazolam, propofol)
Remifentanil	Bolus 0.5 µg/kg IV followed by an infusion of 0.1 µg/kg/min	Infusion can subsequently be titrated by 0.025 µg/kg/min to 0.05 µg/kg/min in 5 min intervals to achieve adequate sedation
Dexmedetomidine	Bolus 1 µg/kg IV over 10 min, followed by an infusion of 0.2–0.7 µg/kg/h	Reduce dose in the elderly and in patients with depressed cardiac function
Ketamine	0.2–0.8 mg/kg IV	Pretreat with antisialagogue Consider administration of midazolam to attenuate undesirable psychological effects.
Diphenhydramine	12.5–50 mg IV	Useful as a substitute for midazolam in the elderly

With Permission from Hagberg and Artime [37]

Benzodiazepines

- Benzodiazepines (BZDs) are commonly used for sedation due to their hypnotic, sedative, anxiolytic, and amnestic properties. The most commonly used BZD OOR sedation is midazolam, followed by lorazepam and diazepam [1].
- The pharmacologic action of BZDs is mediated via $GABA_A$ receptors, leading to opening of GABA-activated chloride channels and hyperpolarization of post-synaptic membranes, inhibiting neurotransmission [2].
- BZDs provide no analgesia, and therefore are frequently used in combination with opioids [3] or are used solely for their amnestic and anxiolytic effects when other sedatives (e.g., dexmedetomidine or ketamine) are chosen as the primary agent [4, 5].

Clinical Effects

- Central Nervous System (CNS): sedation/hypnosis, anterograde amnesia, anti-convulsive, decreased cerebral metabolic rate of oxygen ($CMRO_2$)
- Cardiovascular (CV): mild decrease in systemic vascular resistance (SVR) and arterial blood pressure (BP)
- Respiratory: depressed hypercarbic and hypoxic ventilatory response; synergistic effect with coadministration of opioids

Midazolam

Pharmacokinetics

- Onset: peak effect within 2–3 min of intravenous (IV) administration; 15–30 min after intramuscular (IM) or oral (*per* os [PO]) administration
- Duration of action: 20–40 min after IV administration; 2 h after IM administration; termination of effect of single dose is primarily a result of redistribution to adipose tissue
- Elimination: hepatically metabolized and renally cleared (active metabolites); elimination half-life of 1.7–3.5 h with prolongation in cirrhosis, obesity, and renal failure.

Dosing

- IV: 1–2 mg (0.025–0.1 mg/kg), repeated as needed after 5 min (*pro re nata* [PRN])
- IM: 0.07–0.2 mg/kg
- PO: 0.25–0.5 mg/kg

Uses

- Most commonly used BZD attributable to its rapid onset, easy titratability, and shorter duration of action.
- Can be used as a sole agent for non-stimulating procedures (e.g., imaging) or in combination with topical anesthesia for endoscopic procedures [6, 7].
- Usually combined with an opioid in decreased doses to account for synergistic interactions; the combination is especially useful for painful or stimulating procedures (e.g., cardioversion, endoscopy, and bronchoscopy) [8–10].
- Less likely to produce hypotension as compared to propofol and dexmedetomidine; useful for sedating patients at risk for hypotension (cardiovascular disease, gastrointestinal bleed) [9]
- Amnesia can last as long as 3 h; median duration of amnesia is 30 min with lower total doses (0.07 mg/kg) vs. 75 min with higher doses (0.1–0.13 mg/kg) [11].
- Useful as an anxiolytic premedication; the PO route is commonly used in children.

Diazepam

Pharmacokinetics

- Onset: peak effect within 3–5 min of IV administration
- Duration of action: 1–2 h
- Elimination: hepatically metabolized; elimination half-life of 20–50 h with prolongation in the elderly, obesity, and patients with hepatic dysfunction.

Dosing

- IV: 2–4 mg (0.05–0.2 mg/kg), repeated PRN after 10 min

Lorazepam

Pharmacokinetics

- Onset: peak effect within 10–15 min of IV administration
- Duration of action: 6–8 h
- Elimination: hepatically metabolized; elimination half-life of 8–25 h with prolongation in patients with hepatic dysfunction.

Dosing

- IV: 0.5–1 mg (0.02–0.08 mg/kg), repeated PRN after 10 min

Uses

- Suitable as a sole agent for longer, non-stimulating procedures

Adverse Effects

- Primary adverse effect is dose-dependent respiratory depression; increased incidence when coadministered with opioids.
- Diazepam and lorazepam can cause pain on injection and thrombophlebitis.
- BZDs can be associated with delirium and agitation in the elderly; reduced doses or avoidance are suggested [12].
- Midazolam and diazepam are considered Category D drugs in pregnancy and should be avoided [13].

Reversal

- Flumazenil is a specific BZD antagonist that can be used to reverse the sedative and respiratory effects of BZDs if a patient becomes too heavily sedated.
- Dosing: incremental IV doses of 0.2 mg, repeated PRN to a maximum dose of 3 mg.
- Flumazenil has a half-life of 0.7–1.8 h, so resedation can be a problem if it is being used to reverse high doses or longer-acting agents and patients should be monitored carefully in those circumstances. It is generally safe and devoid of major side effects [14, 15].

Opioids

- Opioids provide analgesia, sedation, and depression of airway reflexes, making them a useful addition to sedating regimens for OOR anesthesia.
- The primary pharmacologic action of opioids is mediated by agonism of μ- (analgesia, respiratory depression) and K- (analgesia, sedation) opioid receptors in the brain and spinal cord [16].
- While any μ-opioid agonist could be used for sedation in OOR anesthesia, the synthetic phenylpiperidine class of opioids – fentanyl, remifentanil, alfentanil, and sufentanil – are particularly useful due to their rapid onset, relatively short duration of action, and ease of titration.

Clinical Effects

- CNS: analgesia, pruritus, muscle rigidity; augmentation of sedative effects of other IV agents
- CV: bradycardia; little effect on myocardial contractility or SVR
- Respiratory: respiratory depression characterized by decreased respiratory rate with an overall decrease in minute ventilation; apnea with higher doses

Fentanyl

- Onset: peak effect in 2–3 min after IV administration
- Duration of action: 20–30 min; termination of effect is primarily a result of redistribution
- Elimination: hepatically metabolized; elimination half-life of 2–4 h
- Sedative dose: 25–100 mcg IV (0.25–1 mcg/kg), repeated PRN
- Most commonly used opioid for sedation; usually used in combination with midazolam.
- Can be combined with propofol sedation for added analgesia; has been shown to reduce the total dose of propofol and provide improved hemodynamic stability [17].
- Has also been used in combination with ketamine and dexmedetomidine [18, 19].

Remifentanil

- Onset: rapid onset in 1–2 min
- Duration of action/elimination: ultrashort-acting opioid with a half life 3–4 min; rapidly metabolized by nonspecific plasma and tissue esterases – independent of hepatic and renal function

- Sedative dose: as a single agent, IV infusion of 0.1 mcg/kg/min titrated by 0.025–0.05 mcg/kg/min in 5 min intervals to achieve adequate sedation; can start with a bolus dose of 0.5 mcg/kg [20]
- Decrease dose by in the elderly by 25–50 % due to increased opioid sensitivity
- May be used in combination with other agents (e.g., midazolam, propofol); decrease dose to account for synergistic effects [19].
- Has been shown to lead to a shorter time to discharge when compared to sedation with midazolam and meperidine [21].

Alfentanil

- Onset: rapid onset in 1–2 min
- Rapid recovery; duration of a single bolus dose is 10–15 min
- Duration of effect is prolonged with repeated boluses due to significant increase in context-sensitive half time
- Sedative dose: 500–1500 mcg IV (10–30 mcg/kg), additional boluses of 5–10 mcg/kg PRN

Sufentanil

- Is ~10 times more potent than fentanyl; has a similar pharmacokinetic profile after a single bolus dose
- Sedative dose: 2.5–10 mcg IV (0.025–0.1 mcg/kg), repeated PRN

Meperidine

- Meperidine has historically been an opioid of choice for sedation, but its use is declining in favor of fentanyl due to its prolonged duration of action and associated tachycardia [22].

Adverse Effects

- Primary adverse effect of opioids is dose-dependent respiratory depression and apnea.
- Hypotension (mild) and bradycardia (may be unsuitable for certain electrophysiological procedures).
- Muscle rigidity resulting in difficulty with mask ventilation. While this is commonly attributed to "chest wall rigidity", studies have shown that vocal cord closure is the primary cause of difficult ventilation after opioid-induced anesthesia. Treatment with small doses of paralytic or topical lidocaine (laryngotracheal

anesthesia) can be effective in relaxing the vocal cords to allow for mask ventilation and/or intubation [23, 24].
- Repeated doses of meperidine are associated with seizures due to accumulation of normeperidine, which decreases the seizure threshold.
- Urinary retention

Reversal

- Naloxone 0.04–0.08 mg IV, repeated every 2–3 min PRN until restoration of spontaneous ventilation
- Onset within 1–2 min; duration of 30–60 min

Dexmedetomidine

- Dexmedetomidine is a centrally-acting, highly-selective, α2-adrenergic receptor agonist.
- It has sedative, analgesic, anxiolytic, antitussive, and antisialagogue properties that are useful for sedation in OOR anesthesia.
- Sedation with dexmedetomidine provides unique conditions in which the patient is asleep, but is easily arousable and cooperative when stimulated [25, 26].

Systemic Effects

- CNS: sedation/hypnosis, analgesia (central α_{2A}-adrenergic receptors)
- CV: bradycardia, decreased SVR, cardiac output, contractility, and arterial BP (peripheral α_{2A}-adrenergic receptors resulting in presynaptic feedback inhibition of norepinephrine release); hypertension and bradycardia during initial loading dose due to direct vasoconstrictive effect (peripheral α_{2B}-adrenergic receptors) [2]
- Respiratory: small reduction in minute ventilation with preservation of hypercarbic ventilatory response

Pharmacokinetics

- Onset of effect in approximately 15 min.
- Elimination half life of 2–3 h.
- Hepatically metabolized; decrease dose in patients with hepatic impairment.
- No change in pharmacokinetic profile in renal failure, though in patients with severe renal disease the sedative effect may be more pronounced due to a lower degree of protein binding [2, 27].

Dose

- Bolus 1 mcg/kg over 10 min, followed by a continuous infusion of 0.2–0.7 mcg/kg/h (some patients may require higher maintenance doses)
- Reduce doses in the elderly, patients with hepatic or renal impairment, or in patients with depressed cardiac systolic function
- Intranasal dose: 0.5–1.5 mcg/kg (3–4 mcg/kg in pediatric patients) [28, 29]

Uses

- As a sole agent, dexmedetomidine can provide sedation but allow patient cooperation and examination of neurologic status; this is particularly useful for certain interventional neuroradiology procedures.
- Can be used in combination with propofol to provide deeper sedation for procedures such as endoscopy [30].
- Can also be used in combination with ketamine for moderate sedation; a benefit of this technique is that ketamine offsets the bradycardia and hypotension of dexmedetomidine, while the antisialagogic effects of dexmedetomidine counteract the increased secretions and emergence phenomena typical of ketamine [31].
- Dexmedetomidine has unreliable amnestic properties and so is frequently combined with midazolam to decrease the incidence of recall [32].
- Intranasal administration can be used for sedation, as an adjuvant to sedation with other agents, or as a pre-sedation anxiolytic.

Adverse Effects

- Bradycardia: can be treated with anticholinergics (e.g., glycopyrrolate).
- Hypotension: can be avoided in high risk patents by decreasing or forgoing the loading dose.
- Hypertension: can be avoided by decreasing the loading dose or administering it over 20 min

Ketamine

- Ketamine, a phencyclidine derivative, is an N-Methyl-D-Aspartate (NMDA) receptor antagonist that produces dissociative anesthesia, which manifests clinically as a cataleptic state with eyes open, nystagmus, and preservation of corneal and laryngeal reflexes [2].
- Ketamine also has potent analgesic effects.

Systemic Effects

- CNS: sedation/hypnosis, dissociative anesthesia, hallucinations, emergence reactions
- CV: increased arterial BP, heart rate, and cardiac output secondary to release of endogenous catecholamines and inhibition of norepinephrine reuptake; direct myocardial depression which may be unmasked in catecholamine-depleted states
- Respiratory: minimal to no respiratory depression; bronchial smooth muscle relaxation; hypersalivation

Pharmacokinetics

- Onset: within 1–2 min after IV administration, 5–10 min after IM
- Duration of sedation: 20–45 min after IV, 30–120 min after IM
- Hepatically metabolized; dosage adjustment not needed in renal failure

Dose

- IV: 0.2–0.5 mg/kg, repeated PRN
- IM: 2–4 mg/kg
- Pretreatment with an antisialagogue (e.g., glycopyrrolate) is recommended to counteract increased secretions.

Uses

- When administering ketamine, treatment with a benzodiazepine (e.g., midazolam) can attenuate undesirable psychological effects.
- As a sole agent, ketamine sedation does not produce immobility or abolish airway reflexes and may increase the risk of laryngospasm; therefore, it may not be suitable for a variety of OOR procedures.
- A combination of ketamine and dexmedetomidine can provide adequate sedation for endoscopic procedures, albeit with a delayed recovery time [33].
- Addition of low-dose ketamine (0.3 mg/kg) to a midazolam-fentanyl-propofol sedative regimen can reduce propofol consumption, provide more stable hemodynamics, and result in fewer adverse respiratory effects [34].
- A ketamine propofol admixture, "ketofol", provides adequate sedation for a variety of procedures; various ketamine to propofol ratios from 1:1 to 1:10 have been studied – a ratio of 1:3 to 1:4 provides maximal benefit without prolonging recovery [35].

Diphenhydramine

- Diphenhydramine is a histamine (H_1) receptor antagonist with central anticholinergic properties that provide sedation.
- It can be used as an adjunct to sedative regimens using other drugs.

Pharmacokinetics and Dose

- IV: 12.5–50 mg
- Rapid onset
- Hepatically conjugated with a portion excreted unchanged in the urine
- Half life: 4–8 h

Adverse Effects

- Dizziness and blurry vision
- Dry mouth and thickening of bronchial secretions
- Urinary retention

Uses

- As an adjunct to midazolam/opioid sedation, has been shown to improve sedation and reduce dosage requirements of other agents without increased adverse effects or prolonged recovery [36].
- Useful for light sedation in non-stimulating procedures when the clinician wishes to avoid BZDs (e.g., in the elderly).

Pharmacokinetic and Pharmacodynamic Considerations for Special Patient Populations

Elderly

- Pharmacodynamically, the elderly show increased sensitivity to sedative agents.
- Pharmacokinetically, clearance is decreased for most agents, including BZDs, propofol, dexmedetomidine, and remifentanil. The clearance of fentanyl is minimally affected.
- The result is that elderly patients need significantly lower doses than healthy adults, and initial dose reductions are warranted.

Obese

- Obese patients and those with obstructive sleep apnea (OSA) are more sensitive to the respiratory effects of sedative drugs such as opioids, BZDs, and propofol; therefore careful titration and dose reduction strategies should be implemented.
- Most sedative agents can be dosed on a corrected body weight, which approximates lean body mass; corrected body weight = ideal body weight + 0.4(total body weight – ideal body weight).

References

1. Shin JY, Lee SH, Shin SM, Kim MH, Park SG, Park BJ. Prescribing patterns of the four most commonly used sedatives in endoscopic examination in Korea: propofol, midazolam, diazepam, and lorazepam. Regul Toxicol Pharmacol. 2015;71(3):565–70.
2. Vuyk J, Sitsen E, Reekers M. Intravenous anesthetics. In: Miller RD, editor. Miller's anesthesia. 8th ed. Philadelphia: Elsevier/Saunders; 2015. p. 821–63.
3. Patatas K, Koukkoulli A. The use of sedation in the radiology department. Clin Radiol. 2009;64(7):655–63.
4. Wakita R, Kohase H, Fukayama H. A comparison of dexmedetomidine sedation with and without midazolam for dental implant surgery. Anesth Prog. 2012;59(2):62–8.
5. Sener S, Eken C, Schultz CH, Serinken M, Ozsarac M. Ketamine with and without midazolam for emergency department sedation in adults: a randomized controlled trial. Ann Emerg Med. 2011;57(2):109–14. e2.
6. Singh R, Kumar N, Vajifdar H. Midazolam as a sole sedative for computed tomography imaging in pediatric patients. Paediatr Anaesth. 2009;19(9):899–904.
7. Laluna L, Allen ML, Dimarino Jr AJ. The comparison of midazolam and topical lidocaine spray versus the combination of midazolam, meperidine, and topical lidocaine spray to sedate patients for upper endoscopy. Gastrointest Endosc. 2001;53(3):289–93.
8. Thomas SP, Thakkar J, Kovoor P, Thiagalingam A, Ross DL. Sedation for electrophysiological procedures. Pacing Clin Electrophysiol. 2014;37(6):781–90.
9. Goudra BG, Singh PM. Propofol alternatives in gastrointestinal endoscopy anesthesia. Saudi J Anaesth. 2014;8(4):540–5.
10. Jose RJ, Shaefi S, Navani N. Sedation for flexible bronchoscopy: current and emerging evidence. Eur Respir Rev. 2013;22(128):106–16.
11. Miller RI, Bullard DE, Patrissi GA. Duration of amnesia associated with midazolam/fentanyl intravenous sedation. J Oral Maxillofac Surg. 1989;47(2):155–8.
12. Moore AR, O'Keeffe ST. Drug-induced cognitive impairment in the elderly. Drugs Aging. 1999;15(1):15–28.
13. Cappell MS. Sedation and analgesia for gastrointestinal endoscopy during pregnancy. Gastrointest Endosc Clin N Am. 2006;16(1):1–31.
14. White PF, Shafer A, Boyle 3rd WA, Doze VA, Duncan S. Benzodiazepine antagonism does not provoke a stress response. Anesthesiology. 1989;70(4):636–9.
15. Amrein R, Hetzel W, Hartmann D, Lorscheid T. Clinical pharmacology of flumazenil. Eur J Anaesthesiol Suppl. 1988;2:65–80.
16. Fukuda K. Opioid analgesics. In: Miller RD, editor. Miller's anesthesia. 8th ed. Philadelphia: Elsevier/Saunders; 2015. p. 864–914.
17. Haytural C, Aydinli B, Demir B, Bozkurt E, Parlak E, Disibeyaz S, et al. Comparison of propofol, propofol-remifentanil, and propofol-fentanyl administrations with each other used for the sedation of patients to undergo ERCP. BioMed Res Int. 2015;2015:465465.

18. Peng K, Liu HY, Liu SL, Ji FH. Dexmedetomidine-fentanyl compared with midazolam-fentanyl for conscious sedation in patients undergoing lumbar disc surgery. Clin Ther. 2016;38(1):192–201. e2.
19. Heidari SM, Loghmani P. Assessment of the effects of ketamine-fentanyl combination versus propofol-remifentanil combination for sedation during endoscopic retrograde cholangiopancreatography. J Res Med Sci. 2014;19(9):860–6.
20. Atkins JH, Mirza N. Anesthetic considerations and surgical caveats for awake airway surgery. Anesthesiol Clin. 2010;28(3):555–75.
21. Manolaraki MM, Theodoropoulou A, Stroumpos C, Vardas E, Oustamanolakis P, Gritzali A, et al. Remifentanil compared with midazolam and pethidine sedation during colonoscopy: a prospective, randomized study. Dig Dis Sci. 2008;53(1):34–40.
22. Childers RE, Williams JL, Sonnenberg A. Practice patterns of sedation for colonoscopy. Gastrointest Endosc. 2015;82(3):503–11.
23. Bennett JA, Abrams JT, Van Riper DF, Horrow JC. Difficult or impossible ventilation after sufentanil-induced anesthesia is caused primarily by vocal cord closure. Anesthesiology. 1997;87(5):1070–4.
24. Abrams JT, Horrow JC, Bennett JA, Van Riper DF, Storella RJ. Upper airway closure: a primary source of difficult ventilation with sufentanil induction of anesthesia. Anesth Analg. 1996;83(3):629–32.
25. Belleville JP, Ward DS, Bloor BC, Maze M. Effects of intravenous dexmedetomidine in humans. I. Sedation, ventilation, and metabolic rate. Anesthesiology. 1992;77(6):1125–33.
26. Ebert TJ, Hall JE, Barney JA, Uhrich TD, Colinco MD. The effects of increasing plasma concentrations of dexmedetomidine in humans. Anesthesiology. 2000;93(2):382–94.
27. Venn RM, Karol MD, Grounds RM. Pharmacokinetics of dexmedetomidine infusions for sedation of postoperative patients requiring intensive caret. Br J Anaesth. 2002;88(5): 669–75.
28. Tug A, Hanci A, Turk HS, Aybey F, Isil CT, Sayin P, et al. Comparison of two different intranasal doses of dexmedetomidine in children for magnetic resonance imaging sedation. Paediatr Drugs. 2015;17(6):479–85.
29. Cheung CW, Qiu Q, Liu J, Chu KM, Irwin MG. Intranasal dexmedetomidine in combination with patient-controlled sedation during upper gastrointestinal endoscopy: a randomised trial. Acta Anaesthesiol Scand. 2015;59(2):215–23.
30. Nonaka T, Inamori M, Miyashita T, Harada S, Inou Y, Kanoshima K, et al. Feasibility of deep sedation with the combination of propofol and dexmedetomidine hydrochloride for esophageal endoscopic submucosal dissection. Dig Endosc. 2016;28(2):145–51.
31. Tobias JD. Dexmedetomidine and ketamine: an effective alternative for procedural sedation? Pediatr Crit Care Med. 2012;13(4):423–7.
32. Bergese SD, Patrick Bender S, McSweeney TD, Fernandez S, Dzwonczyk R, Sage K. A comparative study of dexmedetomidine with midazolam and midazolam alone for sedation during elective awake fiberoptic intubation. J Clin Anesth. 2010;22(1):35–40.
33. Goyal R, Hasnain S, Mittal S, Shreevastava S. A randomized, controlled trial to compare the efficacy and safety profile of a dexmedetomidine-ketamine combination with a propofol-fentanyl combination for ERCP. Gastrointest Endosc. 2016;83(5):928–33.
34. Tuncali B, Pekcan YO, Celebi A, Zeyneloglu P. Addition of low-dose ketamine to midazolam-fentanyl-propofol-based sedation for colonoscopy: a randomized, double-blind, controlled trial. J Clin Anesth. 2015;27(4):301–6.
35. Coulter FL, Hannam JA, Anderson BJ. Ketofol dosing simulations for procedural sedation. Pediatr Emerg Care. 2014;30(9):621–30.
36. Tu RH, Grewall P, Leung JW, Suryaprasad AG, Sheykhzadeh PI, Doan C, et al. Diphenhydramine as an adjunct to sedation for colonoscopy: a double-blind randomized, placebo-controlled study. Gastrointest Endosc. 2006;63(1):87–94.
37. Hagberg CA, Artime CA. Airway management in the adult. In: Miller RD, editor. Miller's anesthesia. 8th ed. Philadelphia: Elsevier/Saunders; 2015. p. 1647–83.

Chapter 2
Pharmacology of Anesthetic Drugs Used in Out of Operating Room Anesthesia

Elizabeth W. Duggan and Kathy L. Schwock

Abstract The number and variety of procedures occurring outside of an operating room environment daily, has challenged anesthesiologists to increasingly use inhaled and intravenous anesthetics in unknown environments. Often, routine anesthetic equipment is not stored in these procedural locations where creating scenarios familiar anesthetic agents require new techniques. Alternatively, there are times where anesthetic medications may more frequently be used in austere environments due to their ease of delivery. The lack of nearby resources, including physician colleagues and anesthesia technicians, the inexperience of procedural teams with anesthetics and delivery machines, and locations that limit the type of equipment available, mean that our specialty is adapting our approach to medication delivery to keep patients comfortable and safe. Additionally, tailoring to the diverse range of procedures across all populations –invasive versus diagnostic interventions, short (<30 min) versus all-day cases, level of sedation needed (MAC versus general anesthetic), pediatric versus elderly – requires an in-depth understanding of the pharmacology of the agents available and evidence regarding best use in these situations.

Keywords Sevoflurane • Isoflurane • Desflurane • Nitrous Oxide • Propofol • Etomidate • Ketamine • Methohexital

Inhaled Anesthetics

- To date, the exact mechanism of inhaled anesthetics (nitrous oxide and the halogenated agents) is unknown. However, there is strong evidence that volatile fluorinated anesthetics enhance activity at the $GABA_A$ receptor subunit which contributes to hypnosis and amnesia [40].

E.W. Duggan, MD (✉)
Department of Anesthesiology, Emory University Hospital,
1364 Clifton Road, Office B-352, Atlanta, GA 30322, USA
e-mail: ewdugga@emory.edu

K.L. Schwock, MD
Department of Anesthesiology, Emory University, Atlanta, GA, USA

© Springer International Publishing Switzerland 2017
B.G. Goudra, P.M. Singh (eds.), *Out of Operating Room Anesthesia*,
DOI 10.1007/978-3-319-39150-2_2

- The operational definition (to guide practitioners and research) of the minimum alveolar concentration of gas is a state of immobility in response to surgical stimulus.
- All inhaled anesthetics provide amnestic effects and a decrease (or complete loss) in sensation to stimuli. A state of unconsciousness is commonly accepted as a component of general anesthesia.
- Inhaled anesthetics are absorbed from the alveoli into the blood. Over time, the partial pressure of the gas in the alveoli (P_A) equilibrates with the arterial blood (Pa), and the anesthetic is delivered to and achieves equilibrium with the tissue in the brain (Pbr).
- A multiple compartment model best describes volatile anesthetic uptake, distribution and elimination. The vessel-rich group (VRG) is comprised of the organs that receive the greatest portion of the body's cardiac output. It is this group that is responsible for the initial large uptake of inhaled anesthetic however, due to its small tissue capacity, rapid (4–8 min) equilibrium is reached between the VRG and plasma. After equilibrium is reached with the VRG, the muscle and skin remove anesthetic, followed by the fat and finally vessel poor tissues [33].
- The solubility, in blood and tissues, of an inhaled anesthetic is defined by a partition coefficient. This describes the concentration of the gas between two compartments when the partial pressures are the same.
- Volatile halogenated anesthetics (sevoflurane, desflurane and isoflurane) cause a dose-dependent depression in cardiovascular function. Mean arterial blood pressure is decreased due to a in systemic vascular resistance (SVR). Nitrous oxide does not result in changes in vascular resistance when administered alone.
- At >0.6 MAC, volatile agents produce cerebral vasodilation and decrease in cerebral metabolic rate for oxygen ($CMRO_2$) [85]. Although the cerebral vasculature remains appropriately responsive to $PaCO_2$ [103], autoregulation of cerebral blood flow (CBF) is impaired in a dose-related manner.
- A dose-dependent increase in respiratory rate is caused by inhaled anesthetics. Tidal volume is however decreased and the overall effect is a decrease in minute ventilation.
- Inhaled anesthetics in NORA may be limited because they require access to a delivery system (in radiology, this may include an MRI suite with compliant equipment), carbon dioxide absorbent and a waste gas line.

Isoflurane

- Isoflurane is a pungent halogenated methyl ethyl ether. The most potent of the volatile anesthetics with a MAC of 1.17 and a blood:gas partition coefficient of 1.46.
- Isoflurane undergoes hepatic oxidative metabolism involving cytochrome P-450 2E1 (CYP2E1). Versus halothane, in which 25 % of administered agent is metabolized into trifluoroacetic acid (TFA), chloride and bromide, only 0.2 % of isoflurane is recovered as TFA components [81].

- Due to the small percentage of oxidative metabolism of isoflurane, the incidence of liver injury following isoflurane exposure is low [95]. However, histopathologic changes, including centrilobular injury and microvesicular fatty changes have been observed in small number of patients [135]. During the 45 years of its clinical use, acute fulminant failure and fatal hepatotoxicity have rarely been reported [10, 135].
- Nephrotoxicity from inorganic fluoride with isoflurane metabolism is unlikely [73] and serum fluoride levels following isoflurane use are not significant [52].
- As alveolar isoflurane concentration increases toward 1 MAC, EEG patterns show increasing voltage and frequency [31]. However as anesthetic levels deepen (1.0 MAC), the EEG demonstrates decreased frequency and maximal voltage. At 1.5 MAC burst suppression occurs, and electrical silence is present at 2.0 MAC [37].
- Isoflurane at 1.1 MAC increases CBF by almost 20% with normal range systemic pressure. $CMRO_2$ is reduced approximately 45% [71].
- Complete suppression of EEG under isoflurane causes a relative reduction in $CMRO_2$ and CBF that is greater in the neocortex than other areas of the brain [104].
- Cortical somatosensory evoked responses to median nerve stimulation are difficult to elicit with 1.5 MAC [104].
- Isoflurane increases heart rate from 0.5 to 1.5 MAC [79]. This increases myocardial work and decreases diastolic filling time however; in animal studies, isoflurane anesthesia increases oxygen content in coronary sinus blood [130].
- Preconditioning with isoflurane anesthesia has been demonstrated to attenuate the deleterious effects of myocardial ischemia and reperfusion injury [115]. Cardiac biomarkers are reduced [62] and left ventricular function is improved (as measured by echocardiography) [75] after anesthetic preconditioning. There may be some benefit in using isoflurane (or sevoflurane) for patients with risks for coronary ischemia undergoing procedures.
- Cardiac contractility is depressed in vivo yet at 0.9–1.4 MAC there is minimal myocardial depression in vitro. At 2 MAC, normal volunteers demonstrate decreasing cardiac output [31].
- Systemic arterial pressure decreases in a dose-dependent manner due to a decrease in total peripheral resistance.
- Isoflurane anesthesia produces a dose dependent prolongation effect on QTc [126].
- Inhaled anesthetics cause a dose dependent decrease in tidal volume and increase respiratory rate, however isoflurane does not increase the respiratory rate above 1.0 MAC [28].
- Isoflurane and desflurane are most irritating to the airway, particularly at >1 MAC concentrations [68].

Sevoflurane

- Sevoflurane is the least pungent halogenated agent. It is often the preferred agent for inhalational induction because it does not cause respiratory irritation. This proves valuable in procedures where preserved spontaneous ventilation is preferred or short procedures not requiring muscle relaxant.

- Despite an increase in respiratory rate, smaller tidal volumes result in a decrease in minute ventilation under sevoflurane anesthesia. Apnea can occur at concentrations between 1.5 and 2.0 MAC [21].
- Sevoflurane inhibits hypoxic pulmonary vasodilation however, at clinically relevant concentrations, it appears to have only minimal effects in vivo [74].
- At clinical concentrations, cardiac output is usually preserved [32].
- Sevoflurane prolongs the QT segment of electrocardiogram [9] and case reports have demonstrated that versus propofol, it may limit procedures evaluating and ablating accessory pathways [11]. However, small studies using 2 % sevoflurane versus conscious sedation with midazolam and alfentanil, do not demonstrate clinically significant changes in accessory pathways and all general anesthesia patients underwent successful ablation [120].
- Given its favorable effects on cerebral blood flow and preservation of autoregulation, sevoflurane is commonly used in neurointerventional procedures. When compared to a comparable depth of anesthesia as provided by propofol, the sevoflurane group showed faster recovery for eye opening, extubation and orientation [12, 14]—all important variables when a rapid post-procedure neurologic exam is desired. However, subdural intracranial pressure has been demonstrated to be lower in propofol anesthetics as compared to sevoflurane in patients with cerebral tumors [105].
- Defluorination occurs through oxidative metabolism, increasing serum fluoride concentrations [81]. There is however, minimal intra-renal defluorination, which may explain its decreased nephrotoxic potential [103]. Large studies have evaluated fluoride levels following 10-h, low-flow (1 L/min), 1 MAC sevoflurane anesthesia; subsequent renal function as measured by BUN, creatinine, urine glucose, urine pH and specific gravity is not significantly changed [46]. Peak fluoride levels were higher in patients following sevoflurane versus isoflurane anesthetics however, no clinically significant difference was found in renal function.
- Concern has been expressed about the formation of compound A (a nephrotoxic) when sevoflurane is defluorinated and exposed to carbon dioxide adsorbent. Varied carbon dioxide absorbents (sodalime, Baralyme, e.g.,) demonstrate varied propensity to form Compound A with sevoflurane contact [64]. Multiple studies evaluating human subjects for renal harm due to compound A exposure during low flow anesthesia (<1L/min) do not demonstrate renal injury despite up to 10-h exposures [7, 8]. Using 2 L fresh gas flow will likely prevent toxic levels of compound A exposure and will minimize the risk of renal injury.
- Hepatic biotransformation of sevoflurane occurs principally by cytochrome P450 and frees fluoride ions [103]. Unlike other halogenated agents that are metabolized into Fluoroacetylate TFA, compound A has been theorized to be the offending agent in liver dysfunction and/or inflammation following sevoflurane anesthetics. Case reports describe both elevations in liver transaminases [113] and acute liver failure following sevoflurane exposure [69, 82, 147].

- It has been suggested that in patients with known hepatic dysfunction, maintenance of adequate blood flow and oxygen supply (via maintenance of cardiac output, normalized perfusion pressures and pulmonary ventilation/oxygenation) may prevent hepatitis or liver failure associated with sevoflurane [123].

Desflurane

- Desflurane, a fluorinated methyl ethyl ether, is a third-generation halogenated anesthetic. With a boiling point of 24 °C and vapor pressure near atmosphere (669 mmHg at 20 °C), desflurane requires a unique heated and pressurized vaporizer [44] that is powered by electricity. The need for specialized equipment can limit its availability in NORA.
- Desflurane has the lowest blood:gas partition coefficient (0.42) and therefore, is the least potent gas. Combined with its low fat:blood partition coefficient (27.2), it undergoes rapid elimination allowing for predictable emergence.
- Of the fluorinated anesthetics, desflurane undergoes the least in vivo metabolism (0.01 %) [95], minimizing the risk of hepatocellular injury with exposure. Rare cases of desflurane liver damage have been reported [2].
- Desflurane induces direct cerebral vasodilation and a decrease in $CMRO_2$. The vasodilation is dose-dependent and more pronounced for desflurane > isoflurane > sevoflurane [20].
- Desflurane induces significant impairment in cerebral autoregulation, with greater effect on the body's ability to maintain appropriate cerebral blood flow at higher gas concentration [20].
- A rapid increase in desflurane concentration stimulates the sympathetic nervous system. A transient surge in systemic blood pressure, heart rate, and pulmonary artery pressure may occur and, can induce myocardial ischemia [48].
- Desflurane has been shown to depress myocardial function [144] however, the sympathetic stimulation of desflurane seems offset the decrease in myocardial contractility in a normal ventricle [100].
- With sympathetic and renin-angiotensin system activation, increased levels of epinephrine, norepinephrine, vasopressin, and renin are released [60]. This activation may be attenuated by opioids [99].
- Desflurane lengthens the cardiac repolarization time and prolongs the QTc interval. Given the impact of other anesthetic drugs and adjuvants on the heart's electrical pathway, as well as the adrenergic stimulus of surgery/stimulation, desflurane appears to be more torsadogenic than sevoflurane [126].
- As the most pungent of the inhaled agents, desflurane can trigger upper airway reactions including coughing, laryngospasm and bronchospasm. Its use is not recommended for mask induction. Consideration of alternative inhaled agents in sensitive asthmatics is prudent [41].
- Compared to both sevoflurane and isoflurane at 1.5 MAC, desflurane causes a 30 % increase in airway resistance above baseline [96].

- Studies suggest that desflurane has beneficial effects on the resumption of adequate ventilation and oxygenation in obese patients [63, 127], which may influence a provider's decision to use in environments where access to post-operative care or anesthesiology colleagues is limited.
- The quicker emergence of desflurane has also been shown to have beneficial effects on the ability to quickly recover protective airway reflexes compared to sevoflurane [83], including in those who are obese [84].

Nitrous Oxide

- Nitrous oxide (N_2O) is currently, the most used non-halogenated anesthetic agent in the United States. However, due to limited wall gas delivery system in non-operating room environments, it is often unavailable as an anesthetic unless delivered via tank system.
- Cannot be delivered at 1 MAC due to the risk of hypoxia. It is most frequently combined with at least 30% oxygen. If the use of oxygen is limited during a procedure due to risk of airway fire or spark with electrocautery during sedation, care needs to be taken using nitrous oxide.
- As a single agent, it may not provide sufficient muscle relaxation or immobility for invasive cases/procedures.
- N_2O is not metabolized in human tissues but instead, is reduced to nitrogen (N_2) in a chemical reaction with Vitamin B_{12} [81]. Due to this reaction, it has been theorized to inhibit methionine synthetase and impair DNA synthesis.
- Prolonged N_2O has been associated with elevated levels of homocysteine; it is unclear however if this is clinically significant. When the hematologic effect of nitrous oxide exposure was examined in pediatric patients, it was not associated with megaloblastic anemia [25].
- Likewise, elevated homocysteine levels have been postulated to place patients at increased perioperative risk for cardiovascular event. However, the recently published ENIGMA-II trial examined >7,000 patients with known or suspected coronary artery disease, undergoing non-cardiac surgery, and found no increased risk for death, cardiac complication or wound infection in those randomized to 70% nitrous oxide [93].
- The blood gas partition of N_2O is 0.47 [33], which facilitates its use for short procedures, including in-office dental work. A recent prospective, randomized trial comparing propofol alone to propofol+N_2O demonstrated a smaller decrease in mean blood pressure in the group given nitrous compared to propofol alone. Patients who received N_2O reported improved amnesia and less pain with propofol injection; there were no differences in recovery characteristics [146].
- The increased solubility of nitrous oxide compared to nitrogen does result in the rapid transfer of N_2O into air-filled spaces. Caution should be used in procedures that entrain air into a non-compliant space (patients with pneumothorax or those undergoing middle ear, intraocular cases) or if there is a possibility of venous air embolism.

- The outpouring of nitrous oxide on the recovery of anesthesia was first described in 1955 as "diffusion hypoxia" [36]. Discontinuing a nitrous anesthetic should be done with 100 % oxygen to minimize the risk of hypoxia resulting from the large volume release of N_2O into the alveoli. Particular care should be provided during the recovery phase for sedation patients exposed to nitrous if they have decreased or impaired minute ventilation.
- Cerebral vasodilation and blood flow is increased with N_2O use and the $CMRO_2$ also demonstrates modest increase when used alone.
- In contrast with volatile anesthetics, nitrous does not cause a decrease in systemic blood pressure. Cardiac output is slightly increased, possibly due to its mild sympathomimetic effects.
- An increase in pulmonary vascular resistance (PVR) may occur in patients with pre-existing pulmonary hypertension [118]. Infants may also be susceptible to the vasoconstrictive activity of N_2O in the pulmonary vascular bed [35].
- An increased risk of post-operative nausea and vomiting has been demonstrated with the use of N_2O [93] however, this appears to be less significant for anesthetic exposure lasting less than 1 h [106] and when anti-emetic prophylaxis is used [92].
- As a single agent for sedation, nitrous oxide has been used for a variety of procedures. Specifically in pediatric patients, it was demonstrated to be safe in non-fasting patients undergoing minor procedures [101].

Intravenous Anesthetics

Propofol

- Propofol is a sedative-hypnotic administered intravenously for induction and/or maintenance of general anesthesia. It can also be used as a sedative for monitored anesthesia care in a great variety of settings and is the most frequently used IV anesthetic.
- Propofol (2, 6-diisopropylphenol) is an alkylphenol compound and is water insoluble. Therefore, it is formulated in a white, oil-in-water emulsion.
- Propofol marketed under the trade name Diprivan contains soybean oil (100 mg/mL), glycerol (22.5 mg/mL), egg lecithin (12 mg/mL), and disodium edetate (0.005 %) with sodium hydroxide to adjust pH. The emulsion is isotonic and has a pH of 6.5–7 [23]. Disodium edetate was added to propofol to retard bacterial growth.
- Patients with an anaphylactic allergy to eggs should not be given propofol. Recent studies however, do not demonstrate that those with other egg allergy, peanut or soy allergy have a cross-reactive allergic reaction when given propofol [4, 47].
- Propofol is a supportive growth medium for both Escherichia coli and Candida albicans and bacteriostatic for Staphyloccoccus aureus [142]. Formulations with EDTA [23], metabisulfite [109], or benzyl alcohol (Hospira) [108] act only as retardants to growth; emulsions still support mircoorganisms and these

are not antimicrobially preserved under the Unites States Pharmaceuticals standards [141].

- The exact mechanism of action explaining propofol's hypnotic effects has yet to be determined however, the GABA receptor mediated chloride channel is clearly linked as one of its primary targets [40].
- Accumulating evidence from functional MRI and PET techniques have demonstrated that at sedative doses of propofol, changes in the brain occur in the occipital, frontal and temporal lobes. During propofol-induced unconsciousness there is an increasing global metabolic reduction in the thalamus and ultimately, the thalomocortical and frontoparietal network [124].
- Following IV bolus administration, propofol's hypnotic actions are terminated in 2–8 minutes by redistribution from the brain to other tissues [24]. The time to peak effect following bolus dose is 90 seconds [27].
- Induction doses range from 1 to 2 mg/kg IV and should be reduced in elderly patients. Higher doses may be needed in patients younger than age 2.
- Propofol is rapidly cleared by hepatic oxidative metabolism by cytochrome P450. Following conjugation in the liver, the inactive water-soluble metabolites are excreted by the kidneys [131].
- Propofol's clearance rate of 23–50 mL/kg/min exceeds hepatic blood flow and extrahepatic metabolism of the drug has been confirmed during the anhepatic phase of liver transplantation [140]. The lungs appear to be the most important site of metabolism outside of the liver and account for up to 30 % of elimination following bolus dose [67].
- Varied dosing schematics have been proposed for infusion rates in obese patients; studies comparing true body weight (TBW) with free fat mass, lean body weight and normal fat mass, suggest that TBW best describes clearance in this subset of patients [18].
- The context-sensitive half-time is approximately 40 min when used for sedation/ anesthesia in procedural settings where cases last less than 8 h [55]. The elimination half-life is 4–7 h [114].
- Propofol elimination after bolus dosing in cirrhotic patients is not significantly changed [119] and renal disease does not alter the drug's pharmacokinetics [58].
- High infusion rates produce burst suppression on EEG but lower doses also achieve seizure control in epileptic patients [80]. Conversely, propofol use has also been associated with seizure-like phenomena (SLP) in both epileptic and non-epileptic patients [143].
- For electroconvulsive therapy (ECT), propofol is associated with shorter seizures than other anesthetics. Using the lowest effective propofol dose to achieve amnesia minimizes its effect on seizure elicitation and duration [110]. Propofol administered in small doses (0.75 mg/kg) is more effective at attenuating the acute hemodynamic responses than etomidate [102].
- ICP is decreased in both normal patients and those with intracranial hypertension. Propofol also decreases $CMRO_2$ [138].

- During deep brain stimulator placement for Parkinson's disease, propofol has been shown to change neuronal activity patterns [70] Microelectrode recording (MER) used to detect and amplify the activity of individual neurons appears to be dampened due to the drug's GABA receptor-mediated activity in the subcortical brain [57]. Propofol is often used for placement of the stereotactic frame and burr holes but discontinued for mapping.
- The most notable cardiovascular effect of propofol is a drop in arterial blood pressure during induction, related to a drop in peripheral resistance [114]. Heart rate does not change significantly even in the setting of hypotension [19].
- Following an induction dose, transient apnea is common with propofol use. Using a continuous infusion with preservation of spontaneous ventilation results in an overall decrease in minute ventilation as both respiratory rate and tidal volume are decreased. Additionally, CO_2 responsiveness is decreased [42].
- Laryngeal reflexes are reduced with propofol more than other IV anesthetic agents, facilitating intubation and decreasing the risk of laryngospasm [49].
- There is a reduction in hypopharyngeal dimensions and relaxation of the upper pharyngeal muscles [73]. Patients with reduced airway diameter restrict air flow and may require intubation with increasing doses of propofol.
- The risk for post-operative nausea and vomiting is significantly reduced with propofol-based anesthetics [3].
- Propofol infusion syndrome (PRIS) is extremely rare but has been described in patients being treated with long durations of the medication (sedation for prolonged mechanical ventilation) or high doses (>4 mg/kg/h or >67 mcg/kg/min) [88]. Symptoms include treatment resistant bradycardia, cardiac failure, rhabdomyolysis and kidney failure.
- Risk factors for PRIS include carbohydrate depletion, severe illness and concomitant administration of catecholamines and glucocorticosteriods. The pathophysiology of this condition includes disruption of the electron transport chain [88] possibly at Coenzyme Q [139].
- Given its ease of delivery and versatility as a sedative-hypnotic, propofol has been used in a variety of NORA settings with great success. Some of the most well accepted uses for propofol in NORA include bronchoscopy, endoscopy/colonoscopy as well as advanced GI procedures (small balloon enteroscopy and ERCP), neurointerventional radiology (angiograms, coiling, embolization), MRI (diagnostic and interventional), and interventional cardiology (electrophysiology and catheterization). Each of these procedures is individually addressed in further chapters.
- In vitro fertilization often requires sedation, neuraxial or general anesthesia due to the discomfort of transvaginal oocyte retrieval. Propofol can be used as a sole agent for sedation or in conjunction with neuraxial anesthesia. Some studies report that propofol has a negative impact on the success of IVF [107], while other studies indicate that there is no difference in fertilization and/or pregnancy rates when propofol is used versus other medications [5, 6, 54]. Propofol does accumulate in follicular fluid [13].

Etomidate

- Etomidate is an intravenous anesthetic used most frequently for the induction of anesthesia. It can also be used to provide a period of unconscious sedation for short procedures or blocks.
- The drug is a carboxylated imidazole-ring that is administered as a single isomer, the R (+) enantiomer. The S(−) enantiomer has only one-fifth of the potency [134] and is therefore not used in prepared formulations of the medication.
- Etomidate selectively binds to sites on the $GABA_A$ receptors, enhancing the affinity of the receptor for the inhibitory neurotransmitter GABA.
- Cardiovascular stability, as measured by blood pressure, stroke volume, cardiac index, and systemic vascular resistance, has been demonstrated with 0.3 mg/kg IV etomidate as used as an induction dose [43].
- Unlike most other sedatives and hypnotics, hemorrhagic shock produces minimal changes in the pharmaco-kinetics/dynamics of etomidate [61].
- Cerebral penetration of the drug occurs in approximately 1 min; the onset-time for effect is rapid. A single bolus induction dose lasts between 6 and 10 min.
- Plasma elimination of etomidate occurs in a three-compartment model. Hepatic microsomal enzymes and plasma esterases hydrolyze the ester side chain resulting in a water-soluble, inactive compound that is predominantly excreted in the urine [112].
- Redistribution is responsible for the loss of the hypnotic effect of etomidate after a single bolus dose. Liver dysfunction does not significantly prolong the drug's alpha half-life, however, in patients with cirrhosis, the elimination (beta) half-life is doubled [136].
- An induction dose (0.2–0.3 mg/kg) reduces CBF and $CMRO_2$ while mean arterial pressure (MAP) remains similar. At doses that cause electroencephalograph (EEG) suppression, etomidate lowers intracranial pressure (ICP) [89].
- Grand Mal seizures have been linked to etomidate use and it increases seizure activity in epileptogenic foci [29]. This suggests that seizure-mapping procedures may benefit from its use as a pre-operative evaluation tool and/or during the ablative surgery [50].
- For procedures requiring somatosensory evoked potentials (SSEPs), etomidate enhances signals [122]. It also decreases motor-evoked potentials (MEPs) less than propofol, thiopental or methohexital [129].
- The duration of epileptiform activity after electroconvulsive therapy (ECT) is longer after etomidate than methohexital [22].
- Involuntary myoclonus is common following an induction dose of etomidate and has also been reported with its use during procedural sedation [137]. Caution should be exercised during procedures where this would be an undesirable side effect.
- To date, the greatest concern regarding etomidate use has been its demonstrated suppression of the hypothalamic-pituitary-adrenal (HPA) axis. Reversible inhibition of the enzyme 11β-hydroxylase prevents the formation of cortisol from its precursors.

- Adrenocortical suppression occurs at blood concentrations of 8 ng/ml whereas hypnosis occurs at 200 ng/ml. Thus, plasma levels achieving anesthesia or sedation cause adrenal suppression lasting for 8 h following a single dose [39].
- Trauma patients and those with sepsis may experience upwards of 24 h of adrenal suppression after a single dose of etomidate [1]. Compared to ketamine for rapid-sequence induction in critically ill patients, a recent RCT did not demonstrate increased mortality in the etomidate group Additionally, the *a priori* subgroup analysis of trauma and sepsis patients did not reveal an increase in organ dysfunction or failure if given etomidate [59]. However, the CORTICUS trial does suggest that those with severe sepsis had a significantly higher 30-day mortality if they received etomidate [125]. Although the data is mixed, consideration for alternative anesthetic agents is prudent when caring for a septic patient outside of the operating room.

Ketamine

- Ketamine is a water-soluble drug derived from phencyclidine. It is a non-competitive antagonist of N-methyl D-aspartate receptors (NMDA) receptors in the central nervous system. This limits the excitatory activation of the receptor by preventing glutamate binding.
- There are two optical isomers of ketamine. Although the most common preparation of the drug includes both enantiomers, the S(+) left-handed isomer produces more potent analgesia [65].
- Peak plasma levels are achieved within 1 min of intravenous administration and 5 min of intramuscular injection. Due to its liposolubility, initial distribution is to VRG organs, followed by redistribution to more poorly perfused tissues.
- Duration of action after an induction bolus dose of ketamine (2 mg/kg IV) is 10–15 min [17]. Concomitant administration of a benzodiazepiene may prolong its action [98].
- Eighty percent of administered ketamine is demethylated by p450 enzymes into the active metabolite norketamine. It is then excreted in the bile or, further conjugated and filtered by the kidneys [87].
- Elimination of ketamine is dependent on liver blood flow. It has a half-life of 2–3 h following single dose [118]. Norketamine, although only one-third as potent as ketamine, persists for up to 5 h [78].
- An advantage of ketamine for use as an anesthetic is its multiple routes of administration: intravenous, intramuscular, oral, rectal or intranasal.
- Ketamine provides an anesthetic state vastly different than other agents. The "dissociative" effects of the drug render a cataleptic state; open eyes, nystagmus, hypertonia and purposeful movement not linked to surgical stimulus are all defining characteristics of the amnestic state [112].
- In addition to binding at NMDA receptors, ketamine has been reported to be an agonist at μ, k and β opioid receptors [56] and an antagonist at both muscarinic and nicotinic acetylcholine receptors [16].

- The relay between nociceptive transmission between the spine and supraspinal level is blocked at the reticularis formation, theorized to be a component in ketamine's analgesic properties [97].
- Ketamine reduces hyperalgesia and allodynia associated with peripheral neurologic lesions so can be an adjunct for those with phantom limb pain [94] or complex regional pain syndrome [121]. Due to the same interaction with NMDA receptors, ketamine has also been used to supplement analgesia or help taper narcotic use in opioid tolerant patients.
- Converging evidence suggests that abnormalities in glutaminergic signaling may play a role in the pathophysiology of major depressive disorders (MDD) [77, 116]. Ketamine now plays a growing role in psychiatric treatment of MDD, particularly in patients who a resistant to other therapies. It has demonstrated antidepressant efficacy when given as a single dose [91] or as repeated infusions over time [111]. This may be an emerging role for anesthesiologists in NORA.
- Ketamine increases $CMRO_2$, CBF and ICP. Cerebrovascular responsiveness to $PaCO_2$ is preserved with ketamine.
- SSEPs are preserved during ketamine anesthesia.
- Psychedelic effects occur with ketamine use both following emergence after a general anesthetic or when used as a sedative. This may include vivid dreaming, illusions, or hallucinations and they are often accompanied by emotional excitement, confusion, euphoria or fear. The incidence is approximately 10–30 % in adults receiving ketamine as a sole anesthetic agent or as part of a balanced anesthetic approach [114]. Benzodiazepines appear to be the most effective class of medication to prevent or attenuate ketamine emergence reactions [26, 66].
- SVR, PVR, HR and CO are increased with ketamine; this also increases myocardial oxygen demand. The hemodynamic changes are not related to dose [148].
- Increases in heart rate and blood pressure can be attenuated with the use of benzodiazepines, alpha and beta-blockers, and inhaled anesthetics.
- Shunt fraction is not increased nor shunt direction changed in those with congenital heart disease [90]; however, in patients with pulmonary hypertension, the increase in PVR is proportionately greater than the increase in SVR [51].
- Minimal effect on the respiratory system; there is no change in responsiveness to $PaCO_2$ with minimal change in ventilation. Following bolus dosing, a transient (2–3 min) decrease in respiratory drive may occur.
- Ketamine is a safe anesthetic adjunct in patients with obstructive sleep apnea (OSA). It abolishes the link between sleep and the reduction in upper airway muscle activity, helping to maintain a patent airway during spontaneous ventilation [34].
- Bronchodilation is a positive effect of ketamine, particularly in asthmatic patients. Increased salivary and tracheobronchial secretion occurs after administration and often an anti-sialogogue is administered pre-operatively.
- Ketamine is often used as a sedative due to its ability to maintain ventilation, respiratory drive and $PaCO_2$ responsiveness. It has been successfully be used for cardiac catheterization, radiation therapy, radiologic studies and dressing changes. It has also been used for dental work and in pediatric sedation.

Methohexital

- Methohexital is an ultra-short acting oxybarbiturate and is easily titrated to effect due to its short onset time and half-life. It is 2.5 times more potent than thiopental [112].
- Sedation and hypnosis are achieved via allosteric action at the $GABA_A$ receptor. Binding at the alpha subunit increases the affinity of GABA and prolongs the duration of chloride conduction though the ion channel, resulting in a hyperpolarized cell membrane. This decreases post-synaptic neuronal firing [128]. At high concentrations, barbiturates can directly activate chloride channels without binding to GABA receptors [133].
- General anesthesia can be obtained in approximately 30 s when administered at a dose of 1–1.5 mg/kg IV. After a single bolus dose, the recovery time is approximately 7 min [86]. Given rectally, methohexital 25 mg/kg produces a hypnotic effect in approximately 10–15 min. Loss of consciousness will occur after rectal administration if plasma concentrations >2 mcg/mL are reached [76]. This can be useful for pediatric cases requiring pre-medication for a procedure or, as an induction agent in uncooperative patients.
- Like thiopental, redistribution of methohexital is responsible for its rapid wake-up time after a single dose. However, methohexital is more rapidly cleared from the body than thiopental resulting in faster emergence and recovery.
- Infusions can be used to maintain hypnosis and at doses of 50–150 mcg/kg/min it will achieve a similar anesthetic effect as propofol [114].
- Methohexital has two asymmetric centers and four stereoisomers. The β-1-isomer is 4–5 times more potent than the α-1-isomer but produces excessive motor responses (myoclonus, e.g.,). Therefore, methohexital is marketed as the racemic mixture of the α-1 isomer [145].
- Methohexital is metabolized to inactive hydroxyderivatives. Clearance (11 mL/kg/min) is dependent upon hepatic blood flow. The byproducts are water soluble and excreted by the kidneys [86]. The elimination half-life is 4 h [145].
- Barbiturates induce other hepatic enzymes, notably δ-aminolevulinic acid synthetase which is involved in the porphyrin production pathway, Methohexital should not be used in patients with acute intermittent porphyria as it may precipitate an attack, manifested by severe abdominal pain, nausea and vomiting.
- Barbituates are cerebral vasoconstrictors and decrease cerebral blood flow, lowering ICP. They also cause a proportional decrease in $CMRO_2$.
- Unlike other drugs in this class, methohexital produces less depression of the electroencephalogram (EEG). It is the preferred agent for electroconvulsive therapy due to its seizure-provoking effects [53]. Methohexital should be used with caution in patients with a history of epilepsy or seizures due to its epileptogenic effects.
- Methohexital is often preferred to propofol for its effectiveness in improving depression scores and increasing seizure duration for ECT. Compared to propofol, methohexital was found to be significantly associated with higher seizure

duration (p = 0.018) and depression scores. Patients who were administered methohexital had significantly improved symptomatology than those who received propofol (p = 0.001) [38].

- Peripheral vasodilation, in addition to a decrease in sympathetic output, occurs on administration of methohexital and results in a drop in arterial blood pressure [30]. A decrease in cardiac output also occurs due to negative inotropy [132]. Caution should be exercised when administering methohexital to hypovolemic patients, as the drop in blood pressure and cardiac preload can be significant.
- Heart rate increases after barbiturate administration and is attributed to the baroreceptor reflex responding to the decrease in blood pressure.
- In patients with coronary heart disease, methohexital has been reported to decrease blood pressure by 15 % with a decrease in cardiac output by 20 %. Compared to propofol, it also increases heart rate [72]. Combined, these cardiovascular changes can decrease coronary perfusion pressure in patients at-risk for coronary ischemia.
- Respiratory depression is a dose-related side effect of all barbiturates. Methohexital decreases the body's respiratory sensitivity to carbon dioxide [15].
- Minute ventilation is reduced and apnea occurs at induction doses. Ventilatory efforts return in approximately 5 min. However, tidal volumes and repiratory rate may take up to 15 min to normalize to pre-drug state [45].
- Laryngeal responses are not well blunted with methohexital; opioids and/or lidocaine may be useful adjuncts prior to airway manipulation.
- Methohexital diffuses across the placenta and has been detected in breast milk [86].

References

1. Absalom A, Pledger D, Kong A. Adrenocortical function in critically ill patients 24 h after a single dose of etomidate. Anaesthesia. 1999;54:861–7.
2. Anderson JS, Rose NR, Martin JL, Eger EI, Njoku DB. Desflurane hepatitis associated with hapten and autoantigen-specific IgG4 antibodies. Anesth Analg. 2007;104:1452–3.
3. Apfel CC, Korttila K, Abdalla M, et al. A factorial trial of six interventions for the prevention of postoperative nausea and vomiting. N Engl J Med. 2004;350(24):2441–51.
4. Asserhoj LL, Mosbech H, Krøigaard M, Garvey LH. No evidence for contraindications to the use of propofol in adults allergic to egg, soy or peanut. Br J Anaesth. 2016;116(1):77–82.
5. Ben-Shlomo I, Moskovich R, Katz Y, Shalev E. Midazolam/ketamine sedative combination compared with fentanyl/propofol/isoflurane anaesthesia for oocyte retrieval. Hum Reprod. 1999;14(7):1757–9.
6. Ben-Shlomo I, Moskovich R, Golan J, Eyali V, Tabak A, Shalev E. The effect of propofol anaesthesia on oocyte fertilization and early embryo quality. Hum Reprod. 2000;15(10):2197–9.
7. Bito H, Ikeda K. Plasma inorganic fluoride and intracircuit degradation product concentrations in long-duration, low-flow sevoflurane anesthesia. Anesth Analg. 1994;79:946–51.
8. Bito H, Ikeda K. Renal and hepatic function in surgical patients after low-flow sevoflurane anesthesia. Anesth Analg. 1996;82:173–6.
9. Booker PD, Whyte PD, Ladusans EJ. Long QT syndrome and anaesthesia. BJA. 2003;90(3):349–66.

10. Brunt EM, White H, Marsh JW, et al. Fulminant hepatic failure after repeated exposure to isoflurane anesthesia: a case report. Hepatology. 1991;13:1017–21.
11. Caldwell JC, Fong C, Muhyaldeen SA. Should sevoflurane be used in the electrophysiology assessment of accessory pathways? Europace. 2010;12(9):1332–5.
12. Castagnini HE, van Eijs F, Salevsky FC, Nathanson MH. Sevoflurane for interventional neuroradiology procedures is associated with more rapid recovery than propofol. Can J Anaesth. 2004;51(5):486–91.
13. Christiaens F, Janssenswillen C, Verborgh C, et al. Propofol concentrations in follicular fluid during general anaesthesia for transvaginal oocyte retrieval. Hum Reprod. 1999;14(2): 345–8.
14. Choi ES, Shin JY, Oh AY, Park HP, Hwang JW, Lim YJ, Jeon YT. Sevoflurane versus propofol for interventional neuroradiology: a comparison of the maintenance and recovery profiles at comparable depths of anesthesia. Korean J Anesthesiol. 2014;66(4):290–4.
15. Choi SD, Spaulding BC, Gross JB, Apfelbaum JL. Comparison of the ventilator effects of etomidate and methohexital. Anesthesiology. 1985;62:442–7.
16. Coates KM, Flood P. Ketamine and its preservative, benzethonium chloride, both inhibit human recombinant alpha7 and alpha4beta2 neuronal nicotinic acetylcholine receptors in *Xenopus* oocytes. Br J Pharmacol. 2001;134:871–9.
17. Corssen G, Domino EF. Dissociative anesthesia: further pharmacologic studies and first clinical experience with the phencyclidine derivative CI-581. Anesth Analg. 1966;45:29–40.
18. Cortinez LI, Anderson BJ, Penna A, Olivares L, Munoz HR, Holford NHG, Struys MMRF, Sepulveda P. Influence of obesity on propofol pharmacokinetics: derivation of a pharmacokinetic model. Br J Anaesth. 2010;105(4):448–56.
19. Cullen PM, Turtle M, Prys-Roberts C, et al. Effect of propofol anesthesia on baroflex activity in humans. Anesth Analg. 1987;66:1115–20.
20. De Deyne C, Joly LM, Ravussin P. Newer inhalational anaesthetics and neuro-anaesthesia; what is the place for sevoflurane or desflurane? Ann Fr Anesth Reanim. 2004;23(4): 367–74.
21. De Hert S, Moerman A. Sevoflurane. F1000Res. 2015;4:626. doi:10.12688/f1000research.6288.1.
22. Ding Z, White PF. Anesthesia for electroconvulsive therapy. Anesth Analg. 2002;94:1351–64.
23. Diprivan [package insert] Lake Zurich: Fresenius Kabi, LLC; 2014.
24. Dolin SJ. Drugs and pharmacology. In: Padfield NL, editor. Total intravenous anesthesia. Oxford: Butterworth Heinemann; 2000. p. 13–35.
25. Duma A, Cartmill C, Blood J, Sharma A, Kharasch E, Nagele P. The hematological effects of nitrous oxide anesthesia in pediatric patients. Anesth Analg. 2015;120(6):1325–30.
26. Dundee JW, Lilburn JK. Ketamine-lorazepam: attenuation of the psychic sequlae of ketamine bylorazepam. Anesthesia. 1977;37:312–4.
27. Dyck J, Varvel J, Hung O. The pharmacokinetics of propofol versus age. Anesthesiology. 1991;75:A315.
28. Ebert TJ, Lindenbaum L. Inhaled anesthetics. In: Barash PG, editor. Clinical anesthesia. 7th ed. Philadelphia: Lippincott Williams & Wilkins; 2013. p. 467.
29. Ebrahim ZY, DeBoer GE, Luders H, Hahn JF, Lesser RP. Effect of etomidate on the electroencephalogram of patients with epilepsy. Anesth Analg. 1986;65:1004–6.
30. Eckstein JW, Hamilton WK, McCammond JM. The effect of thiopental on peripheral venous tone. Anesthesiology. 1961;22:525–8.
31. Eger 2nd EI. Isoflurane: a review. Anesthesiology. 1989;55:559–76.
32. Eger 2nd E. New inhaled anesthetics. Anesthesiology. 1994;80(4):906–22.
33. Eger 2nd EI. Uptake and distribution. In: Miller RD, editor. Miller's anesthesia. 6th ed. Philadelphia: Elsevier; 2005. p. 133–4.
34. Eikerman M, Grosse-Sundrup M, Zaremba S, Henry ME, Bittner EA, Hoffman U, Chamberlin NL. Ketamine activates breathing and abolished the coupling between loss of consciousness and upper airway muscle dysfunction. Anesthesiology. 2012;116(1):35–46.
35. Eisele JH, Milstein J, Goetzman B. Pulmonary vascular resistance to nitrous oxide in newborn lambs. Anesthesia and Analgesia. 1986;65(1):62–4.

36. Fink BR. Diffusion anoxia. Anesthesiology. 1955;16:511–9.
37. Flood P, Shafer S. Inhaled anesthetics. In: Flood P, Rathmell JP, Shafer S, editors. Stoelting's pharmacology and physiology in anesthetic practice. 5th ed. Philadelphia: Wolters Kluwer Health; 2015. p. 118.
38. Fond G, Bennabi D, Haffen E, et al. A Bayesian framework systematic review and meta-analysis of anesthetic agents effectiveness/tolerability profile in electroconvulsive therapy for major depression. Sci Rep. 2016;25:19847.
39. Fragen RJ, Shanks CA, Molteni A, Avram MJ. Effects of etomidate on hormonal responses to surgical stress. Anesthesiology. 1984;61:652–6.
40. Garcia PS, Kolesky SE, Jenkins A. General anesthetic actions on $GABA_A$ receptors. Curr Neuropharmacol. 2010;8(1):2–9.
41. Goff MJ, Arain SR, Ficke DJ, Uhrich TD, Ebert TJ. Absence of bronchodilation during desflurane anesthesia: a comparison to sevoflurane and thiopental. Anesthesiology. 2000;93(2):404–8.
42. Goodman NW, Black AM, Carter JA. Some ventilator effects of propofol as sole anaesthetic agent. Br J Anaesth. 1987;59:1497–503.
43. Gooding JM, Corssen G. Effect of etomidate on the cardiovascular system. Anesth Analg. 1977;56:717–9.
44. Graham SG. The desflurane Tec 6 vaporizer. Br J Anaesth. 1994;72(4):470–3.
45. Gross JB, Zebrowski ME, Carel WD, et al. Time course of ventilator depression after thiopental and midazolam in normal subjects and those with chronic obstructive pulmonary disease. Anesthesiology. 1983;58:540–4.
46. Groudine SC, Fragen, RJ, Kharasch ED, Eisenman TS, Frink EJ, McConell and the Sevoflurane Low-Flow Study Group. Comparision of renal function following anesthesia with low-flow sevoflurane and isoflurane. J Clin Anes. 1999;11(3):201–7.
47. Harper NJ. Propofol and food allergy. Br J Anaesth. 2016;116(1):11–3.
48. Helman JD, Leung JM, Bellows WH, Pineda N, Roach GW, Reeves 3rd JD, Howse J, McEnany MT, Mangano DT. The risk of myocardial ischemia in patients receiving desflurane versus sufentanil anesthesia for coronary artery bypass graft surgery. The SPI Research Group. Anesthesiology. 1992;77(1):47–62.
49. Hemmings Jr HC. The pharmacology of intravenous anesthetic induction agents: a primer. Anesthes News. 2010;Special Edition:9–16.
50. Herrick IA, Gelb AW. Anesthesia for temporal lobe epilepsy surgery. Can J Neurol Sci. 2000;27(S1):S64–7.
51. Hickey PR, Hansen DD, Cramolini GM, et al. Pulmonary and systemic hemodynamic responses to ketamine in infants with normal and elevated pulmonary vascular resistance. Anesthesiology. 1985;62:287–93.
52. Holaday DA, Fiserova-Bergerova V, Latto IP, Zumbiel MA. Resistance of isoflurane to biotransformation in man. Anesthesiology. 1975;43:325–32.
53. Hooten WM, Rasmussen Jr KG. Effects of general anesthetic agents in adults receiving electroconvulsive therapy: a systematic review. J ECT. 2008;24(3):208–23.
54. Huang HW, Huang FJ, Kung F, et al. Effects of induction anesthetic agents on outcome of assisted reproductive technology: a comparison of propofol and thiopental sodium. Chang Gung Med J. 2000;23(9):513–9.
55. Hughes MA, Glass PS, Jacobs JR. Context-sensitive half-time in multi-compartment pharmacokinetic models for intravenous anesthetic drugs. Anesthesiology. 1992;76(3):334–41.
56. Hurstveit O, Maurset A, Oye I. Interaction of the chiral forms of ketamine with opioid, phencyclidine, and muscarinic receptors. Pharmacol Toxicol. 1995;77:355–9.
57. Hutchison WD, Lozano AM. Microelectrode recordings in movement disorder surgery. In: Lozano AM, editor. Movement disorder surgery. Basel: Karger; 2000. p. 103–17.
58. Ickx B, Cockshott ID, Barvais L, Byttebler G, De Pauw L, Vandesteene A, D'Hollander AA. Propofol infusion for induction and maintenance of anaesthesia in patients with end-stage renal disease. Br J Anaesth. 1998;81(6):854–60.

59. Jabre P, Combes X, Lapostolle F, Dhaouadi M, Ricard-Hibon A, Vivien B, Bertrand L, Beltramini A, Gamand P, Albizzati S, Perdrizet D, Lebail G, Chollet-Xemard C, Maxime V, Brun-Buisson C, Lefrant JY, Bollaert PE, Megarbane B, Ricard JD, Anguel N, Vicaut E, Adnet F, KETASED Collaborative Study Group. Etomidate versus ketamine for rapid sequence intubation in acutely ill patients: a multicentre randomised controlled trial. Lancet. 2009;374:293–300.
60. Jokobsson J. Desflurane: a clinical update of a third generation inhaled anesthetic. Acta Anaesthesiol Scand. 2012;56(4):420–32.
61. Johnson KB, Egan TD, Layman J, Kern SE, White JL, McJames SW. The influence of hemorrhagic shock on etomidate: a pharmacokinetic and pharmacodynamic analysis. Anesth Analg. 2003;96(5):1360–8.
62. Julier K, da Silva R, Garcia C, Bestmann L, Frascarolo P, Zollinger A, Chassot PG, Schmid ER, Turina MI, von Segesser LK, Pasch T, Spahn DR, Zaugg M. Preconditioning by sevoflurane decreases biochemical markers for myocardial and renal dysfunction in coronary artery bypass graft surgery: a double-blinded, placebo-controlled, multicenter study. Anesthesiology. 2003;98:1315–27.
63. Juvin P, Vadam C, Malek L, Dupont H, Marmuse JP, Desmonts JM. Postoperative recovery after desflurane, propofol, or isoflurane anesthesia among morbidly obese patients: a prospective, randomized study. Anesth Analg. 2000;91:714–9.
64. Kharasch ED, Powers KM, Artru AA. Comparison of Amsorb, sodalime, Baralyme degradation of volatile anesthetics and formation of carbon monoxide and compound a in swine in vivo. Anesthesiology. 2002;96(1):173–82.
65. Kohrs R, Durieux ME. Ketamine: teaching an old drug new tricks. Anesth Analg. 1998;88:1186–93.
66. Kothary S, Zsigmond E. A double-blind study of the effective anti-hallucinatory doses of diazepam prior to ketamine anesthesia. Clin Pharmacol Ther. 1977;21:108.
67. Kuipers JA, Boer F, Olieman W, et al. First-pass lung uptake and pulmonary clearance of propofol: assessment with a recirculatory indocyanine green pharmacokinetic model. Anesthesiology. 1999;91:1780–7.
68. Lindgren L, Randell T, Saarnivaara L. Comparison of inhalation induction with isoflurane or halothane in children. Eur J Anaesthesiol. 1991;8:33–7.
69. Lehmann A, Neher M, Kiessling AH, Isgro F, Koloska A, Boldt J. Case report; fatal hepatic failure after aortic valve replacement and sevoflurane exposure. Can J Anaesth. 2007;54(11):917–21.
70. Lettieri C, Rinaldo S, Devigili G, Pauletto G, Verriello L, Budai R, et al. Deep brain stimulation: Subthalamic nucleus electrophysiological activity in awake and anesthetized patients. Clin Neurophysiol. 2012;123:2406–13.
71. Lenz C, Rebel A, Klaus V, et al. Local cerebral blood flow, local cerebral glucose utilization, and flow-metabolism coupling during sevoflurane versus isoflurane anesthesia in rats. Anesthesiology. 1998;89:1480–8.
72. Lepage JM, Pinaud ML, Helias J, Cozian AY, Le Normand Y, Souron RJ. Left ventricular performance during propofol or methohexital anesthesia: isotopic and invasive cardiac monitoring. Anesth Analg. 1991;73(1):3–9.
73. Lerman J. Pediatric anesthesia. In: Barash PG, editor. Clinical anesthesia. 7th ed. Philadelphia: Lippincott Williams & Wilkins; 2013. p. 1224.
74. Lesitsky MA, Davis S, Murray PA. Preservation of hypoxic pulmonary vasoconstriction during sevoflurane and desflurane anesthesia compared to the conscious state in chronically instrumented dogs. Anesthesiology. 1998;89:1505.
75. Loveridge R, Shroeder F. Anaesthetic preconditioning. Contin Educ Anaesth Crit Care Pain. 2010;10(2):38–42.
76. Liu LMP, Gaudreault P, Friedman PA, et al. Methohexital plasma concentrations in children following rectal administration. Anesthesiology. 1985;62:567–70.
77. Maeng S, Zarate CA. The role of glutamate in mood disorders: results from the ketamine in major depression study and the presumed cellular mechanism. Curr Psychiatry Rep. 2007;9(6):467–74.

78. Malinovsky JM, Servin F, Cozian A, Lepage JY, Pinaud M. Ketamine and norketamine plasma concentrations after IV, nasal and rectal administration in children. Br J Anaesth. 1996;77:203–7.

79. Marano G, Mauro G, Tiburzi F, Vergari A, Zanghi F. Effects of isoflurane on cardiovascular system and sympathovagal balance in New Zealand white rabbit. J Cardiovasc Pharmacol. 1996;28(4):513–8.

80. Marik PE, Varon J. The management of status epilepticus. Chest. 2004;126:582–9.

81. Martin Jr JL, Njoku DB. Metabolism and toxicity of modern inhaled anesthetics. In: Miller RD, editor. Miller's anesthesia. 6th ed. Philadelphia: Elsevier; 2005. p. 231–72.

81. Martin JL Jr., Njoku DB. Metabolism and Toxicity of Modern Inhaled Anesthetics. In Miller RD (Ed.) Miller's Anesthesia, Sixth Edition. Philadelphia, Pennsylvania. Elsevier. 2005;237–238.

82. Masin-Spasovska J, Dimitrovski K, Stavridis S, Stankov O, Dohcev S, Saidi S, Jokovski K, Balkanov T, Labacevski N, Lekovski L, Spasovski G. Acute fulminant hepatitis in kidney transplant recipience after repeated sevoflurane anesthesia—a case report. Curr Drug Saf. 2013;8(2):141–4.

83. McKay RE, Large MJ, Balea MC, McKay WR. Airway reflexes return more rapidly after desflurane anesthesia than after sevoflurane anesthesia. Anesth Analg. 2005;100:697–700.

84. McKay RE, Malhotra A, Cakmakkaya OS, Hall KT, McKay WR, Apfel CC. Effect of increased body mass index and anaesthetic duration on recovery of protective airway reflexes after sevoflurane vs desflurane. Br J Anaesth. 2010;104:175–82.

85. McKay RE, Sonner J, McKary WR. Inhaled anesthetics. In: Stoelting RK, Miller RD, editors. Basics of anesthesia. 5th ed. Philadelphia: Churchill Livingstone Elsevier; 2007. p. 93.

86. Methohexital [package insert]. Rochster: JHP Pharmaceuticals, LLC; 2014.

87. Mion G, Villevielle T. Ketamine pharmacology: an update (pharmacodynamics and molecular aspects, recent findings). CNS Neurosci Ther. 2013;19:370–80.

88. Mirrakhimov AE, Voore P, Halytskyy O, Khan M, Ali AM. Propofol infusion syndrome in adults: a clinical update. Crit Care Res Pract. 2015;2015.

89. Modica PA, Tempelhoff R. Intracranial pressure during induction of anaesthesia and tracheal intubation with etomidate-induced EEG burst suppression. Can J Anaesth. 1992;39:236–41.

90. Morray JP, Lynn AM, Stamm SJ, et al. Hemodynamic effects of ketamine in children with congenital heart disease. Anesth Analg. 1984;63:895–9.

91. Murrough JW, Iosifescu DV, Chang LC, Al Jurdi RK, Green CE, Perez AM, Iqbal S, Pillemer S, Foulkes A, Shah A, Charney DS, Mathew SJ. Antidepressant efficacy of ketamine in treatment-resistant major depression: a twi-site randomized controlled trial. Am J Psychiatry. 2013;170:1134–42.

92. Myles PS, Chan MTV, Kasza J, Paech MJ, Leslie K, Peyton PJ, Sessler DI, Haller G, Beattie S, Osborne C, Sneyd R, Forbes A. Severe nausea and vomiting in the elimination of nitrous oxide in the gas mixture for anesthesia II trial. Anesthesiology. 2016;124(5):1032–40. doi:10.1097/ALN.0000000000001057.

93. Myles PS, Leslie K, Chan MTV, Forbes A, Peyton PJ, Paech MJ, Beattie WS, Sessler SI, Devereaux PJ, Siblert B, Schricker T, Wallace S; the ANZCA Trials Group for the ENIGMA-II Investigators. Lancet. 2014;384(9952):1446–54.

94. Nikolajsen L, Hansen CL, Nielsen J, Keller J, Arendt-Nielsen L, Jensen TS. The effect of ketamine on phantom pain: a central neuropathic disorder maintained by peripheral input. Pain. 1996;67:69–77.

95. Njoku D, Laster MJ, Gong DH, Eger EI, Reed GF, Martin JL. Biotransformation of halothane, enflurane, isoflurane, and desflurane to trifluoroacetylated liver proteins: association between protein acylation and hepatic injury. Anesth Anal. 1997;84(1):173–8.

96. Nyktari V, Papaioannou A, Volakakis N, Lappa A, Margaritsanaki P, Askitopoulou H. Respiratory resistance during anaesthesia with isoflurane, sevoflurane, and desflurane: a randomized clinical trial. Br J Anaesth. 2011;107:454–61.

97. Ohtani M, Kikuchi H, Kitahata LM, et al. Effects of ketamine on nociceptive cells in the medial medullary reticular formation of the cat. Anesthesiology. 1979;51:414–7.
98. Okamoto GU, Duperon DF, Jedrychowski JR. Clinical evaluation of the effects of ketamine sedation on pediatric dental patients. J Clin Pediatr Dent. 1992;16:253–7.
99. Pacentine GG, Muzi M, Ebert TJ. Effects of fentanyl on sympathetic activation associated with the administration of desflurane. Anesthesiology. 1995;82:823–31.
100. Pagel PS, Kersten JR, Farber NE, Warltier DC. Cardiovascular phamacology. In: Miller RD, editor. Miller's anesthesia. 6th ed. Philadelphia: Elsevier; 2005. p. 192–3.
101. Pasarón R, Burnweit C, Zerpa J, Malvezzi L, Kinght C, Shapiro T, Ramos-Irizarry C, Velis E. Nitrous oxide procedural sedation in non-fasting pediatric patients undergoing minor surgery: a 12-year experience with 1,058 patients. Pediatr Surg Int. 2015;31:173–80.
102. Patel AS, Gorst-Unsworth C, Venn RM, Kelley K, Jacob Y. Anesthesia and electroconvulsive therapy: a retrospective study comparing etomidate and propofol. J ECT. 2006;22(3): 179–83.
103. Patel SS, Goa KL. Sevoflurane: a review of its pharmacodynamics and pharmacokinetic properties and its use in general anesthesia. Drugs. 1996;51(4):658–700.
104. Patel PM, Drummond JC. Cerebral physiology and the effects of anesthetic drugs. In Miller Rd (Ed.) Miller's Anesthesia, Seventh Edition. Philadelphia: Elsevier. 2010, pg. 307.
105. Petersen KD, Landsfeldt U, Cold GE, Petersen CB, Mau S, Hauerberg J, Hoist P, Olsen KS. Intracranial pressure and cerebral hemodynamic in patients with cerebral tumors: a randomized prospective study of patients subjected to craniotomy in propofol-fentanyl, isoflurane-fentanyl, or sevoflurane-fentanyl anesthesia. Anesthesiology. 2003;98(2):329–36.
106. Peyton P, Wu CY. Nitrous Oxide-related postoperative nausea and vomiting depends on duration of exposure. Anesthesiology. 2014;120(5):1137–45.
107. Piroli A, Marci F, Marinangeli F, et al. Comparison of different anaesthetic methodologies for sedation during in vitro fertilization procedures: effects on patient physiology and oocyte competence. Gynecol Endocrinol. 2012;28(10):796–9.
108. Propofol injectable emulsion 1 % [package insert]. Lake Forest: Hospira Pharmaceuticals; 2015.
109. Propofol injectable emulsion 1 % [package insert]. Schaumburg: SAGENT Pharmaceuticals; 2014.
110. Rasmussen KG. Propofol for ECT anesthesia a review of the literature. J ECT. 2014;30(3):210–5.
111. Rasmussen KG, Lineberry TW, Galardy CW, Kung S, Lapid MI, Palmer MJ, Schak KM, Sola CL, Hanson AJ, Frye MA. Serial infusions of low-dose ketamine for major depression. J Psychopharmacol. 2013;27(5):444–50.
112. Rathmell J, Roscow CE. Intravenous sedatives and hypnotics. In: Flood P, Rathmell JP, Shafer S, editors. Stoelting's pharmocology and physiology in anesthetic practice. 5th ed. Philadelphia: Wolters Kluwer Health; 2015. p. 160–203.
113. Ray DC, Bomont R, Mizushima A, et al. effect of sevoflurane anaesthesia on plasma concentrations of glutathione S-transferase. Br J Anaesth. 1994;73:590–5.
114. Reves JG, Glass PSA, Lubarsky DA, Mcevoy MD. Intravenous non-opiod anesthetics. In: Miller RD, editor. Miller's anesthesia. 6th ed. Philadelphia: Elsevier; 2005. p. 347.
115. Riess ML, Stowe DF, Warltier DC. Cardiac pharmacological preconditioning with volatile anesthetics: from bench to bedside? Am J Physiol. 2004;286(5):H1603–7.
116. Sanacora G, Zarate CA, Krystal JH, Manji HK. Targeting the glutamatergic system to develop novel, improved therapeutics for mood disorders. Nat Rev Drug Discov. 2008;7:426–37.
117. Schulte-Sasse U, Hess W, Tarnow J. Pulmonary vascular responses to nitrous oxide in patient with normal and high pulmonary vascular resistance. Anesthesiology. 1982;57(1):9–13.
118. Schuttler J, Stanski DR, White PF, et al. Pharmacodynamic modeling of the EEG effects of ketamine and its enantiomers in man. J Pharmacokinet Biopharm. 1987;15:241–53.

119. Servin F, Desmonts JM, Haberer JP, Cockshott ID, Plummer GF, Farinotti R. Pharmacokinetics and protein binding of propofol in patients with cirrhosis. Anesthesiology. 1988;69(9): 887–91.
120. Sharpe MD, Cuillerier DJ, Lee JK, Basta M, Krahn AD, Klein GJ, Yee R. Sevoflurane has no effect on sinoatrial node function or on normal atrioventricular and accessory pathway conduction in Wolff-Parkinson-White syndrome during alfentanil/midazolam anesthesia. Anesthesiology. 1999;90(1):60–5.
121. Sigtermans MJ, van Hilten JJ, Bauer MCR, Arbous S, Marinus J, Sarton EY, Dahan A. Ketamine produces effective and long-term pain relief in patients with complex regional pain syndrome type I. Pain. 2009;145(3):304–11.
122. Sloan TB, Ronai AK, Toleikis JR, Koht A. Improvement of intraoperative somatosensory evoked potentials by etomidate. Anesth Analg. 1988;67:582–5.
123. Solelmanpour H, Safari S, Rahmani F, Ameli H, Alavian SM. The role of inhalational anesthetic drugs in patients with hepatic dysfunction: a review article. Anesth Pain Med. 2015;5(1):e23409. doi:10.5812/aapm.23409.
124. Song XX, Yu BW. Anesthetic effects of propofol in the healthy human brain: functional imaging evidence. J Anesth. 2015;29(2):279–88.
125. Sprung CL, Annane D, Keh D, Moreno R, Singer M, Freivogel K, Weiss YG, Benbenishty J, Kalenka A, Forst H, Laterre PF, Reinhart K, Cuthbertson BH, Payen D, Briegel J, CORTICUS Study Group. Hydrocortisone therapy for patients with septic shock. N Engl J Med. 2008;358:111–24.
126. Staikou C, Stamelos M, Stavroulakis E. Impact of anaesthetic drugs and adjuvants on ECG markers of torsadogenicity. Br J Anaesth. 2014;11(2):217–30.
127. Strum EM, Szenohradszki J, Kaufman WA, Anthone GJ, Manz IL, Lumb PD. Emergence and recovery characteristics of desflurane versus sevoflurane in morbidly obese adult surgical patients: a prospective, randomized study. Anesth Analg. 2004;99:1848–53.
128. Tanelian DL, Kosek P, Mody I, MacIver MB. The role of the GABA$_A$ receptor/chloride channel complex in anesthesia. Anesthesiology. 1993;78:757–76.
129. Taniguchi M, Nadstawek J, Langenbach U, Bremer F, Schramm J. Effects of four intravenous anesthetic agents on motor evoked potentials elicited by magnetic transcranial stimulation. Neurosurgery. 1993;33:407–15.
130. Tarnow J, Eberlein HJ, Oser G, et al. Influence of modern inhalation anaesthetics on haemodynamics, myocardial contractility, left ventricular volumes and myocardial oxygen supply. Anaesthesist. 1977;26:220–30.
131. Takizawa D, Hiraoka H, Goto F, Yamamoto K, Horiuchi R. Human kidneys play an important role in the elimination of propofol. Anesthesiology. 2005;102(2):327–30.
132. Todd MM, Drummond JC, U HS. The hemodynamic consequences of high-dose thiopental anesthesia. Anesth Analg. 1985;64:681–7.
133. Tomlin SL, Jenkins A, Lieb WR, Franks NP. Preparation of barbiturate optical isomers and their effects on GABA(A) receptors. Anesthesiology. 1999;90:1714–22.
134. Tomlin SL, Jenkins A, Lieb WR, et al. Stereoselective effects of etomidate on optical isomers on gamma-butyric acid type A receptors and animals. Anesthesiology. 1998;88(3): 708–17.
135. Turner GB, O-Rourke D, Scott GO, Beringer TR. Fatal hepatotoxicity after re-exposure to isoflurane anesthesia: a case report and review of the literature. Eur J Gastroenterol Hepatol. 2000;12:955–9.
136. Van Beem H, Manger FW, van Boxtel C, van Bentem N. Etomidate anaesthesia in patients with cirrhosis of the liver: pharmacokinetic data. Anaesthesia. 1983;38(Suppl):61–2.
137. Van Keulen SG, Burton JH. Myoclonus associated with etomidate for ED procedural sedation and analgesia. Am J Emerg Med. 2003;21(7):556–8.
138. Vandesteene A, Trempont V, Engelman E, et al. Effect of propofol on cerebral blood flow and metabolism in man. Anaesthesia. 1988;43(supple):42–3.
139. Vanlander AV, Okun JG, de Jaeger A, Smet J, De Latter E, De Paepe B, Dacremont G, Wuyts B, Vanheel B, De Paepe P, Jorens PG. Possible pathogenic mechanism of propofol infusion syndrome involves coenzyme q. Anesthesiology. 2015;122(2):343–52.

140. Veroli P, O'Kelly B, Betrand F, et al. Extrahepatic metabolism of propofol in man during the anhepatic phase of orthotopic liver transplantation. Br J Anaesth. 1992;68:183–6.
141. Vu N, Lou JR, Kupiec TC. Quality control analytic methods: microbial limit tests for nonsterile pharmaceuticals, part 1. Int J Pharm Compd. 2014;18(3):213–21.
142. Wachowski I, Jolly DT, Hrazdil J, Galbraith JC, Greacen M, Clanachan AS. The growth of microorganisms in propofol and mixtures of propofol and lidocaine. Anesth Analg. 1999;88(1):209–12.
143. Walder B, Tramer MR, Seeck M. Seizure-like phenomena and propofol: a systematic review. Neurology. 2002;58:1327–32. cd.
144. Weiskoph RB, Cahalan MK, Eger II EI, et al. Cardiovascular actions of desflurane on normocarbic volunteers. Anesth Analg. 1991;73:143–56.
145. White P, Eng MR. Intravenous anesthetics. In: Barash PG, editor. Clinical anesthesia. 7th ed. Philadelphia: Lippincott Williams & Wilkins; 2013. p. 485.
146. Yokoe C, Hanamoto H, Sugimura M, Morimoto Y, Kudo C, Niwa H. A prospective, randomized controlled trial of conscious sedation using propofol combined with inhaled nitrous oxide for dental treatment. J Oral Maxillofac Surg. 2015;73(3):402–9.
147. Zizek D, Ribnikar M, Zizek B, Ferlan-Marolt V. Fatal subacute liver failure after repeated administration of sevoflurane anaesthesia. Eur J Gastroenterol Hepatol. 2010;22(1):112–5.
148. Zsigmond E, Domino E. Clinical pharmacology and current uses of ketamine. In: Aldrete J, Stanley T, editors. Trends in intravenous anesthesia. Chicago: Year Book; 1980. p. 283.

Chapter 3
Principles of Delivery of Sedatives and Intravenous Anesthetics in Out of Operating Room Anesthesia

Jean Gabriel Charchaflieh, Monica Ganatra, and Erin Springer

Abstract Safe and effective delivery of IV sedatives and anesthetics for Out of Operating Room Anesthesia (OORA) is based on the same principles that govern delivery of these medications in the OR settings, while taking into account the unique conditions imposed by the diverse environments of each of the procedural locations. This entails understanding, and implementing, all applicable scientific, technological, regulatory, and organizational principles in order to enhance patient safety and operational efficiency. Delivering OORA poses physical and operational constraints, in the forms of limited lighting; excessive noise; limited access by the clinician to the patient; and limited devise allowance into OORA sites, e.g., MRI suite; disorganized scheduling and inadequate patient preparation.

The benefits of understanding operational principles of OORA extend to OR and ICU settings as many OR suites are becoming increasingly hybrid environments, e.g., OR MRI or OR-bi-plane angiography, and OR electrophysiology; and as many procedures are performed in ICU settings, e.g., percutaneous tracheotomy tube insertion and percutaneous endoscopic gastrostomy (PEG) tube insertions. The portability and versatility of IV anesthetics and sedatives make them particularly suitable choices for OORA. Technological advances in drug delivery of IV anesthetic and sedatives, in the forms of programmable drug delivery devices, and target-controlled infusion (TCI) systems, enhance the utility of IV anesthetics and sedatives in the OORA environment and extends as well to the OR and intensive care units (ICU).

J.G. Charchaflieh, MD, PhD (✉)
Department of Anesthesiology, Yale University School of Medicine,
333 Cedar Street, TMP 3, New Haven, CT 06510, USA
e-mail: jean.charchaflieh@yale.edu

M. Ganatra, MD, MPH • E. Springer, MD
Department of Anesthesiology, Yale New Haven Hospital,
333 Cedar Street, TMP 3, P.O. Box 208051, New Haven, CT, USA
e-mail: monica.ganatra@yale.edu; erin.springer@yale.edu

© Springer International Publishing Switzerland 2017
B.G. Goudra, P.M. Singh (eds.), *Out of Operating Room Anesthesia*,
DOI 10.1007/978-3-319-39150-2_3

Keywords Pharmacokinetics (PK) • Pharmacodynamics (PD) • Pharmacogenomics • Bioavailability • Variability • Half-life (T1/2) • Context sensitive halftimes • Apparent volume of distribution (Vd) • Elimination rate (ER) • Drug clearance (CL) • Target blood concentration (TBC) • Drug infusion rate (DIR) • Target-controlled infusion (TCI) • Manually controlled infusion (MCI) • Bispectral Index (BIS)

Introduction

Safe and effective delivery of IV sedatives and anesthetics for Out of Operating Room Anesthesia (OORA) is based on the same principles that govern delivery of these medications in the OR settings, while taking into account the unique conditions imposed by the diverse environments of each of the procedural locations. This entails understanding, and implementing, all applicable scientific, technological, regulatory, and organizational principles in order to enhance patient safety and operational efficiency. Delivering OORA poses physical and operational constraints, in the forms of limited lighting, excessive noise, limited access by the clinician to the patient, and limited devise allowance into OORA sites, e.g., MRI suite, disorganized scheduling and inadequate patient preparation.

The benefits of understanding operational principles of OORA extend to OR and ICU settings as many OR suites are becoming increasingly hybrid environments by including OR MRI or OR-bi-plane angiography, and OR electrophysiology; and as many procedures are performed in ICU settings, e.g., percutaneous tracheotomy tube insertion and percutaneous endoscopic gastrostomy (PEG) tube insertions. The portability and versatility of IV anesthetics and sedatives make them particularly suitable choices for OORA. Technological advances in drug delivery of IV anesthetic and sedatives, in the forms of programmable drug delivery devices, and target-controlled infusion (TCI) systems, enhance the utility of IV anesthetics and sedatives in the OORA environment and extends as well to the OR and intensive care units (ICU).

Basic Pharmacokinetics and Pharmacodynamics, Variability, Blood and Effect Site Concentrations, Context Sensitive Halftimes

Pharmacokinetics (PK) is the study of drug movement in the body, while pharmacodynamics (PD) is the study of drug effects on the body. PK studies indicate that the IV route is the fastest route of delivering anesthetics and sedatives to their target site of action in the CNS, where they can exert their PD effect. However before reaching the CNS, the IV injected medication has to pass by the lung and the heart, which can affect drug bioavailability and side effects.

In the lungs, the enzymatically active pulmonary vascular endothelium can reduce the bioavailability of certain drugs, such as propofol, by metabolizing the medication. Also in the lungs, the large surface area of the pulmonary alveolar endothelium provides a high rate of uptake of lipophilic drugs, such as fentanyl, with later reinfusion of the drug into the blood. The process of pulmonary first-pass uptake of a drug slows both the rate of delivering the drug to its site of action in the CNS, and the rate of termination of its action if enough amount of drug is stored in the pulmonary endothelium and later re-infused into the blood. Pulmonary first pass uptake is increased in cigarette smokers, and decreased by co-administration of other lipophilic drug, including inhalation agents.

In the heart, cardiac side effects can be aggravated by rapid delivery of a large bolus of an IV injected medication that has low therapeutic index for cardiac side effects, such as propofol. Decreased cardiac function aggravates the hemodynamic side effects of IV sedatives and anesthetics both by decreasing the reserve function of the heart and by slowing the delivery of drug into its site of action in the CNS, which might lead the clinician into injecting a repeated dose, in order to achieve a faster CNS response, resulting in greater cardiac side effects. In patients with decreased cardiac function, cardiac side effects of IV anesthetics can be ameliorated, by slow, incremental administration of the IV drug, allowing extra time for CNS effects to manifest, (the rule of giving half the dose and double the time), while providing frequent (every 1 min), if not continuous, measurement of blood pressure (BP), and having appropriate pressors available for the treatment of detected cardiac side effects.

From the blood, the drug moves to the interstitial space and its receptor site, most commonly, by a process of passive diffusion, which is based on the concentration gradient across the diffusion membrane, and enhanced by small drug molecular weight, decreased binding to plasma proteins, decreased drug ionized/nonionized fraction, and increased drug lipophilicity. For certain drugs, diffusion is facilitated by a carrier molecule that facilitates drug diffusion into the cell along concentration gradient, in a non-energy requiring process (facilitated diffusion). Carrier molecules can also actively transport a drug into the cell, against a concentration gradient, in an energy-requiring process (active transport), or actively transport a drug out of the cell by energy-driven pumps known as ATP-binding cassettes transporters (ABC transporters).

Bioavailability refers to the portion of the drug that is present in a form that can exert a PD effect at the site of action. Some drugs are administered in a non-active, or less-active, pro-drug form that has better pharmacokinetic profile, but poorer pharmacodynamic effect and is bio-transformed in the body into a more active form. For example, in vitro, at pH < 6, the benzodiazepine midazolam is hydrophilic and therefore less irritant to the vein upon injection, but is also less active; while in vivo, at pH > 6, it is bio-transformed, by closing its imidazole ring, into a more active lipophilic form. The opioid drugs codeine, oxycodone, and hydrocodone, are administered as pro-drugs that are bio-transformed in the body into their active forms of morphine, oxymorphone and hydromorphone, respectively.

The time lag between reaching a certain drug level in the plasma and achieving a certain drug effect in the CNS is called hysteresis, which manifests clinically as the speed of onset of action of a drug, and is influenced by factors that affect drug diffusion into its site of action. For example, the opioid drug alfentnail has a faster hysteresis, i.e., faster onset of action than fentanyl, because, at physiologic pH, alfentnayl has a higher non-ionized fraction in the plasma than fentanyl, which results also in shorter duration of action than fentanyl, as diffusion from the site of action is also faster for alfentanil.

Once the drug reaches its site of action, and exerts its PD effect, its termination of action is achieved by dissociation from the site of action, redistribution from the central (vessel rich) compartment into peripheral (vessel poor) compartment, and final elimination by inactivation and/or excretion.

The PK process is influenced by physiologic factors that affect drug distribution between compartments, such as hydration status and plasma protein levels of the patient; drug metabolism, such as enzymatic activity; and drug elimination, such as organ dysfunction of organs involved in drug elimination such as the liver and the kidney. Drug metabolism in the liver can eliminate drug action by transforming the drug into an inactive form and/or by facilitating its excretion by the kidney through the processes of polarization, conjugation and increased hydrophilicity.

The effect of liver dysfunction on drug elimination is a function of both hepatic blood flow and hepatic extraction ratio. For drugs that have high hepatic extraction ratio, such as propofol, clearance from plasma is dependent on hepatic blood flow (flow limited elimination). However, in the case of propofol, the rate of elimination exceeds the rate of hepatic blood flow, which indicates the presence of extra-hepatic sites of drug elimination. For drugs that have low hepatic extraction ratio, such as alfentanil, clearance from plasma is dependent on the capacity of hepatic function (capacity limited elimination).

Besides the liver and the kidney, drug elimination can occur by enzymatic hydrolysis or by spontaneous (Hofmann) degradation. Enzymatic hydrolysis can occur by plasma esterases or tissue esterases. Drugs that are cleared by plasma esterases include the muscle relaxants succinylcholine, and mivacurium and the local anesthetic chloroprocaine. For these medications, quantitative or qualitative decrease in function of plasma esterases results in delayed drug clearance from the plasma, manifesting as prolonged duration of action of the drug. The ultra-short acting opioid remifentanil is cleared mainly by tissue esterases of muscles and intestines and to a much less extent by tissue esterases of lung, liver, kidney and blood, which makes clearance of remifentanil independent of decreased plasma esterase activity. The muscle relaxant cisatracurium is cleared primarily by Hofmann degradation, which is pH- and temperature-dependent spontaneous degradation of the drug, which makes clearance of this drug independent of liver or kidney function or plasma enzymatic activity but decreased by hypothermia and acidosis.

The rise and decline in plasma levels after drug administration, is presented in pharmacodynamic models, as a curve of steep linear rise during the infusion, followed by an inverse exponential curve of elimination that can be divided to three phases: rapid decline due to initial distribution, intermediate decline due to later re-distribution and slower decline due to elimination. The inverse exponential curve of drug elimination is based on the conceptual two-compartment model of drug distribution: the central (vessel rich) compartment and the peripheral (vessel poor) compartment, with the initial rapid decline in plasma level representing the initial rapid distribution of the drug from the central compartment to the peripheral compartment. When modeling drug elimination from the body as one compartment, a distinction is made between first-order and zero order kinetics, where first-order kinetics refers to fractional (percentage) drug elimination from the plasma per unit of time, while zero-order kinetics refers to constant amount of drug elimination from the plasma per unit of time.

Serial measurements of drug plasma concentrations after administering a certain dose of a drug, allows calculating the apparent volume of distribution of the drug, (Vd), elimination rate (ER) of the drug, drug clearance (CL), and half-life (T1/2) of the drug. These calculations form the basis of designing TCI systems that predict drug concentration using these parameters.

The apparent (Vd) of a drug is the calculated conceptual volume of a body compartment that is required to produce the measured concentration (C) from the measured dose (D) of the drug (Vd = D/C). The calculated Vd is expressed in liters (L) and can be expressed per body compartment such as blood (b), plasma (p) or water (w). Depending on drug properties that govern drug distribution in between the two compartments, the apparent Vd can actually exceed the actual plasma volume. This occurs in cases of drugs that produce low plasma concentrations due to any or combination of factors such as low binding to plasma proteins, low ionized fraction, high lipophilicity and high binding to tissues outside the plasma, (e.g., fentanyl Vd = 350 L). Thus, Vd can be considered an index of the factors that affect drug distribution between the compartments in a two-compartment model. Since the Vd is a calculated number based on measuring C after a certain D was administered, the calculated Vd varies based on the time interval between administering D and measuring C. Therefore the Vd is dynamic and it changes with drug redistribution between compartments and eventual elimination. The calculated Vd of a drug is obtained immediately after drug administration and is thought to reflect C after the initial phase of drug distribution. Knowing the Vd of a drug, allows calculating the D of drug that is needed to produce a certain C, based on rearranging Vd formula to read: D = Vd × C.

Drug clearance (CL) is defined as the volume, in liters (L), that is cleared of the drug per unit of time, in hours (h), and is calculated by dividing drug elimination rate (ER) by drug concentration (C), CL = ER/C. The conceptual CL can be calculated for specific body compartment: blood (b), plasma (p) or water (w), or organs: liver (L), kidney (K), lung (L) or other (O), with the total systemic clearance being the sum of individual organs clearances, CL systemic = CL (L) + CL (K) + CL (O). Using the calculated conceptual Vd and CL, the half-life (T1/2) of a drug can be calculated as: T1/2 = 0.7 × Vd/CL, where 0.7 is used as an approximation to the natural logarithm of 2, which is expressing a two-fold decrease in drug concentration per T1/2. In a static model, following a single bolus drug administration, after five T1/2 have elapsed, the concentration of a drug would be 1/32 (3.125%) of its original concentration, which would be considered negligible for most drugs. However, with continuous drug infusion, the T1/2 of a drug, becomes sensitive to the duration of infusion, since drug uptake into, and redistribution from, inert tissues, affects concentration at the target effect site.

For most drugs, continuous infusion produces a longer T1/2 than that following a single bolus, and is called context-sensitive T1/2, where the context is the duration of infusion. This is an important concept when aiming for reliable emergence from drug effects after continuous infusion over hours. Among currently available IV opioids, only remifentanyl has a T1/2 that is independent of duration of infusion, because it is metabolized by tissue esterase. Recovery from remifentanyl is usually within 3–5 min regardless of duration of infusion, and its terminal elimination T1/2 is 9 min.

PD studies explain how a drug achieves its effects at the targeted site of action, and elsewhere. The PD process can be complicated by the level of activity of the targeted receptor, which can be affected either by physiologic status of the patient or by the presence of other drugs that interact either with the target receptor or even with other receptors that affect the function of the target receptor.

Drug receptors are generally cell membrane proteins that are activated by binding to the administered drug, and, when activated, they can activate a G-protein, open an ion channel or activate an enzyme. Opening an ion channel can be done by binding the drug to its ligand or by changing the voltage across cell membrane. Examples of the former include the GABA receptor, which is the site of action for benzodiazepines, propofol, etomidate and barbiturates; and the nicotinic acetylcholine receptor, which is the site of action of non-depolarizing neuromuscular blocking agents (NMBA); while an example of the latter is the sodium channel which is the site of action of local anesthetics.

IV anesthetics and sedatives, acting at different receptors, can have synergistic effects. The IV opioid alfentanil, which activates the opioid receptors, has synergistic effect with the IV anesthetic propofol, which activates the GABA receptor. Moderate plasma levels of alfentnail 100–400 (ng/ml) have been shown to decrease the required plasma level of propofol that is associated with 50% probability of no response to surgical incision, i.e. effective dose 50% (ED50), the equivalent of minimal alveolar concentration (MAC); and the required plasma level of propofol that is associated with 50% probability of awakening, i.e. the equivalent of MAC awake [1].

Variability in drug response among individual patients occurs due to genetic factors, physiologic state (including age), co-morbidities and co-medications. Genetic factors affect both the PK and PD of a drug. It is likely that variability in drug response reflects variability in multiple factors affecting both PK and PD.

Genetic factors affect PK, mainly by affecting activity of drug metabolizing enzymes. Examples of genetic factors affecting PK include genetic variants of CYP3A4 (cytochrome p450), CYP2C19, CYP2D6, and butyrylcholinesterase.

Genetic variant CYP3A4*18 of CYP3A4, has decrease activity, which affects metabolism of opioids, benzodiazepines, local anesthetics, steroids, calcium channel blockers, haloperidol and halothane; while genetic variant CYP3A4*19 has increased activity. Genetic variants of CYP2C19 that have decreased activity are found predominantly in African Americans and can affect the metabolism of diazepam. Inactive genetic variants of CYP2D6 are found in 70–100 % of Caucasians, which leads to inability to convert the pro-drugs codeine, oxycodone, and hydrocodone, to their active forms of morphine, oxymorphone and hydromorphone respectively, and thus render the parent drug devoid of analgesic activity in such patients. This common enzyme variance can explain variance in analgesic response among patients, and it could possible form the basis for variance in side effects, e.g., delirium, to certain opioids. Genetic variants of butyrylcholinesterase that have decreased activity, are more common in people of Middle Eastern descent, and can result in decreased metabolism of succinylcholine and ester local anesthetics, which manifests as longer paralysis with the former and more systemic effects with the latter.

Genetic factors affect PD by affecting drug receptors, second messenger system or ion channels. The metabolic syndrome of malignant hyperthermia (MH) represents an altered PD response to halogenated vapors and succinylcholine, and could be due to either mutations in the ryanodine receptor gene RYR1, (>50 % of cases of MH), or due to altered voltage gated dihydropyridine receptor, either of which results in altered calcium regulation in the muscular sarcoplasm, which leads to altered response to the triggering drug, which manifests as hyperthermia, hypercapnea, hyperkalemia, metabolic acidosis and muscle rigidity.

Physiologic changes in the elderly that affect PK include:

1. Decreased total body water, which decreases initial volume of distribution, which leads to higher peak concentration, manifesting as increased sensitivity to the CNS effects of anesthetics and sedatives.
2. Increased body fat, which increases the likelihood of accumulating lipophilic drugs, manifesting as increased duration of action of these drugs.
3. Decreased both hepatic blood flow and metabolic capacity, which decreases clearance of many drugs, manifesting as increased sensitivity and duration of action of many anesthetics and sedatives including, opioids, hypnotics, benzodiazepines and muscle relaxants.
4. Decreased plasma albumin, which increases free fraction of albumin-bound drugs such as diazepam, manifesting as increased sensitivity to these drugs.
5. Increased plasma α_1-acid glycoproteins (α_1-GP), which decreases the free fraction of α_1-GP-bound drugs, such as lidocaine, and might lead to decreased clearance.

Physiologic changes in the elderly that affect PD are not well defined but are likely to include decreased number of drug receptors due to decreased brain mass, resulting in increased sensitivity to anesthetics and sedatives.

Co-morbidities can affect PK and PD of IV anesthetics and sedatives. Congestive heart failure (CHF) affects PK by decreasing hepatic blood flow resulting in decreased hepatic clearance of IV anesthetics and sedatives. Similarly, decreased liver function decreases hepatic metabolic capacity resulting in decreased hepatic clearance. Renal failure decreases the elimination of drugs or their active metabolites resulting in prolonged or altered effects. For example the accumulation of opioids and their active metabolites can result in increased and prolonged respiratory depression effects of these drugs, while the accumulation of mepiridine's active metabolite, nor-mepiridine, can result in seizure activity in patients with renal failure.

Co-morbidities affect PD by affecting drug receptor pathways. Myasthenia gravis (MG) is an autoimmune disorder in which antibodies against post-synaptic nicotinic acetylcholine receptors decrease their number and results in increased sensitivity to muscle relaxants. Spinal cord injury results in chronic muscle denervation, which results in increased density (number) of the nicotinic acetylcholine receptors at the neuromuscular junction, which results in increased sensitivity to the exogenous nicotinic acetylcholine receptor agonist, succinylcholine, manifesting clinically as life-threatening hyperkalemia.

CHF is associated with compensatory chronic increase in endogenous norepinephrine which results in decreased density (number) of β-adrenergic receptors, (75 % decrease in β_1 and 25 % in β_2), which decreases sensitivity to exogenous catecholamines (desensitization). In CHF patients, administration of chronic low-dose β-adrenergic receptor blockers can help re-sensitize β-adrenergic receptors to endogenous, as well as exogenous, catecholamines resulting in improved function and survival.

Co-medications can affect PK and PD of IV anesthetics and sedatives. Co-medications can affect PK by affecting hepatic enzymes or blood flow. The hepatic enzyme system CYP3A4 is responsible for the metabolism of about 50 % of all drugs and can be inhibited or induced by certain drugs, supplements and nutrients. Agents that inhibit the CYP3A4 include grapefruit juice, ketoconazole, itraconazole, ritonavir, indinavir, saquinavir, troleandomycin, clarithromycin, erythromycin, fluoxetine, sertraline and propofol. Agents that induce the CYP3A4 include rifampin, rifabutin, tamoxifen, glucocorticoids, carbamazepine, barbiturates, and St. John's Wort. The CYP2D6 enzyme is responsible for the conversion of the pro-drugs codeine, oxycodone, and hydrocodone, to their active forms of morphine, oxymorphone and hydromorphone respectively. CYP2D6 is significantly inhibited by certain drugs including quinidine, fluoxetine and paroxetine, which significantly decrease the conversion of the parent drugs to their active forms. Anesthetic agents, by decreasing cardiac output, decrease hepatic blood flow, which decreases hepatic drug clearance, which increases the sensitivity to drugs, metabolized by the liver.

Co-medications can affect PD by affecting drug receptor pathways. Chronic administration of β-adrenergic receptor blockers results in increased density (number) of β-adrenergic receptors, which increases sensitivity to endogenous and exogenous catecholamines (sensitization). If this sensitization is coupled with abrupt withdrawal of chronic beta-blockers, then the patient becomes vulnerable to myocardial ischemia and infarction during periods of sympathetic discharge in response to laryngoscopy, or intubation or surgical stimulation.

Planning Administration of IV Anaesthetics and Sedatives with Particular Reference to Addressing Variability in Broad Spectrum of Patients: From Those Presenting for EGD (Young and Fit) to Those Undergoing Cardiac Ablation Procedures (with Very Low EF)

In planning the administration of IV anesthetics and sedatives, the goals are to achieve pharmacologic specificity, precision and adjustability. Specificity refers to achieving the desired effect of the medication at the desired site of action, the central nervous system (CNS), while minimizing undesirable side effects at other sites of action, particularly the cardiovascular and respiratory systems. Precision refers to achieving the desired level of the effect of the drug at the desired site of action, i.e., the desired level of sedation or depth of anesthesia. Adjustability (ability to titrate) refers to the ability of rapidly change the level of the desired effect of the medication by changing the rate of the administration of the IV medication.

The desired effects of the administration of IV anesthetics and sedatives include all, or part of, the 6 A's of anesthesia, which are: analgesia, amnesia, anxiolysis, anesthesia, akinesia and adrenergic blockade. For non-surgical procedures, achieving analgesia and anxiolysis, might be sufficient, while for more invasive surgical procedures, additional components of the 6 A's may be required. As more components of the 6 A's are achieved, the side effects on the respiratory and cardiovascular systems are expected to become more evident. A prudent approach would be to choose the least invasive anesthetic approach that would allow safe conduct of the planned procedure while achieving the desired level of comfort for the patient. Seeking more invasive levels of anesthesia for minimally invasive procedures might complicate the conduct and recovery from the anesthetic procedure, without necessarily enhancing the safety of the anesthetic procedure. Planning an anesthetic procedure should include all phases of anesthesia, namely the pre-operative, the intra-operative and post-operative periods, including patient disposition and follow-up.

According to the American Society of Anesthesiologists (ASA) Practice Advisory on Pre-anesthetic Evaluation (PAE), the timing of PAE should be based on the degree of invasiveness of the planned procedure, the severity of illness of the patient, and resource availability within the specific health care system or practice. The ASA Advisory recommends that for highly invasive procedures or for patients with high severity of illness, PAE should be performed before the day of the procedure, taking into consideration the resources of the healthcare system or practice. While for procedures of less invasiveness and illnesses of less severity, PAE can be performed either before or on the day of the procedure [2]. Contents of the PAE should always include evaluation of the patient's airway and, in almost all patients, evaluation of the cardiovascular and respiratory systems.

Planning for the intra-operative period of the anesthetic procedure include, securing the availability of personnel with skills and qualifications in accordance with the planned level of anesthesia or sedation, appropriate monitoring, supplemental oxygen, airway management devices including suction source, respiratory management devices including the ability to provide positive pressure ventilation (PPV) by the use bag-valve-mask (BVM) device, and cardiovascular management drugs and devices including vasopressors and defibrillator. Nonanesthesia personnel administering moderate sedation should be able to rescue the patient from deep sedation and those administering deep sedation should be able to rescue the patient from general anesthesia [3]. The ASA Standards for Basic Anesthetic Monitoring should be applied whenever general, regional or monitored anesthesia care is provided. The same ASA standards for monitoring should also be applied when deep sedation is provided since readiness to rescue the patient from general anesthesia should be maintained whenever deep sedation is administered. The ASA considers the use of propofol to require level of care consistent with deep sedation, even if moderate sedation is intended. Also the ASA recommend monitoring of ventilation by the detection of end-tidal CO_2 (ETCO2), or similar means, even when moderate sedation is provided, whenever access is impeded for direct monitoring of ventilation.

The decision to use invasive blood pressure monitoring (BP) should be based on considerations of severity of systemic illness, invasiveness of the surgical procedure, the degree of expected perturbation in cardiovascular function during cardiac electrophysiology procedures, and the practice setting in terms of ease of access to the patient and supportive personnel. Continuous monitoring of BP allows rapid detection of perturbation in cardiovascular function, and rapid assessment for therapeutic interventions. Besides providing continuous monitoring of BP, arterial catheters allow sampling of arterial blood gases (ABGs), electrolytes and hemoglobin levels, which allows rapid assessment of metabolic derangements and rapid assessment of their therapeutic interventions. The use of central venous catheters (CVC) should be based more on the need to access a large central vein than the need to monitor central venous pressure (CVP), since such monitoring is of little clinical utility in most settings. The need to access a large central vein is based on the need to infuse vasopressors, which might compromise peripheral arterial circulation if infused through a small peripheral vein, or the need to infuse hyperosmolar agents, such as hypertonic saline, that could be irritating to a small peripheral vein. In addition, CVC might be indicated when peripheral venous access is inadequate for infusion of fluids, medications, and blood products.

The risk of fire in OORA procedures might be small but not negligible. Supplemental oxygen should be provided to the patient as needed. The Anesthesia Patient Safety Foundation (APSF) Algorithm recommends that if supplemental oxygen is provided at concentrations greater than 30%, then a closed delivery system such as laryngeal mask airway (LMA) or endotracheal tube (ETT) be used rather than an open system such as nasal cannula (NC) or face mask (FM). Alcohol based surgical field preparation solutions should be allowed to be completely dried (3 min on shaved skin and 60 min on hair) before application of electrocautery surgical unit (ESU). Heat sources such as laser sources and fiberoptic scopes should be directed away from surgical drapes as the generated heat might ignite the surgical drape. An OR fire prevention and management protocol such as that developed by the APSF or the ASA should be in place for OORA procedures as well [4].

In planning the administration of OORA, physical access to the patient by personnel and well-functioning resuscitative devices should be kept a high priority by the anesthesiologist since physical and operational designs of most practice settings of OORA tend to emphasize procedural priorities rather than resuscitative needs that anesthesiologists are much more in-tuned to. Resuscitative priorities should be emphasized not only during the procedure period but also during the entire peri-procedure period, including the recovery area and during transport to the recovery area.

Safe and effective administration of OORA requires knowledge of the pharmacology of not only IV anesthetics and sedatives, but also their antagonist drugs, and drugs used to treat the cardiovascular side effects of these medications. Scientific and technological advancements enhance the safety and efficacy of OORA, but do not completely eliminate biologic variability among patients, which can be compensated for by thorough understanding of physiologic, pharmacologic, and pathophysiologic processes as well as through personal experience.

Manual and Target Controlled Infusion (TCI) Systems with Their Pros and Cons

The underlying principle of TCI systems is the greater ability, or availability, of a computer than the clinician to perform frequent, and possibly complex, mathematical calculations, using PK-PD, principles to set and adjust drug infusion rate (DIR) to achieve the desired PD response at various stages of a procedure, to individuals with various PK-PD characteristics. TCI systems set DIR based on clinician-selected target blood concentration (TBC), taking into consideration input patient's PK-PD characteristics such as weight, age, ASA status, etc. The process of using TBC to guide DIR is the process performed by the anesthesiologist when using exhaled concentrations of inhalational anesthetics to guide DIR from a vaporizer.

In the 1980's, TCI systems were used in clinical research under different acronyms such as, Computer-Assisted Total IV Anesthesia (CATIA), Titration of IV Agents by Computer (TIAC), and Computer–Assisted Continuous Infusion (CACI). These systems were used with multiple IV anesthetic agents, including etomidate, fentnayl, alfentanil, sufentanil, midazolam and propofol [5]. In 1986, propofol (Diprivan) was introduced into clinical practice as the first truly total intravenous anesthesia (TIVA) agent. In 1996, Diprifusor, a Diprivan-specific TCI system was introduced into clinical practice in many countries around the world, but failed to get approval by the US Food and Drug Administration (FDA). In 2003, second generation TCI devices were introduced that were programmed to utilize with different anesthetic agents, open TCI devices, including propofol, fentanyl, sufentanil, alfentanil and remifentanil, while others are being developed to allow the administration of dexmedetomidine, ketamine and various benzodiazepines [4]. Further development in TCI systems consists in developing closed-loop TCI systems, in which PD data, in addition to PK data, are used in the form of processed electroencephalogram (EEG), such as Bispectral Index (BIS), to guide setting the DIR [6]. Paedfusor TCI device is designed for use in children 1-year-old or older, but the use of TCI technique in children is limited [7].

The safety of TCI technique is well established. In an estimated 20,000,000 use over 22 years, there has been only 7 reported incidents of technical incidents, not related to PK-based TCI algorithm, with no resulting adverse outcome [8]. A Cochrane review comparing TCI vs. manually controlled infusion (MCI), which included 20 trials of poor quality, and high heterogeneity, involving 1759 patients, found that TCI was associated with higher total doses of propofol, higher propofol drug costs, fewer interventions by the anesthetist with no differences in quality of anesthesia or adverse events [9]. Lack of difference in outcome, between TCI and MCI, could indicate true lack of difference, or lack of sensitivity and specificity of applied methods to detect a difference.

True lack of difference in outcome, could be understood on the basis, that in actual clinical practice, whether using MCI or TCI technique, the anesthesiologist ends up delivering to the patient a DIR that is set and adjusted, using all available information, including PK-PD, patient characteristics, co-morbidities, co-medications, desired level of sedation or anesthesia, varying levels of procedural stimulation, varying level of sedation or anesthesia, and monitored vital functions. Some factors involved in TCI might be difficult to assess, such the time involved in setting the TCI system or the advantage obtained by freeing the anesthesiologists, once the TCI system is set, to focus on tasks other than infusion-pump operation. The higher overall drug use and drug cost, when using TCI, could be understood on the basis that TCI technique involves greater number of changes in DIR than the MCI technique. Also to be considered, when using TCI, is the higher cost of TCI devices than MCI devices. Many studies demonstrated softer outcome differences favoring TCI over MCI.

One study found that propofol TCI, vs. MCI, was associated with faster induction, earlier insertion of a laryngeal mask airway (LMA), less movement during surgery, and more propofol use [10]. A study in spontaneously breathing patients undergoing colonoscopy under propofol/remifentanil anesthesia, found TCI-administered remifentanil, to be associated with fewer episodes of respiratory depression than MCI-administered remifentanil (7 vs. 16) [11]. Closed loop TCI technique, compared to MCI technique, has been shown to result in better precision in achieving target BIS and in maintaining heart rate within 25 % of the baseline [12]. During endoscopy procedures, TCI of propofol and alfentanil, compared to MCI technique, resulted in shorter recovery time, less hypotension, shorter period of bradypnea, and lower relative risk of desaturation [13]. Propofol TCI for general anesthesia (GA) was associate with increased total dose mainly due to higher rate of propofol administration in the first 30 min, and lower BIS scores were lower during the first 15 min of anaesthesia [14]. In dental patients with intellectual disability, BIS-guided TCI propofol sedation vs. MCI was associated with reduced propofol dose and recovery time [15].

Summary

Safe and effective delivery of IV sedatives and anesthetics for Out of Operating Room Anesthesia (OORA) requires accommodating the unique conditions imposed by the diverse environments of each of the procedural locations. Some OORA-specific constraints include environments of limited lighting, excessive noise, limited access to patient, limited devise allowance, limited patient preparation and disorganized scheduling. Scientific, technological, regulatory, and organizational principles should be implemented to enhance patient safety and operational efficiency.

The benefits of understanding operational principles of OORA extend to the OR and the ICU as many OR suites are becoming hybrid environments, and many procedures are being performed in ICU. The portability and versatility of IV anesthetics and sedatives make them particularly suitable choices for OORA. Technological advances such as target-controlled infusion (TCI) systems, are well suited for application in OORA as well as OR and ICU settings.

References

1. Vuyk J, Lim T, Engbers FH, Burm AG, Vletter AA, Bovill JG. The pharmacodynamic interaction of propofol and alfentanil during lower abdominal surgery in women. Anesthesiology. 1995;83(1):8–22.
2. Committee on Standards and Practice Parameters, Apfelbaum JL, Connis RT, Nickinovich DG, American Society of Anesthesiologists Task Force on Preanesthesia Evaluation, Pasternak LR, Arens JF, Caplan RA, Connis RT, Fleisher LA, Flowerdew R, Gold BS, Mayhew JF, Nickinovich DG, Rice LJ, Roizen MF, Twersky RS. Practice advisory for preanesthesia evaluation: an updated report by the American Society of Anesthesiologists Task Force on Preanesthesia Evaluation. Anesthesiology. 2012;116(3):522–38.
3. American Society of Anesthesiologists Task Force on Sedation and Analgesia by Non-Anesthesiologists. Practice guidelines for sedation and analgesia by non-anesthesiologists. Anesthesiology. 2002;96(4):1004–17.
4. Apfelbaum JL, Caplan RA, Barker SJ, Connis RT, Cowles C, Ehrenwerth J, Nickinovich DG, Pritchard D, Roberson DW, Caplan RA, Barker SJ, Connis RT, Cowles C, de Richemond AL, Ehrenwerth J, Nickinovich DG, Pritchard D, Roberson DW, Wolf GL, American Society of Anesthesiologists Task Force on Operating Room Fires. Practice advisory for the prevention and management of operating room fires: an updated report by the American Society of Anesthesiologists Task Force on Operating Room Fires. Anesthesiology. 2013;118(2): 271–90.
5. Struys MM, De Smet T, Glen JI, Vereecke HE, Absalom AR, Schnider TW. The history of target-controlled infusion. Anesth Analg. 2016;122(1):56–69.
6. Short TG, Hannam JA, Laurent S, Campbell D, Misur M, Merry AF, Tam YH. Refining target-controlled infusion: an assessment of pharmacodynamic target-controlled infusion of propofol and remifentanil using a response surface model of their combined effects on bispectral index. Anesth Analg. 2016;122(1):90–7.
7. Absalom AR, Glen JI, Zwart GJ, Schnider TW, Struys MM. Target-controlled infusion: a mature technology. Anesth Analg. 2016;122(1):70–8.

8. Schnider TW, Minto CF, Struys MM, Absalom AR. The safety of target-controlled infusions. Anesth Analg. 2016;122(1):79–85.
9. Leslie K, Clavisi O, Hargrove J. Target-controlled infusion versus manually-controlled infusion of propofol for general anaesthesia or sedation in adults. Cochrane Database Syst Rev. 2008;(3):CD006059.
10. Russell D, Wilkes MP, Hunter SC, Glen JB, Hutton P, Kenny GN. Manual compared with target-controlled infusion of propofol. Br J Anaesth. 1995;75(5):562–6.
11. Moerman AT, Herregods LL, De Vos MM, Mortier EP, Struys MM. Manual versus target-controlled infusion remifentanil administration in spontaneously breathing patients. Anesth Analg. 2009;108(3):828–34.
12. Puri GD, Mathew PJ, Biswas I, Dutta A, Sood J, Gombar S, Palta S, Tsering M, Gautam PL, Jayant A, Arora I, Bajaj V, Punia TS, Singh G. A multicenter evaluation of a closed-loop anesthesia delivery system: a randomized controlled trial. Anesth Analg. 2016;122(1):106–14.
13. Chiang MH, Wu SC, You CH, Wu KL, Chiu YC, Ma CW, Kao CW, Lin KC, Chen KH, Wang PC, Chou AK. Target-controlled infusion vs. manually controlled infusion of propofol with alfentanil for bidirectional endoscopy: a randomized controlled trial. Endoscopy. 2013;45(11):907–14.
14. Breslin DS, Mirakhur RK, Reid JE, Kyle A. Manual versus target-controlled infusions of propofol. Anaesthesia. 2004;59(11):1059–63.
15. Sakaguchi M, Higuchi H, Maeda S, Miyawaki T. Dental sedation for patients with intellectual disability: a prospective study of manual control versus Bispectral Index-guided target-controlled infusion of propofol. J Clin Anesth. 2011;23(8):636–42.

Part II
Patient Safety in Procedures Outside the Operating Room

Chapter 4
Preoperative Assessment: General Principles

Radha Arunkumar and Pascal Owusu-Agyemang

Abstract The number of diagnostic and interventional procedures performed outside the operating room (OR) has increased dramatically over the last several years. There are multiple challenges involved in anesthesia provided to patients outside the OR. With improvements in technology for interventional procedures outside the OR, older, younger and sicker patients who may be inoperable are scheduled for these procedures. Appropriate preoperative assessment and optimization of medical status are important aspects of our practice. Safe patient care can be enhanced by adequate patient assessment in the preoperative period, appropriate patient selection and use of targeted interventions to improve outcomes.

Keywords Preoperative • Pre-anesthesia • Assessment • Evaluation • Guidelines • Co-morbidities

Introduction

The number of diagnostic and interventional procedures performed outside the operating room (OR) has increased dramatically over the last several years. There are multiple challenges involved in anesthesia provided to patients outside the OR. Due to the different organizational aspects and hazards outside the OR, providing well tolerated anesthesia with the same standard of care as in the OR remains challenging.

The **limitations** faced while providing anesthesia outside the OR include the following but are not limited to:

- Inadequate space and lighting,
- Not all equipment may be available,
- Different organization compared to the OR,

R. Arunkumar, MD (✉) • P. Owusu-Agyemang, MD
Department of Anesthesiology and Perioperative Medicine, The University of Texas MD Anderson Cancer Center, 1400 Holcombe Blvd, Unit 409, Houston, TX 77030, USA
e-mail: rarunkum@mdanderson.org; poagyemang@mdanderson.org

© Springer International Publishing Switzerland 2017
B.G. Goudra, P.M. Singh (eds.), *Out of Operating Room Anesthesia*,
DOI 10.1007/978-3-319-39150-2_4

53

- Lack of direct access to patient (depending on location),
- Inexperienced personnel unfamiliar with possible anesthesia complications and hence inability to assist when the necessity arises, and
- The need for remote monitoring (as in MRI and radiation therapy suites).

Appropriate preoperative assessment and optimization of medical status are important aspects of our practice that lead to safe patient care. Yet, when it comes to procedures outside the OR, there is a question for the need for a thorough assessment for a supposedly minor procedure. On the other hand, it is important not to forget that with improvements in technology for interventional procedures outside the OR, older, younger and sicker patients who may be inoperable are scheduled for these procedures. Hence, the importance of adequate preoperative evaluation cannot be stressed enough.

The **US closed claims' analysis** for anesthesia in remote locations identified respiratory damaging events (44 vs. 20 %, $P<0.001$) especially with inadequate oxygenation and ventilation (21 vs. 3 % in OR claims, $P<0.001$) being more common in out of OR locations than in the OR [1]. The **4th National Audit Project** of the Royal College of Anaesthetists and Difficult Airway Society is the first prospective study of all major airway events occurring throughout the UK during anesthesia, in the intensive care unit and emergency department [2, 3]. Problems with tracheal intubation were the most frequently recorded primary airway problem in all areas. Repeated gaps in care that were identified included **poor identification of at-risk patients** and poor and/or inadequate planning and monitoring, all potentially avoidable. This emphasizes the importance of adequate preoperative assessment not only for the OR patients but also for patients undergoing out of OR procedures.

The **Practice Advisory** by the American Society of Anesthesiologists (**ASA**) provides guidelines for pre-anesthesia evaluation [4]. It applies to patients of all ages having general anesthesia, regional anesthesia or sedation for procedures, both surgical and nonsurgical. It includes the assessment of information from the following:

- Patient's medical records, especially previous anesthetic records if available
- Patient interview with regards to their medical history and medications
- Physical examination of the patient, and *at a minimum*, directed at the assessment of the airway, lungs and heart, with documentation of vital signs
- Preoperative testing as indicated and findings from test results
- Other consultations as appropriate
- Timing of the evaluation is guided by the combination of factors such as surgical invasiveness and severity of disease
- For patients with high severity of disease and/or high surgical invasiveness, it is recommended that the evaluation be done at least the day before surgery/procedure
- For patients with low severity of disease and low invasiveness of procedure, the evaluation may be done on or before the day of surgery

History- Important Aspects to Consider

- Previous surgical and anesthesia history, especially with regards to personal and family history to elicit malignant hyperthermia, succinylcholine apnea from pseudocholinesterase deficiency, airway difficulty, severe postoperative nausea and vomiting etc.
- Allergies- to medications, latex, food etc.
- Medications
- Use of tobacco, alcohol and illicit drugs
- Cardiovascular – hypertension, previous heart attacks, angina, arrhythmias, congestive heart failure (CHF), valvular disease, any interventions such as stent placements, pacemakers, valve replacement surgery, coronary bypass surgery etc., and mainly *effort tolerance*. If patients are unable to perform average levels of exercise as measured by metabolic equivalents (METS), they are at risk for postoperative complications [5]. 4 METS would approximate to the ability to walk 4 blocks or go up 2 flights of stairs.
- Respiratory – recent cough, smoking, asthma, chronic obstructive pulmonary disease (COPD), use of inhalers, snoring and obstructive sleep apnea (OSA)
- Neurologic – strokes, transient ischemic attacks (TIA), seizures, deficits
- Gastrointestinal- reflux, hiatal hernia
- Endocrine- diabetes, thyroid
- Hematological- anemia, bleeding or clotting problems
- Renal- failure, dialysis, transplant
- Liver- cirrhosis, hepatitis
- Possibility of pregnancy
- History of chemotherapy and radiation therapy
- Pertinent airway history- problems with teeth such as loose or chipped, dentures, caps, crowns, braces etc., problems opening mouth or moving neck or swallowing, *history of radiation to head and neck (patients may have good mouth opening but will be difficult laryngoscopy)*
- Relevant testing done previously and their results
- Other relevant history to specific procedures- for e.g., history of claustrophobia or pain in MRI and CT areas, history of rectal bleeding for prostate MRI's (in view of placement of rectal coil), presence of metal and/or stents and drug patches for MRI's (risk of burns, artifacts, incompatibility), issues related to positioning (fractures, rotator cuff injury etc.)

Physical Examination

Important aspects of physical examination include demographics, vital signs, examination of the lungs and heart, and last but not the least, an airway examination.

- Demographics: height, weight, calculated BMI
- Vital signs: heart rate, blood pressure (BP), respiratory rate, oxygen saturation, pain score

- Airway examination: dental check, mouth opening, range of motion of neck, thyromental and sternomental distances- identification of challenging airways will require careful planning of optimal positioning of patient, availability of additional equipment and appropriately skilled personnel.
- Cardiovascular examination includes auscultation of the heart, examination of peripheral pulses, cyanosis, clubbing and pedal edema
- Respiratory examination includes auscultation of the lungs for breath sounds, rales, wheezing, and presence of tachypnea and pattern and effort of breathing
- Neurologic examination to look for any pre-existing neurologic deficits to establish a baseline and to plan for positioning

Patients with **extremes of age** may require special considerations when undergoing procedures out of OR. It may be safer to perform such procedures in the OR if feasible, and if not, require skilled personnel to care for them, with additional specialized equipment as needed immediately available to deal with any complications.

The following sections will outline the assessment of individual systems as relevant to anesthesia outside the OR.

Cardiovascular System

Coronary Artery Disease (CAD)

Cardiovascular risk assessment for optimal patient management is an integral part of pre-anesthesia evaluation. The most recently published 2014 American College of Cardiology/American Heart Association ACC/AHA Task Force guideline on Perioperative Cardiovascular Evaluation and Management of Patients Undergoing Noncardiac Surgery [6], favors preoperative risk stratification based on clinical assessment of patient rather than routine cardiac testing [6–8].

The risk stratification depends on the urgency and risk of the surgical procedure. The guideline defines a *low-risk* procedure as one in which the combined patient and surgical characteristics predict the risk of a major adverse cardiac event (MACE) such as death or myocardial infarction (MI) as <1 %. When the risk is ≥1 %, it is considered *elevated risk*. The current guideline combines the moderate and high risk procedures used in other risk stratification indices into one group for simplification since the recommendations are similar for moderate and high risk procedures [6].

A stepwise approach is used for perioperative cardiac assessment in patients with CAD.

- Step 1: Determine the urgency; if an emergency surgery, clinical risk stratification and proceed with surgery with appropriate clinical monitoring and management as necessary
- Step 2: If procedure is urgent or elective, determine if the patient has an acute coronary syndrome (ACS), if YES, refer patient to cardiology for further evaluation and management. A recent MI, defined as within 6 months of noncardiac

or non-neurologic surgery, increases the risk of perioperative stroke with an eight fold increase in perioperative mortality within 30 days [9]. So it may be prudent to postpone elective noncardiac procedures to at least ≥60 days after an MI [10].

- Step 3: If no ACS, determine the risk of MACE based on the combined clinical/ surgical risk
- Step 4: If low risk of MACE (<1 %), no further testing needed and patient may proceed with surgery. Most of the out of OR procedures fall into this category, such as MRI, CT scans and radiation therapy under sedation, and several endoscopic procedures, since most of the procedures are non-invasive and very little risk of blood loss and fluid shifts.
- Step 5: If elevated risk, then determine functional capacity. If patient has moderate or greater functional capacity (≥4 METS), no further testing needed and proceed to surgery
- Step 6: If poor (<4 METS) or unknown functional capacity, determine if further testing will impact decision making or perioperative care. If YES, pharmacologic stress testing should be considered. If it is normal, proceed with surgery. If abnormal, coronary revascularization may be considered.
- Step 7: If further testing will not affect decision making or care, proceed with surgery or consider alternative strategies such as palliation or noninvasive treatment modalities.

To summarize, any cardiac testing is unlikely to alter management for low risk surgery, which would be the case in most out of OR procedures. It is essential to evaluate for unstable cardiac conditions (such as unstable angina, acute heart failure, significant arrhythmias, symptomatic valvular heart disease, acute or recent MI with residual myocardial ischemia) [11], which may warrant postponement of procedure until stabilization and optimization. Prophylactic coronary revascularization is rarely indicated simply to lower the risk of surgery [12, 13].

Patients with Cardiovascular Implantable Electronic Devices (CIED)

CIEDs (pacemakers and implantable cardioverter defibrillators [ICD]) are being placed in increasing numbers worldwide. In addition to obtaining patient history and information from medical records, patient registration card for the CIED (with manufacturer's name) should be sought out. Pacemakers should have been interrogated within 12 months and ICDs within 6 months of procedure.

Pre-procedure considerations include:

- Type of device,
- Manufacturer and model,
- Date of last interrogation,
- Indication for device,
- Battery longevity (should have at least 3 months),

- If patient is pacemaker dependent, and the underlying rhythm and rate,
- Any alert status on the CIED generator and lead, and
- Last pacing threshold.

   Other aspects to consider include:

- Procedure venue,
- Post procedure plan,
- Type and site of surgery,
- Patient position, and
- Electromagnetic interference (EMI) with type of cautery, if any is to be used.

   If EMI is unlikely, proceed with surgery. If EMI is likely, and procedure is below umbilicus, proceed with surgery. If EMI is likely and procedure is above umbilicus, and if the patient is pacemaker dependent, reprogram the ICD. If the patient is not pacemaker dependent, plan to use a magnet [14].

- Keep magnet immediately available
- Keep external defibrillation equipment in the OR and immediately available
- May need to place defibrillation pads prophylactically
- ECG monitor with a pacing mode set to recognize pacing stimuli
- Return pad as close to the surgical site as possible
- Use bipolar cautery
- If monopolar cautery, use short bursts
- Plan for post procedure re-interrogation and reprogramming as needed

   It is essential for anesthesiologists to become familiar with the response to magnet application or reprogramming on ICD function and to also understand the situations in which magnet use is not advisable [15]. In order to ensure patient safety and reduce adverse outcome, perioperative communication with the patient's cardiologist and surgeon is critical.

Respiratory System

Postoperative pulmonary complications (PPC) occur as commonly as cardiac complications and increase morbidity, mortality and length of stay. Risk factors include patients with COPD, age >60 years, ASA class II or more, poor functional capacity, OSA and congestive heart failure [16, 17]. Patients with mild or moderate asthma do not appear to have a higher risk of PPC. Preoperative chest X-ray and spirometry should not be used routinely to predict the risk of PPC. Preoperative strategies to reduce PPC would include [18]:

- Preoperative smoking cessation- has to happen at least 2 months prior; may not be feasible in out of OR procedures unless planned well ahead
- Strategies to maximize airflow in obstructive disease
- Incentive spirometry

- Chest physical therapy including percussion and deep breathing exercises
- Intermittent and continuous positive airway pressure
- Treating respiratory infections and CHF

Hypertension

Hypertension, depending on severity and duration, can cause comorbidities such as coronary artery disease, renal failure and cerebrovascular disease. Recent guidelines state that hypertension is a risk factor, but not a very strong independent risk factor for cardiovascular complications in non-cardiac surgery [19]. In general, there is strong evidence to support a BP goal of <150/90 mm Hg for persons 60 years or older and for those younger than 60, the recommendation is a goal of 140/90 mm Hg [20]. Anesthesia and surgery should not be cancelled on the grounds of elevated preoperative BP, and intraoperative monitoring is essential to maintain within 20 % of the estimated preoperative arterial pressure [21].

Diabetes

Patients with diabetes, especially if long-standing and uncontrolled are at risk for end-organ dysfunction such as renal failure, strokes, retinopathy, and cardiovascular disease. It is not proven that tight control of glucose confers benefit in the perioperative period but may increase the risk of hypoglycemia. The goals of management should be avoidance of hypoglycemia and adequate blood glucose control. There should be minimal disruption in the patients' antidiabetic treatment, appropriate blood glucose monitoring and resumption of oral intake as soon as feasible after the procedure [22].

Preoperative Testing

The ASA task force on pre-anesthesia assessment does not recommend routine preoperative testing [4]. The patterns of preoperative testing and their association with postoperative complications were evaluated in the National Surgical Quality Improvement Program (NSQIP) database (2005–2010) review of 73,596 patients who underwent elective hernia repair, using multivariate analyses. Major complications such as reintubation, pulmonary embolus, stroke, renal failure, coma, cardiac arrest, myocardial infarction, septic shock, bleeding, or death occurred in 0.3 % of patients and neither testing nor abnormal results were found to be associated with postoperative outcomes [23].

- Testing should be done selectively to guide and optimize perioperative management.
- Test results within 6 months may be acceptable if patient's medical status has not changed.

- More recent testing may be required if there is a change in the patient's medical condition or if the results would facilitate decision making as to the anesthetic technique (e.g. Coagulation studies for regional anesthesia).
- The currently available scientific literature does not help unequivocally define what specific tests or what timing of the tests would help decision making on perioperative management
- Hence selective tests should be timed based on individual patients, after assessing their medical records, interviewing and physically examining them, and their procedure's type and invasiveness.

Specific Tests for Certain Patient Populations

Electrocardiogram (ECG)

- Indicated for patients with cardiac disease, respiratory disease, and for older patients with multiple risk factors
- No minimum age recommendation for ECG
- In our institution, men and women 50 years and over get an ECG, and younger patients get one if they have cardiac risk factors

Cardiac Evaluation Other Than ECG

- This is based on risk stratification as described earlier in the section on cardiovascular system.

Chest X-ray

- No unequivocal indications but patient populations to consider would include smokers, patients with recent respiratory infections, COPD, and cardiac disease.

Other Pulmonary Function Evaluation

- Pulmonary function tests, arterial blood gas analysis depending on individual patient assessment

Blood Tests

- Testing should be done based on individualization
- Tests to consider as indicated are as follows:
  - Hemoglobin
  - Hematocrit
  - Complete blood count
  - Coagulation studies
  - Serum chemistries- especially important to know serum potassium in renal failure patients and if patient is on dialysis
  - Blood glucose
  - Kidney function tests- blood urea nitrogen (BUN) and creatinine especially when performing CT scans and MRI scans for dosing of contrast
  - Pregnancy testing

The ABIM Foundation is a not-for-profit foundation established by the American Board of Internal Medicine in 1999. *Choosing Wisely®* is an initiative launched by the foundation in 2012, and several specialty societies have partnered to create lists of things providers and patients should question, in order to avoid wasteful or unnecessary medical tests, treatments and procedures. The ASA became a partner in 2013 and generated a list after a multi-step survey of anesthesiologists in both the academic and private sector and the ASA Committees of Jurisdiction [24]. The top two recommendations are:

- Don't obtain baseline laboratory studies in patients without significant systemic disease (ASA I or II) undergoing low-risk surgery – specifically complete blood count, basic or comprehensive metabolic panel, coagulation studies when blood loss (or fluid shifts) is/are expected to be minimal.
- Don't obtain baseline diagnostic cardiac testing (trans-thoracic/esophageal echocardiography – TTE/TEE) or cardiac stress testing in asymptomatic stable patients with known cardiac disease (e.g., CAD, valvular disease) undergoing low or moderate risk non-cardiac surgery.

Medication Instructions to Patients

It is important to give instructions to patients about which medications to stop and which ones to continue. This decision is based on the class of medication, indication for the medication, and the type of procedure that needs to be done. The following is a list of most of the commonly used medications:

- Aspirin: should be continued unless the risk of bleeding outweighs the benefit
- Antihypertensives: all antihypertensives should be continued except for angiotensin-converting enzyme inhibitors and angiotensin receptor blockers for risk of hypotension

- Antidiabetic agents: to be discontinued on morning of surgery- risk of hypoglycemia
- Antiplatelet agents: important to continue especially when patients have recent stent placements (<12 months) for most out of OR procedures, except when neuraxial block is planned or for procedures with risk of bleeding (discontinue 5–7 days before), cardiologist should be consulted and prompt resumption as feasible
- Asthma medications: to be continued
- Antiseizure medications: to be continued
- Acid reflux medications: to be continued
- Antipsychotic and antidepressant medications: to be continued, caution with drug interactions with monoamine oxidase inhibitors
- Pain medications: narcotics should be continued, non-steroidals are generally stopped 48 h before surgery if there is risk of bleeding
- Statins: to be continued
- Supplements and herbals: generally discontinued
- Thyroid medications: should be continued
- Warfarin: should be discontinued 5 days before if there is risk of bleeding

After a complete preoperative assessment based on the above principles, the patient is assigned an ASA physical status score [25]. The anesthetic plan is formulated and discussed with the patient or a responsible adult and the consent is obtained.

Patient Selection for Out of OR Procedures

In a review of 244,397 day case eligible surgeries in the American College of Surgeons' NSQIP database (2005–2010), early perioperative morbidity and mortality (within 72 h) occurred in 232 (0.1 %), which approximates to 1 in 1000 patients. The risk factors associated were overweight or obesity, COPD, history of TIA/stroke, hypertension, previous cardiac surgical intervention, and prolonged operative time [26]. This information can be extrapolated to out of OR procedures in patient selection and optimization. There are not many studies delineating the risks and safety of out of OR anesthesia unlike those of OR or in ambulatory anesthesia [27]. Safety can be enhanced by adequate patient assessment in the preoperative period, appropriate patient selection and use of targeted interventions to improve outcomes.

References

1. Metzner J, Posner KL, Domino KB. The risk and safety of anesthesia at remote locations: the US closed claims analysis. Curr Opin Anaesthesiol. 2009;22(4):502–8.
2. Cook TM, Woodall N, Harper J, Benger J. Major complications of airway management in the UK: results of the Fourth National Audit Project of the Royal College of Anaesthetists and the

Difficult Airway Society. Part 2: intensive care and emergency departments. Br J Anaesth. 2011;106(5):632–42.

3. Cook TM, Woodall N, Frerk C. Major complications of airway management in the UK: results of the Fourth National Audit Project of the Royal College of Anaesthetists and the Difficult Airway Society. Part 1: anaesthesia. Br J Anaesth. 2011;106(5):617–31.

4. Apfelbaum JL, Connis RT, Nickinovich DG, Pasternak LR, Arens JF, Caplan RA, et al. Practice advisory for preanesthesia evaluation: an updated report by the American Society of Anesthesiologists Task Force on Preanesthesia Evaluation. Anesthesiology. 2012;116(3):522–38.

5. Morris CK, Ueshima K, Kawaguchi T, Hideg A, Froelicher VF. The prognostic value of exercise capacity: a review of the literature. Am Heart J. 1991;122(5):1423–31.

6. Fleisher LA, Fleischmann KE, Auerbach AD, Barnason SA, Beckman JA, Bozkurt B, et al. 2014 ACC/AHA guideline on perioperative cardiovascular evaluation and management of patients undergoing noncardiac surgery: executive summary: a report of the American College of Cardiology/American Heart Association Task Force on Practice Guidelines. Circulation. 2014;130(24):2215–45.

7. Roberts JD, Sweitzer B. Perioperative evaluation and management of cardiac disease in the ambulatory surgery setting. Anesthesiol Clin. 2014;32(2):309–20.

8. Fleisher LA, Fleischmann KE, Auerbach AD, Barnason SA, Beckman JA, Bozkurt B, et al. 2014 ACC/AHA guideline on perioperative cardiovascular evaluation and management of patients undergoing noncardiac surgery: a report of the American College of Cardiology/American Heart Association Task Force on Practice Guidelines. Circulation. 2014;130(24):e278–333.

9. Mashour GA, Shanks AM, Kheterpal S. Perioperative stroke and associated mortality after noncardiac, nonneurologic surgery. Anesthesiology. 2011;114(6):1289–96.

10. Livhits M, Ko CY, Leonardi MJ, Zingmond DS, Gibbons MM, de Virgilio C. Risk of surgery following recent myocardial infarction. Ann Surg. 2011;253(5):857–64.

11. Schiefermueller J, Myerson S, Handa AI. Preoperative assessment and perioperative management of cardiovascular risk. Angiology. 2013;64(2):146–50.

12. Garcia S, McFalls EO. Need for elective PCI prior to noncardiac surgery: high risk through the eyes of the beholder. J Am Heart Assoc. 2014;3(3):e001068.

13. Garcia S, McFalls EO. Perioperative clinical variables and long-term survival following vascular surgery. World J Cardiol. 2014;6(10):1100–7.

14. Crossley GH, Poole JE, Rozner MA, Asirvatham SJ, Cheng A, Chung MK, et al. The Heart Rhythm Society (HRS)/American Society of Anesthesiologists (ASA) Expert Consensus Statement on the perioperative management of patients with implantable defibrillators, pacemakers and arrhythmia monitors: facilities and patient management this document was developed as a joint project with the American Society of Anesthesiologists (ASA), and in collaboration with the American Heart Association (AHA), and the Society of Thoracic Surgeons (STS). Heart Rhythm. 2011;8(7):1114–54.

15. Joshi GP. Perioperative management of outpatients with implantable cardioverter defibrillators. Curr Opin Anaesthesiol. 2009;22(6):701–4.

16. Smetana GW, Pfeifer KJ, Slawski BA, Jaffer AK, Dutta S, Cohn SL. Risk factors for postoperative pulmonary complications: an update of the literature. Hosp Pract (1995). 2014;42(5):126–31.

17. Qaseem A, Snow V, Fitterman N, Hornbake ER, Lawrence VA, Smetana GW, et al. Risk assessment for and strategies to reduce perioperative pulmonary complications for patients undergoing noncardiothoracic surgery: a guideline from the American College of Physicians. Ann Intern Med. 2006;144(8):575–80.

18. Sweitzer BJ, Smetana GW. Identification and evaluation of the patient with lung disease. Med Clin North Am. 2009;93(5):1017–30.

19. Kristensen SD, Knuuti J, Saraste A, Anker S, Botker HE, De Hert S, et al. 2014 ESC/ESA Guidelines on non-cardiac surgery: cardiovascular assessment and management: The Joint Task Force on non-cardiac surgery: cardiovascular assessment and management of the

European Society of Cardiology (ESC) and the European Society of Anaesthesiology (ESA). Eur J Anaesthesiol. 2014;31(10):517–73.

20. James PA, Oparil S, Carter BL, Cushman WC, Dennison-Himmelfarb C, Handler J, et al. 2014 evidence-based guideline for the management of high blood pressure in adults: report from the panel members appointed to the Eighth Joint National Committee (JNC 8). JAMA. 2014;311(5):507–20.

21. Howell SJ, Sear JW, Foex P. Hypertension, hypertensive heart disease and perioperative cardiac risk. Br J Anaesth. 2004;92(4):570–83.

22. Joshi GP, Chung F, Vann MA, Ahmad S, Gan TJ, Goulson DT, et al. Society for Ambulatory Anesthesia consensus statement on perioperative blood glucose management in diabetic patients undergoing ambulatory surgery. Anesth Analg. 2010;111(6):1378–87.

23. Benarroch-Gampel J, Sheffield KM, Duncan CB, Brown KM, Han Y, Townsend Jr CM, et al. Preoperative laboratory testing in patients undergoing elective, low-risk ambulatory surgery. Ann Surg. 2012;256(3):518–28.

24. ASA-5things-List_102013.pdf. http://www.choosingwisely.org/wp-content/uploads/2015/01/Choosing-Wisely-Recommendations.pdf.

25. American Society of Anesthesiologists – ASA Physical Status Classification System.pdf. .http://www.asahq.org/resources/clinical-information/asa-physical-status-classification-system#.

26. Mathis MR, Naughton NN, Shanks AM, Freundlich RE, Pannucci CJ, Chu Y, et al. Patient selection for day case-eligible surgery: identifying those at high risk for major complications. Anesthesiology. 2013;119(6):1310–21.

27. Metzner J, Domino KB. Risks of anesthesia or sedation outside the operating room: the role of the anesthesia care provider. Curr Opin Anaesthesiol. 2010;23(4):523–31.

Chapter 5
Fasting Guidelines: Do They Need to Be Different?

Pascal Owusu-Agyemang and Radha Arunkumar

Abstract The purpose of fasting guidelines is to reduce the incidence of aspiration during induction and maintenance of anesthesia. Although the traditional dogma of 'nothing by mouth for 8 hours' has been accepted for years, there is a lack of scientific evidence in support of this practice. Furthermore, preoperative fasting has been shown to be associated with some unintended unfavorable metabolic and psychological consequences. As a result, patients may be better served if fasting guidelines were approached from a patient and/or procedure specific perspective. Differences in fasting recommendations may therefore have to be accepted as the norm, rather than an exception.

Keywords Fasting • Preoperative • Guidelines • Metabolism • Aspiration

Introduction

Due to the evolving nature of the literature, several societies continue to publish updated versions of their own fasting guidelines, and recommendations continue to vary [1, 2]. For example, while the American Society of Anesthesiologists (ASA) recommend a fasting time of 8 h for a meal that includes fried or fatty foods, the Scandinavian Society of Anesthesiologists make no such exemptions, and recommend a 6 h fast for all solid food [2, 3]. A recent systematic review of fasting guidelines concluded that in the absence of obvious contraindications, preoperative fasting should be minimized and fasting from midnight is unnecessary in most patients. The review also concluded that patients can consume solids up to 6 h before anesthesia and drink clear fluids or an unlimited amount of water up to 2 h before anesthesia [4]. Despite the available evidence, studies show that patients

P. Owusu-Agyemang, MD (✉) • R. Arunkumar, MD
Department of Anesthesiology and Perioperative Medicine, The University of Texas MD Anderson Cancer Center, 1400 Holcombe Boulevard, Unit 409, Houston, TX, USA
e-mail: poagyemang@mdanderson.org; rarunkum@mdanderson.org

© Springer International Publishing Switzerland 2017
B.G. Goudra, P.M. Singh (eds.), *Out of Operating Room Anesthesia*,
DOI 10.1007/978-3-319-39150-2_5

continue to experience prolonged fasting times and that the majority of fasting guidelines are non-compliant with recommended fasting standards [5, 6].

The following chapter will describe some of the unintended consequences of prolonged preoperative fasting and attempt to explain why patients may be better served if fasting guidelines were patient and/or procedure specific.

Metabolic Consequences of Preoperative Fasting

- Fasting for greater than 10 h has been associated with a greater increase in basal metabolic rate [7].
- This increased metabolic rate has been shown to be associated with a catabolic state and the depletion of glycogen storage before the start of surgery.
- The preoperative stress response, as measured by serum levels of cortisol and C-reactive protein are higher in patients who have fasted for 8 h or more [8].
- In a prospective clinical observational study of children undergoing elective surgery, prolonged fasting times were associated a higher concentration of ketone bodies, a higher serum osmolality and anion gap, and a significantly lower base excess [9].
- Patients requiring repeat procedures over a prolonged duration of time may experience malnutrition as a consequence of the observation of strict fasting guidelines.
- Malnutrition has been associated with poorer outcomes especially in cancer patients [10].

Psychological Consequences of Preoperative Fasting

- Prolonged preoperative fasting may be associated with increased preoperative anxiety [11].
- Patient comfort and satisfaction is negatively impacted by prolonged fasting times.
- In a single center prospective randomized control trial of patients undergoing ophthalmologic surgery, patients drinking 200 ml of a carbohydrate drink before surgery had better postoperative satisfaction scores than patients who fasted for at least 8 h [12].

Current Evidence Suggests the Following

- Solid food intake may be safe for up to 6 h before surgery [13].
- Clear liquids may be safe for up to 2 h before surgery [2].

- Obese adults have been shown to have acceptably low gastric fluid volume 2 h after the ingestion of clear liquids [14].
- Two hours after the ingestion of clear liquids, gastric fluid volumes of obese children were identical to that of children with lower body mass indices [15].
- The preoperative consumption of carbohydrate drinks up to 2 h prior to outpatient surgery has not been shown to be associated with additional complications [16].
- There is currently no evidence that children who are denied oral fluids for more than 6 h benefit in terms of gastric fluid pH and volume, when compared to children who are permitted to ingest a liberal amount of fluids for up to 2 h before anesthesia [17].
- Emesis upon induction of anesthesia has been shown to be associated with increased ASA physical status, but not with the duration of fasting [15].
- Ingestion of oral contrast within 2 h of ketamine sedation may be associated with a higher incidence of emesis [18].
- However, the administration of oral contrast within 2 h of Propofol sedation was not associated with any differences in outcome measures [19].
- Patients who chewed gum prior to endoscopic procedures were found to have a statistically significant higher volume of gastric fluid. However, the authors questioned the clinical relevance of such a small difference [20].

While compliance with the 'nothing by mouth for 8 hours' rule may be safer for patients with a higher ASA status, and in those at a higher risk of aspiration, current literature suggests that relatively healthy and low risk patients may benefit from fluid intake up to 2 h before anesthesia.

For example:

- The preoperative stress response is better regulated in patients who are permitted to have oral intake of fluids up to 2 h before surgery [8].
- A shorter fasting time of less than 8 h and the administration of carbohydrate supplements has been shown to suppress the preoperative stress response [7, 21].
- A recent Cochrane review concluded that preoperative oral carbohydrate treatment with carbohydrate rich fluids up to 2 h before surgery was associated with a lower postoperative insulin resistance and a significantly reduced length of hospital stay [22].
- In order to avoid dehydration, children undergoing elective procedures may benefit from the liberal oral intake of fluids for up to 2 h before anesthesia.
- In smaller children, deviation of fasting guidelines should be as short as possible and not longer than 2 h [9].
- The latter may be particularly important in cancer patients who may require repeat procedures over several days or weeks.

Due to the current absence of a universal consensus, fasting guidelines continue to vary. There is also a paucity of literature on fasting recommendations in the setting of comorbidities such as diabetes and gastro-esophageal reflux disease. Compounded by the lack of scientific evidence supporting older guidelines and the continued publication of data implying that current fasting times may be excessive, anesthesiologists may have to rely on clinical judgment when deciding on the appropriate duration of preoperative fasting. It may therefore have to be accepted that fasting guidelines may vary from patient to patient. Differences in fasting recommendations may therefore have to be accepted as the norm, rather than an exception.

References

1. Smith I, Kranke P, Murat I, Smith A, O'Sullivan G, Soreide E, et al. Perioperative fasting in adults and children: guidelines from the European Society of Anaesthesiology. Eur J Anaesthesiol. 2011;28(8):556–69.
2. American Society of Anesthesiologists C. Practice guidelines for preoperative fasting and the use of pharmacologic agents to reduce the risk of pulmonary aspiration: application to healthy patients undergoing elective procedures: an updated report by the American Society of Anesthesiologists Committee on Standards and Practice Parameters. Anesthesiology. 2011;114(3):495–511.
3. Soreide E, Eriksson LI, Hirlekar G, Eriksson H, Henneberg SW, Sandin R, et al. Pre-operative fasting guidelines: an update. Acta Anaesthesiol Scand. 2005;49(8):1041–7.
4. Lambert E, Carey S. Practice guideline recommendations on perioperative fasting: a systematic review. JPEN J Parenter Enteral Nutr. 2015
5. Williams C, Johnson PA, Guzzetta CE, Guzzetta PC, Cohen IT, Sill AM, et al. Pediatric fasting times before surgical and radiologic procedures: benchmarking institutional practices against national standards. J Pediatr Nurs. 2014;29(3):258–67.
6. Buller Y, Sims C. Prolonged fasting of children before anaesthesia is common in private practice. Anaesth Intensive Care. 2016;44(1):107–10.
7. Yoshimura S, Fujita Y, Hirate H, Kusama N, Azami T, Sobue K. A short period of fasting before surgery conserves basal metabolism and suppresses catabolism according to indirect calorimetry performed under general anesthesia. J Anesth. 2015;29(3):453–6.
8. Zelic M, Stimac D, Mendrila D, Tokmadzic VS, Fisic E, Uravic M, et al. Preoperative oral feeding reduces stress response after laparoscopic cholecystectomy. Hepatogastroenterology. 2013;60(127):1602–6.
9. Dennhardt N, Beck C, Huber D, Nickel K, Sander B, Witt LH, et al. Impact of preoperative fasting times on blood glucose concentration, ketone bodies and acid–base balance in children younger than 36 months: a prospective observational study. Eur J Anaesthesiol. 2015;32(12):857–61.
10. Loeffen EA, Brinksma A, Miedema KG, de Bock GH, Tissing WJ. Clinical implications of malnutrition in childhood cancer patients – infections and mortality. Support Care Cancer. 2015;23(1):143–50.
11. Tosun B, Yava A, Acikel C. Evaluating the effects of preoperative fasting and fluid limitation. Int J Nurs Pract. 2015;21(2):156–65.
12. Bopp C, Hofer S, Klein A, Weigand MA, Martin E, Gust R. A liberal preoperative fasting regimen improves patient comfort and satisfaction with anesthesia care in day-stay minor surgery. Minerva Anestesiol. 2011;77(7):680–6.
13. Brady M, Kinn S, Stuart P. Preoperative fasting for adults to prevent perioperative complications. Cochrane Database Syst Rev. 2003;(4):CD004423.
14. Maltby JR, Pytka S, Watson NC, Cowan RA, Fick GH. Drinking 300 mL of clear fluid two hours before surgery has no effect on gastric fluid volume and pH in fasting and non-fasting obese patients. Can J Anaesth. 2004;51(2):111–5.

15. Cook-Sather SD, Gallagher PR, Kruge LE, Beus JM, Ciampa BP, Welch KC, et al. Overweight/obesity and gastric fluid characteristics in pediatric day surgery: implications for fasting guidelines and pulmonary aspiration risk. Anesth Analg. 2009;109(3):727–36.
16. Singh BN, Dahiya D, Bagaria D, Saini V, Kaman L, Kaje V, et al. Effects of preoperative carbohydrates drinks on immediate postoperative outcome after day care laparoscopic cholecystectomy. Surg Endosc. 2015;29(11):3267–72.
17. Brady M, Kinn S, Ness V, O'Rourke K, Randhawa N, Stuart P. Preoperative fasting for preventing perioperative complications in children. Cochrane Database Syst Rev. 2009;(4):CD005285.
18. Teshome G, Braun JL, Lichenstein R. Ketamine sedation after administration of oral contrast: a retrospective cohort study. Hospital Pediatr. 2015;5(9):495–500.
19. Kharazmi SA, Kamat PP, Simoneaux SF, Simon HK. Violating traditional NPO guidelines with PO contrast before sedation for computed tomography. Pediatr Emerg Care. 2013;29(9):979–81.
20. Goudra BG, Singh PM, Carlin A, Manjunath AK, Reihmer J, Gouda GB, et al. Effect of gum chewing on the volume and pH of gastric contents: a prospective randomized study. Dig Dis Sci. 2015;60(4):979–83.
21. Torgersen Z, Balters M. Perioperative nutrition. Surg Clin North Am. 2015;95(2):255–67.
22. Smith MD, McCall J, Plank L, Herbison GP, Soop M, Nygren J. Preoperative carbohydrate treatment for enhancing recovery after elective surgery. Cochrane Database Syst Rev. 2014;(8):CD009161.

Chapter 6
Organization of a Sedation Suite: Setting the Standards

Rajiv R. Doshi and Mary Ann Vann

Abstract Regulations surrounding the care of patients sedated in remote areas as well as by anesthesia and non-anesthesia trained providers are established by federal, state, local, and institutional guidelines. The guidelines established by the American Society of Anesthesiologists for the minimum setup and equipment for anesthetizing locations outside of the operating room provide a rational framework for setting up and maintaining a sedation suite. Establishing safety standards within the framework of a sedation suite may minimize the incidence of preventable errors during procedural sedation or during the procedure itself performed at remote locations.

Keywords Sedation suite • Guidelines • Policies • Regulations • American Society of anesthesiologist • Equipment • Space • Layout • Safety • Communication • Checklists • Cognitive aids • Documentation • Staff development

Introduction

The number of sedation cases performed outside of the operating room continues to increase at a rapid rate. As cases continue to move out of the operating room to accommodate the equipment required to perform complex procedures on sicker, complicated medical patients, formulating regulations and requirements for the physical layout of the sedation suite ensures uniformity of care and maximizes safety for the patient. Federal, state, local, and institutional guidelines are combined with current local policies to improve care by regulating the necessary equipment, monitoring, and practice that maximize safety, mitigate risk, provide optimal working conditions for the proceduralist, and contribute to improved patient satisfaction.

R.R. Doshi, MD (✉) • M.A. Vann, MD
Department of Anesthesia, Critical Care, and Pain Medicine, Beth Israel Deaconess Medical Center, 330 Brookline Avenue, Boston, MA 02215, USA
e-mail: rdoshi@bidmc.harvard.edu; mavann@earthlink.net

© Springer International Publishing Switzerland 2017   71
B.G. Goudra, P.M. Singh (eds.), *Out of Operating Room Anesthesia*,
DOI 10.1007/978-3-319-39150-2_6

Sedation Suite Locations

• Given the explosive growth of procedures performed outside of the operating room, the number of suites providing sedation services has grown tremendously over the last decade.
• As technological advances continue to improve patient care, the need to perform procedures on patients in remote locations that have specialized equipment will continue to increase.
• The number and scope of remote locations that require anesthesia and sedation services include, but not limited to:

  – Radiology- CT/MRI suites, interventional radiologic procedures
  – Cardiology- cardiac catheterization, pacemaker/automated internal cardiac defibrillator implantation, cardioversion, electrophysiologic procedures
  – Radiation Oncology- PET, Proton Beam, Gamma Knife
  – Gastroenterology- colonoscopy, esophagogastroduodenoscopy (EGD), Endoscopic retrograde cholangiopancreatography (ERCP), Endoscopic Ultrasound (EUS), Small Bowel Enteroscopy,
  – Psychiatry- electroconvulsive therapy (ECT)
  – OB/GYN- in vitro fertilization
  – Plastic surgery procedures
  – Anesthesia- interventional pain management
  – Dentistry-Dental procedures

Patient Selection

• The need to provide sedation services for procedures outside of the operating room is based on the requirements for the procedure, the invasiveness of the procedure, and specific patient factors that may require more profound sedation that is customarily practiced in the suite. Additionally, there may be comorbid medical issues that may make conscious sedation or local anesthesia only procedures difficult (if not impossible) or make the required level of sedation difficult enough to warrant more specialized care and monitoring.
• Not all patients are appropriate for sedation or anesthesia outside of the operating room. Severe systemic disease, difficult airway or other comorbidities without present and functional rescue equipment, and lack of appropriate monitoring during and after the procedure requires discussion with the proceduralist before the procedure and discussion of transfer to a hospital based environment.
• Guidelines should be established prior to the administration of any anesthetic of specific patient selection criteria agreed upon by anesthesia, procedural specialist, and nursing and codified in the facility policies and procedures as to the types of patients who should NOT be done in that facility.

- Patients whom the proceduralist has specific concerns about safety should be addressed with the anesthesia provider as early as possible before the procedure is scheduled.
- Anesthesia, nursing, and procedural specialist all have the responsibility to identify patients who may be at risk or require more services than can be provided at the remote location.
- Certain procedures already in progress may require anesthesia services emergently, such as cardiac catheterization, in order to prevent patient injury. Emergent anesthetic services are often performed with limited medical history known to the anesthesia provider and care should proceed cautiously. Every effort should be taken to obtain clinical history, medications administered including sedation, and procedural clinical course about the patient in these non-ideal situations.

Guidelines for Minimum Standards for a Sedation Suite

- The Standards and Practice committee of the American Society of Anesthesiologists released "Statement on Nonoperating Room Anesthetizing Locations" which lays out the minimum guidelines for a suite in which an anesthetic is delivered outside an operating room [1]. A summary of the guidelines is found in Table 6.1.
- Inter-individual variability in response to sedative medications, related to acute or chronic illness, concomitant medications, or procedural requirements, may require rescue from inadvertent conversion to a more profound state of anesthesia than intended [2].
- These minimum standards ensure that current non-operating room locations as well as future procedural locations conform to the basic requirements for a sedation suite.
- These minimum standards do not replace adequate clinical skills and periodic reassessment of those clinical skills of the practitioner administering sedation, be it an anesthesia provider or non-anesthesia provider.

Policies and Procedures

- Every surgical and procedural society that performs procedures outside of the operating room has developed policies governing the requirements around the use of conscious sedation and moderate sedation in their procedural suites. Society-specific guidelines may also mention the use of general anesthesia; these guidelines make reference to anesthesia-specific guidelines (i.e. American Society of Anesthesiologists in U.S. based practices) when general anesthesia is used within their suites. These also need to be compliant with federal, state, and local statutes [3].

Table 6.1 Summary of minimum guidelines for anesthesia care for out-of-operating room locations

Policies and procedures
Compliance with building codes, safety codes, and facility standards, and minimum requirements for safe care of patients in that location
Space
Adequate space for equipment and personnel and to allow for quick access to patient, monitors, and anesthesia machine (when applicable)
Communication
Adequate staff trained to support anesthesiologist; two-way communication to request assistance should be available to call for assistance
Equipment
Reliable oxygen source with backup supply adequate for procedure duration
Reliable source of suction
Waste anesthetic gas scavenging (when applicable)
Self-inflating resuscitation bag capable of delivering positive pressure ventilation and high concentration of oxygen
Adequate supply of anesthetic drugs, anesthesia equipment, and supplies
Adequate patient monitoring equipment (meeting minimum requirements for "Standards for Basic Anesthetic Monitoring"). Anesthesia machine maintained to current operating room standards should be used if inhalational agents are administered
Sufficient electrical outlets for anesthetic machines and monitoring
Adequate lighting to monitor patient, monitors, and anesthesia machine (when applicable). Backup battery powered lighting should be available
Immediate access to emergency cart, defibrillator, emergency drugs, and ancillary emergency aids
Post-anesthesia care
Appropriate post-anesthesia management should be available with appropriately trained staff and equipment, protocols and resources to facilitate transfer to a different recovery location

Adapted from Ref. [1]

- Each individual institution also has established standards for care of their operating room and non-operating room anesthesia locations. These standards are reviewed periodically to reflect changes in equipment/technology, personnel/staffing, and to remove outdated or time-limited information.
- Facilities located outside of the hospital environment should have a governing body or medical director who has developed metrics to determine staff competencies in sedation management. Additionally, they can develop risk mitigation strategies and quality improvement activities.
- There should be clear guidelines and credentialing requirements for sedation provided by non-anesthesia personnel. An example of such a policy is provided by the American Society of Anesthesiologists [4]. These detailed guidelines stress the importance of developing ongoing systems to check education and training, licensure, practice pattern, and performance improvement [3].

Space

- If possible, anesthesia personnel should be involved in the planning and layout phases of any new procedural area that may require sedation and/or general anesthesia services.
- Similar to operating rooms, considerations around room design should include (1) room size, (2) room orientation (the procedure table is along the long axis of the room), (3) location of medical gases, (4) location and number of electric and gas outlets, (5) points of entry and egress, and (6) location of the procedure room relative to other facilities (if applicable) [5].
- Many non-operating room anesthesia facilities in other departments have procedure tables that are restricted in terms of full mobility. With some procedures, table positioning may preclude easy access to the patient and may require alteration of the anesthetic plan (general anesthesia versus deep sedation for patients in the prone position in small rooms with a significant amount of procedural equipment).
- Many procedure rooms require a significant amount of equipment which may be on mobile carts which further decreases the available floor space available in cases of emergency (e.g. for additional staff, a bed to facilitate transfer to perform cardiopulmonary resuscitation or intubation)

Communication

- Telephone or other two-way communication for the anesthesia provider is necessary in order to mobilize assistance in the event of an emergency, equipment failure, or the need for additional supplies from outside of the sedation suite.
- Access to such devices should be readily available to all other providers in the room if the person performing the sedation is unavailable for direct communication.
- Access to printed/digital lists of commonly used phone numbers is very useful. Numbers for anesthesia technician assistance, pharmacy, and other medical ancillary personnel (in cases of emergency) should be available.

Equipment [1]

- The standards for anesthesia equipment, supplies, and patient monitoring should match the standards for monitoring in operating rooms conducting similar procedures.
- The ASA recommends that wall oxygen, whenever possible, should be used as the primary oxygen supply. Backup systems should include oxygen equivalent to a full E cylinder.

- Wall suction should be reliable and accessible; if no wall suction is available, a functioning portable suction device must be present.
- If anesthesia machines and monitors are present in the sedation suite, competency on that particular machine should be verified. Troubleshooting checklists should be developed to allow the provider to correct common mechanical issues.
- At minimum, the standards that would apply to an operating room anesthesia machine should apply to remote anesthesia machines, including gas analyzers, end-tidal carbon dioxide monitoring, temperature monitoring and reserve oxygen tanks.
- Anesthesia machine check and equipment check of monitors, laryngoscopes, airway devices, self-inflating resuscitation bag and monitors is mandatory prior to performing sedation or general anesthesia. If intubation is likely, difficult airway devices should be available.
- Equipment noise and room acoustics can make alarm recognition difficult. All monitoring alarms must be readily audible and volume should be adjusted to allowing for recognition over ambient noise. If necessary, two-way mobile devices may be utilized to ensure clear staff-to-staff communication.
- Anesthesia supply carts need to have basic anesthesia supplies as well as additional supplies for urgent/emergent situations depending on the availability of ancillary support and the time required to transport those supplies to a remote location.
- Vasopressor, antihypertensive, anticholinergic drugs and other likely necessary medications should be stocked and readily available depending on the type of procedure and location.
- Infusion pumps to allow for continuous administration of propofol or vasopressors are preferred in remote settings for procedures lasting longer than 5 min. This frees the anesthesia provider to focus on monitoring and identifying potential problems related to patient, positioning, or the procedure.
- If general anesthesia is required at a remote location, staff should be educated on anesthesia-specific emergencies (e.g., malignant hyperthermia) and where to locate the emergency resources (e.g., dantrolene).
- Electrical outlets should be clearly identified and marked as to whether they are connected to the facility's backup generator (when available). Most commercial anesthesia machines have at least a 30 minute backup battery to drive the ventilator but may not provide all functions; personnel should become familiar with these limited functions.
- Smaller spaces and procedural requirements can decrease ambient room light and make visualization of the patient, clinical monitor, and the procedure difficult. Light should be made available either with portable sources or increases in ambient room light to allow for visualization of the patient, monitors, and the procedure. Backup battery-powered light should be available in case of power outages.
- Unencumbered access to emergency resuscitation equipment including a defibrillator should be possible at any time during a remote procedure. All staff should be trained in basic life support. Advanced cardiac life support training

is strongly encouraged for all nurses and physicians caring for patients in remote areas.

- Regularly scheduled drills for the most commonly or most likely anticipated emergencies should be performed on a regular basis as determined by the remote site's medical director, local governing body, or accrediting organization.

Post-anesthesia Care

- There should be appropriate numbers of trained staff to recover patients in the remote location or assist in transport of the patient to the post-anesthesia care unit. Appropriate transfer equipment, such as a transport monitor, should also be available.
- Standards for post-anesthesia care should be clear to the personnel delivering sedation (or to the anesthesia provider) and recovery from sedation or general anesthesia should be documented. The American Society of Anesthesia has published guidelines for standards for postanesthesia care to provide the basic framework for care after performance of monitored anesthesia care or general anesthesia [6].

Documentation

- Legible and accurate (real-time) charting of patient's vital signs and anesthesia drugs is mandatory in the sedation suite. The person delivering sedation should have no other responsibilities other than patient monitoring, anesthetic monitoring, and documentation.
- If electronic medical records are utilized, checking computer systems and networks to ensure data transfer can occur should be done before a patient is brought in for the procedure.
- Backup paper documentation should be available at anytime in case of computer failure or power disruption.

Staff Development

- Non-anesthesia staff should be aware of the periprocedural requirements of the anesthesia provider. They should be readily available to assist the anesthesia provider.
- Anesthesia providers must remain calm and patient when utilizing staff in remote environments. Lack of familiarity with routine operating room procedures, such as videolaryngoscopy to facilitate intubation can make complex anesthetic care

stressful for all involved persons. Discussion of specific roles and specific actions should happen prior to the delivery of the anesthetic if personnel assistance is required.

- Because anesthesia-provider directed cases may take longer, realistic expectations for the sedation suite staff and the proceduralist about time for emergence, transport to PACU, handoff time, and potentially anesthesia turnover time should be discussed at the beginning of the day if patients requiring general anesthesia have been previously identified.

- Lectures, simulations, and updates on sedation and airway management should be performed for training purposes and for continuing education and performance improvement.

Unique Non-operating Room Anesthesia Locations

- Radiation oncology

  - Anesthetic management is primarily for children, non-cooperative patients, or patients where anxiety-related increases in respiratory rates can interfere with therapy (e.g., liver, lung)
  - The setup of the suite for sedation is identical to that of the operating suite. No additional equipment is required.
  - During treatments, the anesthesiologist must leave the suite. Remote monitoring and charting must be functional and available during treatment.
  - While sedation protocols with propofol can be successful, treating potential airway obstruction delays treatment. Many centers will secure the airway with a supraglottic airway.

- Magnetic resonance imaging [7]

  - All equipment used for anesthesia in the MRI suite must be non-ferromagnetic (not susceptible to a magnetic field). This includes the anesthesia machine, anesthesia cart, and all related supplies. Detailed protocols for equipment, monitoring, and emergency procedures should be established and readily available to all personnel in the suite.
  - Ferromagnetic materials can become a projectile when drawn toward the MRI magnet and potentially injure the patient, sedation provider, or ancillary staff.
  - All personnel involved in stocking the anesthesia cart should only utilize MRI-safe supplies.
  - Anesthesia personnel providing sedation services should have completed MRI education prior to administration of any anesthetic.
  - There is significant noise within the MRI machine during a scan; audible detection of anesthesia machine alarms and patient monitor alarms is nearly impossible. The patient and the provider should have ear protection during the scan. Remote viewing of patient monitors outside of the MRI machine and remote viewing of the patient is mandatory to assess for issues with anesthetic delivery.

- Angiography/fluoroscopy/computerized tomography

  - There is considerable amount of radiation exposure in these suites. Practitioners who are not directly involved in the procedure but cannot move due to space constraints should wear personal radiation protection of the chest, gonads, thyroid, and eyes (when applicable).
  - Anesthesia machines are usually placed at a distance from the patient. Anesthesia circuit extensions, electrical cord extensions, and infusion set extensions should be available.
  - Monitors used in these suites are also shared by other non-anesthesia providers. Acquisition of data for the appropriate level of sedation, particularly capnography, should be functional prior to the initiation of the anesthetic.

- Cardiac catheterization

  - For cases where anesthesia has already been requested, access to vasopressor drugs is mandatory, and working infusion pumps for drug delivery is preferable.
  - Cases where anesthesia has been requested during emergent changes in patient condition, excessive movement, or respiratory compromise require rapid assessment of patient's condition.
  - Intubation equipment may only be present from the emergency code cart; subsequent anesthetic management may require placement of a portable anesthesia machine and cart. This will require additional personnel and equipment. An interim sedation plan should be initiated until formal anesthetic management can be established.

- Gastrointestinal procedures

  - Standard monitoring in addition to capnography should be used in patients receiving deep sedation or general anesthesia and recommended in patients with certain medical conditions such as sleep apnea even when they are receiving moderate sedation.

Setting the Standards for Safety in the Sedation Suite [8]

- A number of high-profile deaths in the United States during procedures in non-operating room suites has led to intense scrutiny of practices outside of the traditional operating room environment [9].
- There is data to suggest that experienced individuals who routinely perform remote site procedures may decrease the risk of adverse events and may even improve workflow in these areas [10].
- Improving safety in the sedation suite begins with a clear delineation of roles of the anesthesia provider, the proceduralist, and the ancillary staff.
- Open and unrestricted communication amongst all providers participating in the care of the patient must occur to decrease the chance of events occurring due to lack of information.

- There must be a clear and unambiguous description of the procedure that will be performed that is written on the patient's procedural informed consent.
- A "Time Out" or procedural pause should be performed prior to a procedure to confirm the correct patient, procedure, and presence of required equipment. Identification of relevant medical/equipment issues or other information that would improve patient care or procedural success is also shared at this time.
- Implementation of checklists in remote procedural suites may improve care by improving information exchange and providing confidence in unfamiliar environments, such as sites outside the operating room [11]. These checklists would also incorporate the main points included in "Statement on Nonoperating Room Anesthetizing Locations" in order to ensure minimum equipment necessary to deliver a safe anesthetic.
- Cognitive aids could potentially improve care in remote sites by providing up-to-date information at the point of care during urgent or emergent medical issues that may not be seen on a routine basis (code blue emergencies, local anesthetic toxicity). A large high fidelity simulation study showed significant improvement managing operating room crises with use of cognitive aids [12].
- After completion of the procedure and anesthetic, there should be a quality assessment and performance improvement system in place to identify, monitor, and reduce medical errors and to improve patient outcomes [13].

References

1. The American Society of Anesthesiologists. Statement on nonoperating room anesthetizing locations, last amended. 2013. Available at: http://www.asahq.org/~/media/Sites/ASAHQ/Files/Public/Resources/standards-guidelines/statement-on-nonoperating-room-anesthetizing--locations.pdf.Accessed 1 Dec 2015.
2. American Society of Anesthesiologists Task Force on Sedation and Analgesia by Non-Anesthesiologists. Practice guidelines for sedation and analgesia by non-anesthesiologists. Anesthesiology. 2002;96(4):1004–17.
3. Revised Appendix A, Interpretive Guidelines for Hospitals, 42 C.F.R. § 482.52(2011) [regulation on the Internet]. [cited 4 Dec 2015]. Available from: https://www.cms.gov/Regulations-and-Guidance/Guidance/Transmittals/downloads/R74SOMA.pdf.
4. The American Society of Anesthesiologists. Policies and Procedures Governing Anesthesia Privileging in Hospitals. Appendix A: Statement On Granting Privileges For Administration Of Moderate Sedation To Practitioners Who Are Not Anesthesia Professionals, last amended. 2013. Accessed 1 Dec 2015. Available at: http://www.asahq.org/~/media/sites/asahq/files/public/resources/practice%20management/policies%20and%20procedures%20governing%20anesthesia%20privileging%20policy.pdf.
5. Shine TSJ, Leone BJ, Martin DL. Specialized operating rooms. In: Block FE, Helfman S, editors. Operating room design manual. Accessed 2 Dec 2015. Available at: https://www.asahq.org/~/media/legacy/for%20members/practice%20management/ordm/or%20chapter%2013%20specialized%20operating%20rooms.pdf?la=en.

6. The American Society of Anesthesiologists. Standards for Postanesthesia Care, last amended October 15, 2014. Accessed 2 Dec 2015. Available at: http://www.asahq.org/~/media/Sites/ASAHQ/Files/Public/Resources/standards-guidelines/standards-for-postanesthesia-care.pdf.

7. Youn AM, Ko Y-K, Kim Y-H. Anesthesia and sedation outside of the operating room. Korean J Anesthesiol. 2015;68(4):323–9.

8. Mason KP, Mahmoud M (American Society of Anesthesiologists). Establishing and reinforcing a culture of safety in anesthesia outside of the O.R. ASA Newsletter [Internet]. 1 Aug 2015 [cited 8 Dec 2015]. Available from: http://www.asahq.org/resources/publications/newsletter-articles/2015/august-2015/establishing-and-reinforcing-a-culture-of-safety-in-anesthesia-outside-of-the-or.

9. Department of Health and Human Services Centers for Medicare & Medicaid Services. Statement of deficiencies and plan of correction: yorkville endoscopy. 5 Sep 2014 [cited 8 Dec 2015]. Available from: http://documents.latimes.com/report-clinic-treated-joan-rivers/.

10. Goudra BG, Singh PM, Sinha AC. Anesthesia for ERCP: impact of anesthesiologist's experience on outcome and cost. Anesthesiol Res Pract. 2013;2013(1):1–5.

11. Thomassen Ø, Brattebø G, Heltne J-K, Søfteland E, Espeland A. Checklists in the operating room: help or hurdle? A qualitative study on health workers' experiences. BMC Health Serv Res BioMed Central. 2010;10(1):342.

12. Arriaga AF, Bader AM, Wong JM, Lipsitz SR, Berry WR, Ziewacz JE, et al. Simulation-based trial of surgical-crisis checklists. N Engl J Med. 2013;368(3):246–53.

13. Conditions for coverage—Quality assessment and performance improvement, 42 C.F.R. § 416.43 (2015) [regulation on the Internet]. [cited 2015 Dec 10]. Available from: http://www.ecfr.gov/cgi-bin/text-idx?node=pt42.3.416&rgn=div5#se42.3.416_125.

Part III
Anesthesia for Endoscopic Procedures

Chapter 7
Anesthesia for Upper GI Endoscopy Including Advanced Endoscopic Procedures

Mary Elizabeth McAlevy and John M. Levenick

Abstract One of the most frequent locations for providing out of operating room anesthesia is the endoscopy suite. In 2009 an estimated 6.9 million upper endoscopy procedures were performed according to the American Society for Gastrointestinal Endoscopy (ASGE). Utilization of anesthesia services for these procedures has risen to 30–35 % of patients nationwide (Goulson and Fragneto, Anesthesiology Clin 27:71–85, 2009). Sedation offered by anesthesia providers has been shown to play a crucial role in safety, efficiency, patient satisfaction and throughput.

Anesthesia providers are increasingly consulted to provide sedation for newer, more complex endoscopic procedures. The basic principles and guidelines for evaluating and preparing a patient for a screening upper endoscopy are applicable to the anesthetic management of these advanced endoscopic procedures. In addition, the anesthesia provider must be knowledgeable of the indication, technique, complexity and length of these new procedures. Understanding the risks, complications and patient comorbidities is crucial to providing safe sedation.

Upper endoscopic procedures are done for either diagnostic, prognostic, and/or therapeutic purposes. The interventions discussed in this chapter include: standard endoscopy (EGD), endoscopic ultrasound (EUS), endoscopic cystenterostomy, pancreatic necrosectomy and Per oral endoscopic myotomy (POEM).

Keywords EGD • Endoscopic Ultrasound (EUS) • Pancreatic Necrosectomy • Cystgastrostomy • Endoscopic cystenterostomy • Per Oral Endoscopic Myotomy (POEM) • Achalasia • Topicalization • Benzocaine • Capnothorax • Capnomediastinum • Air Embolism • Perforation

M.E. McAlevy, MD (✉) • J.M. Levenick, MD
Department of Anesthesiology and Perioperative Medicine, Penn State Milton
S. Hershey Medical Center, 500 University Drive – HU33, PO Box 850, Hershey, PA, USA
e-mail: mmcalevy@hmc.psu.edu; jlevenick@hmc.psu.edu

© Springer International Publishing Switzerland 2017   85
B.G. Goudra, P.M. Singh (eds.), *Out of Operating Room Anesthesia*,
DOI 10.1007/978-3-319-39150-2_7

Introduction

One of the most frequent locations for providing out of operating room anesthesia is the endoscopy suite. In 2009 an estimated 6.9 million upper endoscopy procedures were performed according to the American Society for Gastrointestinal Endoscopy (ASGE). Utilization of anesthesia services for these procedures has risen to 30–35 % of patients nationwide [1]. Sedation offered by anesthesia providers has been shown to play a crucial role in safety, efficiency, patient satisfaction and throughput.

Anesthesia providers are increasingly consulted to provide sedation for newer, more complex endoscopic procedures. The basic principles and guidelines for evaluating and preparing a patient for a screening upper endoscopy are applicable to the anesthetic management of these advanced endoscopic procedures. In addition, the anesthesia provider must be knowledgeable of the indication, technique, complexity and length of these new procedures. Understanding the risks, complications and patient comorbidities is crucial to providing safe sedation.

Upper endoscopic procedures are done for either diagnostic, prognostic, and/or therapeutic purposes. The interventions discussed in this chapter include: standard endoscopy (EGD), endoscopic ultrasound (EUS), endoscopic cystenterostomy, pancreatic necrosectomy and Per oral endoscopic myotomy (POEM).

EGD

A flexible forward viewing endoscope is passed through a mouth piece, over the tongue with visual access to the esophagus, stomach, and duodenum.

Through a working channel, instruments can be passed through the scope to perform biopsies, treat bleeding, or deploy instruments including luminal stents.

Common indications for EGDs include:

Evaluation of reflux disease and its sequelae
Evaluate and possibly treat causes of dysphagia, odynophagia, including acute food impaction
Dyspepsia and peptic ulcer disease
Iron deficiency anemia
Assess for celiac disease or other proximal small bowel mucosal pathology
Screen for and/or treat esophageal varices
Diagnosis and possibly palliate luminal foregut tumors

EUS (Endoscopic Ultrasound)

- As in EGD, a flexible forward viewing endoscope is passed through a mouth piece, over the tongue allowing visual access to the esophagus, stomach, and duodenum.

EUS technologyuses an oblique angled luminal camera making visualization of the lumen difficult

Two different echoendoscopes:

Radial: gives a 360° ultrasound images perpendicular to the scope tip, used for esophageal cancer, subepithelial masses, etc. Biopsy cannot be taken through it.

Linear: gives a focused ~170° image along the access of the probe used to guide fine needle aspiration under direct visualization.

Used primarily to locally stage foregut tumors as well as diagnose non-luminal foregut tumors (pancreas, liver, abdominal and mediastinal lymph nodes) and pancreatic cysts using fine needle aspiration [2] Has the highest sensitivity for choledocholithiasis and small pancreatic masses of any imaging modality

Endoscopic Cystenterostomy (Cystgastrosomy)

Usually performed using a linear EUS followed by needle aspiration of the cyst cavity. After this a wire is coiled in the cyst under fluoroscopy, and then the tract is sequentially dilated up 10–20 mm in size. Following this, trans-luminal stent(s) are placed to allow ongoing drainage and formalize an enterocystic fistula [2].

Creation of a trans-luminal ostomy between the lumen and a cyst, usually either symptomatic walled off pancreatic necrosis or pseudocyst, to facilitate drainage and possible access for debridement (necrosectomy).

Endoscopic Necrosectomy

After creation or revision of a cystenterostomy, an endoscope is driven through the enteric lumen into the cyst cavity to perform direct necrosectomy of necrotic solid material

Material is gently pulled free from the cavity walls and deposited usually in the stomach or duodenum, but if a large piece exists, it can be removed per os [3]

Frequently these are long (>90–120 min) procedures.

POEM (Per Oral Endoscopic Myotomy)

Utilizes a standard upper endoscope and advanced per oral cavity as in normal EGD.

Treatment of choice now for achalasia

An incision is made through the mucosa into the submucosa of the esophagus ~10–15 cm proximal to the gastroesophageal junction, and using endoscopic dissection, a tunnel is made distally extending 2–3 cm into the stomach [4]

The esophageal muscles, preferentially the circular muscles, are incised. The incision is about 2 cm into the stomach and 7 cm proximal into the esophagus [4]. At the end, the incision site into the tunnel is closed with multiple clips or sutures.

Focused History and Physical Findings for Patients Presenting for Upper GI Endoscopy

The same principles used for pre-anesthetic evaluation of surgical cases should be applied to pre-evaluation of GI endoscopy procedures. Includes review of medical, anesthetic and medication history and completion of a focused physical examination with review of any pertinent diagnostic studies [5].

- Requires a well-defined process in order to prevent the presentation of patients with inadequate work up on the day of the procedure.
- Majority of endoscopy centers perform a phone history and triage patients prior to procedure date. Any concerning findings are flagged and reviewed by a physician to determine if further workup is indicated.
- It is critical to determine during the preanesthetic evaluation the most appropriate location for performing the procedure (Endoscopy suite versus Operating Room). The anesthesia provider must take into account patient comorbidities and complication risk of procedure to ensure the availability of specialized monitoring, airway equipment and additional personnel in case more serious anesthesia complications arise.

Pertinent Approach to Taking the History

- Obtain prior anesthetic history to determine if patient had known complications, difficult airway or family history of malignant hyperthermia.
- Many of the indications for performing an upper GI endoscopy include signs and symptoms that are associated with increased risk of aspiration.
- Past medical history predisposing to *increased aspiration risk* includes: severe gastroesophageal reflux disease, delayed gastric emptying (diabetes, chronic opioid use, pregnancy), dysphagia, achalasia, increased intraabdominal pressure (ascites, obesity) [6].
- Determination of aspiration risk will dictate need for protection of airway with endotracheal intubation.
- Past medical history that is indicative of *increased risk of airway obstruction* include: history of snoring, obstructive sleep apnea (OSA), excessive daytime sleepiness.
- Past medical history indicative of *increased incidence of hypoxia* during sedation include: history of OSA, obesity, tobacco use, shortness of breath, asthma,

COPD, home oxygen use, reactive airway disease or recent upper respiratory infection [7].
- Patients with the aforementioned medical history may exhibit increased volume of secretions which could predispose to coughing, bronchospasm and laryngospasm during procedure.
- Past medical history suggesting an *increased risk of bleeding*: liver disease, esophageal varices, prior GI bleeding, anticoagulation, known coagulopathies (e.g. Hemophilia)

Pertinent Approach to Performing the Physical Examination

A focused physical exam on day of the procedure should evaluate for factors increasing the risk of obstruction/hypoxia, aspiration and cardiopulmonary depression. The skilled anesthesiologist will document all of the following prior to the procedure.

Vital signs
Body Mass Index
Airway exam: Modified Mallampati score, neck circumference, thyromental distance, presence of craniofacial anomalies, neck range of motion

- Pulmonary auscultation with documentation baseline breath sounds and added sounds (if any).
- Visual inspection and palpation of abdomen for ascites in patients with history of liver disease. Paracentesis may be required pre procedure if there is respiratory compromise due to compression of the diaphram.
- Cardiac auscultation with documentation of new murmurs or other abnormal findings.
- Dental examination for any loose teeth that may become dislodged due to bite block, endoscope or instrumentation of the airway.
- Obtain current hemoglobin levels in patients with history of GI bleed and anemia

Patient Optimization

- As with any preoperative evaluation, the goal is to determine whether the patient's medical problems are optimized prior to delivery of an anesthetic.
- These same principles apply to anesthesia out of the operating room for endoscopic procedures.
- The severity of the patient's comorbidities is weighed against the procedure risk.
- EGD is considered a minimally invasive low risk procedure.
- EUS, Pancreatic Cyst Gastrostomy, Necrosectomy, and POEM are considered higher risk procedures.

- Emergent or urgent procedures may not allow time for complete patient optimization and as a result are considered to be higher risk.
- Cardiac optimization should follow 2014 ACC/AHA guidelines on perioperative cardiovascular evaluation and management of patients undergoing noncardiac surgery.
- Patients with Cardiac Implantable Electronic Device (Pacemaker and AICD) should be optimized per consensus guidelines published in July 2011 as a joint project involving the Heart Rhythm Society, American Society of Anesthesiologists, American Heart Association and the Society of Thoracic Surgeons.
- Respiratory symptoms should be at baseline without recent increase in oxygen requirements, dyspnea, and hospitalizations or emergency room visits for pulmonary disease exacerbations.
- Anticoagulant management and recommendations should be determined by the most recent guidelines from the ASGE. These are formulated by determination of the risk of bleeding versus the risk of thromboembolic event.
- Confirmation and documentation of NPO status. NPO guidelines for general anesthesia per American Society of Anesthesiology.
- Patients presenting with achalasia for POEM procedure should be given strict guidelines for clear liquid diet 2 days prior to procedure to reduce aspiration risk [4].

Commonly Used Anesthetic Techniques and Sedative Medications for Standard and Advanced Upper Endoscopy

Selection of Appropriate Sedation Level

- Sedation requirements for upper endoscopic interventions are dependent on patient demographics and the exact procedure to be performed. Sedation may range from light/moderate sedation to general anesthesia [8]. General anesthesia may be provided with or without endotracheal intubation.
- Determination of appropriate sedation technique must take into account medical history, sedation history, patient preference, and level of discomfort anticipated by procedure.
- EGDs are short in duration and less invasive; typically, general anesthesia is not required.
- Conversely, EUS is more complex and stimulating. The EUS scope is larger in caliber, needle aspiration is performed to obtain biopsies and duration of procedure is longer. All of these factors necessitate deep sedation/general anesthesia for patient comfort and optimal operating conditions for the endoscopist.
- Pancreatic Cystgastrostomy and Necrosectomy require general anesthesia with or without endotracheal intubation. These procedures are the longest and most complex. They carry a higher risk of aspiration and complication rate compared to EGD.
- POEM procedures require general anesthesia with endotracheal intubation. The population with achalasia is at high risk of aspiration. General anesthesia with

endotracheal intubation is favored as it allows a still patient and a controlled airway in case of pneumothorax, pneumomediastinum or pneumoperitoneum.
- Moderate sedation for EGD is achieved by combination of opioid and benzodiazepine administration. This level of sedation may be conducted by any physician licensed to administer moderate sedation who may or may not be a trained anesthesia professional.
- Anesthesia providers may choose to provide moderate sedation based on criteria above or may be consulted based on complex patient medical history.
- General anesthesia for EGD may be indicated due to factors which include but are not limited to failed moderate sedation, patient preference, procedure requirement, and need for endotracheal intubation for airway protection.
- Patients with higher risk of aspiration as detailed above in preprocedure evaluation will require airway protection with endotracheal tube placement. Induction of general anesthesia by rapid sequence induction must be considered to further prevent aspiration. Medications used for induction are chosen based on the patient's medical history. Due to the short duration of most endoscopy procedures, a short acting neuromuscular blocking agent may be preferred to facilitate endotracheal intubation. Maintenance of general anesthesia is achieved with inhalational agents or intravenous infusion.
- Fortunately in the majority of cases for upper endoscopy endotracheal intubation is not required and general anesthesia is safely administered via intravenous infusion and supplemental oxygen.

Monitoring

All patients require continuous monitoring following the ASA minimum monitoring recommendations: pulse oximetry, arterial blood pressure monitoring, continuous ECG, temperature, and capnography.

- Many devices for supplemental oxygen delivery have been modified to also allow for carbon dioxide sensing. Oxygen delivery devices most commonly used for upper endoscopy procedures are nasal cannulas or a bite block with an oxygen delivery system incorporated. In addition, facemasks have been developed that provide oxygen delivery/carbon dioxide sampling modified with a port to allow endoscope passage.

Sedative Medications

- Most commonly used medications for moderate sedation include midazolam and fentanyl.
- Another opioid to consider for sedation includes Meperidine, but has become less popular over last decade. Alfentanil may also be considered in place of fentanyl. Benefits of alfentanil include faster onset and shorter duration of action when administered in small bolus doses.

- Most popular agent and technique used to achieve general anesthesia for endoscopy is via Propofol infusion [9].
- Propofol may be administered alone or in combination with a benzodiazepine or opioid depending upon patient sedation requirements.
- Propofol may be given either as an intermittent bolus to achieve desired effect for procedures of short duration or as an infusion for longer procedures.
- Benefits of providing general anesthesia using Propofol include, faster onset of desired level of sedation, quicker recovery time, and improved quality of examination. Propofol has been shown to facilitate the performance of higher volume of procedures compared with moderate sedation [9].
- Other intravenous agents that have been studied and used to provide sedation for endoscopy include; dexmetatomidine, ketamine, and remifentanil.
- Dexmetatomidine infusionprovides sedation with less risk of respiratory depression. There has been conflicting data published on its use for endoscopy. Sedation quality, patient and endoscopist satisfaction are comparable to midazolam and fentanyl [10]. Potential concerns include delayed onset to achieve level of sedation, hypotension, bradycardia and longer recovery time.
- Ketamine has been investigated for use as a sole agent or for use in conjunction with other sedatives. The majority of studies have been in pediatric patients. Benefits include the ability to administer intramuscularly in a combative patient or patient in with difficult intravenous access. Ketamine does not cause respiratory depression and has minimal effect on hemodynamics. An antisialagogue should be co-administered to prevent excess secretions. Increased secretions during upper endoscopy require frequent suctioning to prevent excess cough and laryngospasm.
- Remifentanil provides profound analgesia and sedation with a very short recovery time. However in studies evaluating its use for endoscopy at doses to achieve optimal sedation there was frequent apnea necessitating positive pressure ventilation [11].
- Topicalization with local anesthetic of the posterior oropharynx may be used as an adjunct to sedation. Topicalization may improve endoscope passage by depressing gag reflex and decrease patient coughing and straining [12]. Benzocaine and lidocaine are local agents most commonly used. Caution with Benzocaine sprays as it has risk of causing methemoglobinemia. Metered single dose benzocaine sprays are available to aid in preventing overdose and side effect of methemoglobinemia. Lidocaine is available in various preparations for topicalization including, liquid, viscous and ointment. Lidocaine topicalization is applied with use of atomizers or by direct application [13].

Anticipated Adverse Events and Procedure Complications

Anesthetic complications for endoscopy are no different from those that may occur in the operating room. Risks of moderate sedation and general anesthesia apply to all patients regardless of procedure type and location. However there are specific complications that are more common while providing anesthesia for upper endoscopic procedure. Providers much have awareness of these events which include: aspiration, obstruction, apnea, hypoxia, and laryngospasm. In addition, it is important to also be knowledgeable of the common complications that may occur as a direct result of the procedure itself.

Procedural Complications

Standard EGD [14]

Aspiration
Perforation 1/5–10,000 for diagnostic EGD
Bleeding
Missed lesion

EUS (with FNA*) [2]

Same as EGD
Slightly increased perforation risk with more rigid scope tip and oblique view, especially in the oropharynx or duodenal sweep
Pancreatitis* (1 % if biopsying the pancreas)
Autonomic instability* during celiac plexus neurolysis/block

Cystenterostomy/Necrosectomy [3]

Same as EGD
Air/CO_2 embolus (up to 2 %)
Perforation (at the cyst-enteric fistula) or cyst wall dehiscence (5 %)
Massive bleeding

POEM [15]

Same as EGD
Capnomediastinum, capnothorax, capnoperitoneum (small ones are common)
Bleeding (1–2 %)
Infection (mediastinitis, <1 %)

Sedation Complications

- Sedation and general anesthesia provided without placement of a definitive airway puts patients at risk for aspiration, upper airway obstruction, laryngospasm and apnea.

  Many of the indications for performing EGD include patients with signs and symptoms worrisome for aspiration including but not limited to GERD, dysphagia, achalasia, and gastroparesis.

Medications administered to achieve appropriate levels of sedation lead to relaxation and collapse of tissue in the oropharynx promoting obstruction of upper airway. Laryngospasm may be caused by direct stimulation by secretions or the endoscope. This is more common if the patient has not reached an adequate level of sedation or presence of inadequate topicalization. Apnea is caused by upper airway obstruction, laryngospasm or as a side effect of excess administration of sedative medications.

Dental injury is increased during EGD, even in the absence of direct laryngoscopy and ETT placement. In order to prevent damage to endoscope an oral plastic bite block is placed between the patient's teeth and fastened around the back of the neck with an elastic band. During the procedure the patient may bite down with excessive force or manipulation of the endoscope may cause the bite block to cause dental dislodgement or chipping.

Injury and swelling of the lips has also been described. The lip may be entrapped between teeth and bite block leading to ischemic or mechanical trauma.

Prevention and Management of Adverse Events

Knowledge and awareness of the above mentioned common adverse events during upper endoscopy allows the anesthesia provider to better prepare and manage these potential complications. The principles for management of these complications do not differ from management in the operating room, but anesthesia providers must appreciate that the resources available to handle these problems may not be as readily accessible in the endo suite. This includes not only equipment but also experienced personnel comfortable in managing patient with acute cardiopulmonary depression.

After obtaining a thorough preoperative evaluation and taking into consideration the procedural risk and sedation requirements the anesthesia provider must determine the most appropriate location for performing procedure. The operating room may be preferred over Endoscopy suite based on patient comorbidities and complexity of procedure.

Airway Obstruction

One of the common complications encountered during upper endoscopy and if not managed appropriately can ultimately lead to a fatal cardiopulmonary event.

Airway obstruction can be minimized due to placement of patient in left lateral position for the procedure.

Upper airway obstruction can be first managed by simple maneuvers like neck extension and jaw thrust. If the airway continues to obstruct a nasal trumpet may be inserted. Placement of nasal airway must be done cautiously as to not cause trauma or epistaxis.

Failure of these attempts to relieve obstruction with ensuing signs of hypoxia will necessitate communication with endoscopist to abort procedure to allow definitive airway management.

Patient may require placement of oral airway, face mask, supraglottic airway or ETT for positive pressure ventilation.

Patient's who are deemed high risk for obstruction after preoperative evaluation may require endotracheal intubation at induction of anesthesia.

Hypoxia

- May be witnessed in the absence of airway obstruction.
- Result of multiple physiologic factors that occur during sedation including but not limited to change in tidal volume, functional residual capacity, minute ventilation, and ventilation perfusion mismatch, and apnea during sedation.
- Initial management is to increase amount of supplemental oxygen provided and rule out other causes e.g. obstruction and aspiration. Endotracheal intubation with positive pressure ventilation may be required if hypoxia does not improve.

Aspiration

- Serious complication leading to hypoxia and potential unplanned admission.
- Aspiration can be minimized by adherence to the American Society of Anesthesiology NPO guidelines.
- Patient positioning on left side not only lowers the risk of obstruction but also aspiration. In addition, considerations should be given to place the patient in reverse Trendelenburg.
- If gastric contents are observed after placement of endoscope there are two management options. (1) Suction under direct visualization through the endoscope when volume is small and not viscous. (2) Removal of endoscope and placement of an endotracheal tube via rapid sequence induction technique. This should be done when gastric contents are large volume and thick in consistency.
- General anesthesia with endotracheal intubation via rapid sequence induction should be considered in patients with known history of gastroparesis, achalasia and food impaction.

Air Embolism

- Rare but a potentially fatal complication of upper endoscopic procedures.
- The use of carbon dioxide for insufflation decreases the risk of air embolism as it is easily absorbed due to high solubility coefficient.

- Patient's at higher risk for air embolism include – history of previous interventions or surgeries of the bile duct system, (Transjugular intrahepatic portosystemic shunt) TIPS, inflammation of the digestive system, post-surgical gastrointestinal fistula, gastrointestinal tumors and certain interventional techniques [16].
- Presents with cardiopulmonary and neurologic symptoms and is difficult to diagnose as may be attributed to sedation related complications.
- Remain as differential diagnosis in patients with sudden cardiopulmonary instability and neurologic changes especially during EUS, pancreatic necrosectomy and cystgastrostomy.
- Simple maneuvers to perform to decrease impact of air embolism while definitive diagnosis is established include: stopping procedure, administer high flow 100% oxygen, initiate high volume normal saline infusion, place patient in Trendelenburg and left lateral decubitus position to minimize air migration to brain and force air from the Right Ventricular Outflow Track.
- Definitive diagnosis requires a bedside echocardiogram [16].

Hemorrhage

- Possible in all procedures but most common complication of endoscopic necrosectomy
- Occur during access to the collection, particularly if a vessel is punctured during dilation of the transmural tract or during the direct debridement of the necrotic cavity [17].
- Hemorrhage may also occur from retroperitoneal vessels such as the portal vein during the direct debridement of the necrotic material, representing a sometimes drastic complication that may require emergent angiography or even surgery.
- Ensure adequate IV access and consider type and screen for possible administration blood products.

Perforation

- During upper endoscopy most commonly occurs with dilation of esophageal strictures or achalasia, removal of foreign bodies or application of esophageal endoprostheses [18].
- Perforation causes leakage of gastrointestinal contents into mediastinum or peritoneum resulting in mediastinitis and severe sepsis.
- Patients most commonly present with pain in the recovery area. Subcutaneous emphysema may also be palpated. Fever, sepsis and pneumothorax are later findings. Any patient with worsening pain after instrumentation and interventional procedures during upper endoscopy should be evaluated for perforation. The gastroenterologist should be notified and patient should be sent for barium swallow study.

Capnothorax and Capnomediastinum

- Occurs with esophageal insufflation during POEM procedures.
- General anesthesia with endotracheal intubation and positive pressure ventilation is recommended [19].
- Observation of sudden increase in end tidal carbon dioxide tension may be a sign of subcutaneous emphysema while a sudden increase in peak inspiratory pressures may point to capnothorax.
- Severe cases of capnothorax leading to cardiopulmonary instability, needle decompression may be required.

Preferred Technique

Our preferred technique and recommendation for providing sedation and anesthesia for upper endoscopic procedures takes into consideration all of the above referenced material, preoperative evaluation/optimization, knowledge of anesthetic risks, and known procedural complications. This is then applied to each patient encounter and anesthetic plan is determined based on three main factors: (1) Procedure type, (2) Aspiration Risk, and (3) Individual patient comorbidities.

EGD/EUS performed on patients with a low aspiration risk and no other major medical comorbidities.

- Procedure may be performed safely in an Endoscopy suite with MAC IV sedation or IV general anesthesia. This author's preferred method for this patient population is to provide general anesthesia with intravenous infusion of Propofol.
- Use of IV general anesthesia using Propofol infusion is most preferred as it will provide optimal conditions for endoscopy procedure with more rapid recovery compared to IV sedation with opioids and benzodiazepines. This is especially important during EUS, as these procedures are lengthier and require the patient to be still during needle biopsies. In addition, the specialized ultrasound endoscope is larger than a standard endoscope, and insertion may cause more patient discomfort requiring deeper levels of sedation or general anesthesia.
- Always ensure that there are adequate supplies and medications available in case of rare need for urgent conversion to general endotracheal anesthesia for airway protection or cardiopulmonary collapse.
- After appropriate preoperative evaluation the patient is brought to the endoscopy procedure room. Standard monitors are placed and supplemental oxygen is provided by a carbon dioxide sensing nasal cannula.
- A single metered dose spray of cetacaine spray is applied to posterior oropharynx. This will aid in blunting gag reflex which is especially helpful during EUS.

- Another adjunct to consider is the administration of 0.2 mg IV glycopyrrolate preprocedure. We find it beneficial to aid in decreasing amount of oral secretions that may interfere leading to excessive cough, obstruction and laryngospasm.
- The patient is positioned in left lateral decubitus position to comfort with the head elevated and bed in slight reverse Trendelenburg. This positioning helps to further decrease aspiration risk. The protective bite block is placed carefully prior to administration of sedative medications as to not cause any dental injury.
- Propofol is administered via infusion or incremental bolus to achieve desired level of sedation in order to allow easy passage of the endoscope from posterior oropharynx into esophagus.
- Continuous monitoring for obstruction and apnea and suctioning of secretions is frequent.

EGD/EUS performed on patients with a low aspiration risk and severe medical comorbidities.

- Determination of appropriate location for performing these procedures. Patient safety is improved by providing anesthesia care in an operating room or endoscopy suite within the hospital.
- Patients with known difficult airways will require the availability of various airway adjuncts and personnel comfortable with aiding anesthesia providers in case of emergency.
- Serious medical issues especially those putting patient's at high risk for cardiopulmonary complications also mandate a higher level of monitoring during and after the procedure that may not be able to be safely provided in an outpatient endoscopy suite.
- The anesthesia provider must make this determination based on the available resources provided in their facility.
- MAC sedation or IV general anesthesia may be administered as described earlier with healthy patients, to these patients depending on individual requirements, concern for loss of airway, and hemodynamic side effects.

EGD/EUS performed on patients with high aspiration risk and have no other major medical comorbidities.

- Recommend general anesthesia with placement of endotracheal tube for airway protection.
- Common pathology that increases risk of aspiration includes but not limited to, achalasia, food bolus, and gastroparesis.
- Rapid sequence induction should be considered.
- Procedure may be performed in any location as long as appropriate equipment and personnel for management and recovery of GETA are available.

EGD/EUS in patients with both high aspiration risk and major medical problems.

- Recommend procedure to be performed in a location with immediate access to invasive monitoring supplies, personnel trained to aid anesthesia providers in management of severe cardiopulmonary complications and difficult airway management.

- General endotracheal anesthesia for airway protection is necessary.

Endoscopic cystenterostomy (cystgastrosomy) and pancreatic necrosectomy.

- Primary cystenterostomy and necrosectomy carry the highest complication risk.
- Cyst fluid and necrotic debris from the pancreas will be drained into the stomach and may be snared by endoscope and removed via oral cavity.
- Recommend GETA for airway protection.
- Depending on patient's medical comorbidities and complexity of procedure consider performing in an OR versus outpatient endoscopy suite.
- Hemorrhage risk is elevated especially during primary necrosectomy when the tract is being established with the endoscope for the first time. Recommend obtaining a type and screen and ensure adequate IV access.
- Confirm that antiplatelet and other anticoagulation medications have been held preprocedure.
- Elevated risk of inducing bacteremia during access of infected necrotic pancreatic fluid and tissue. Monitor for hypotension, tachycardia and fever.
- Patient will likely require admission for observation if not already an inpatient.
- Return patients for repeat necrosectomy still require ETT for airway protection. Bleeding less likely than compared to primary necrosectomy however must still be considered.

POEM

- Recommend rapid sequence induction for GETA to provide airway protection from aspiration due to achalasia. Intubation allows for controlled ventilation, and close monitoring of end tidal carbon dioxide during dissection and insufflation.
- To date there have been no studies suggesting clinical importance of anesthetic agent use during POEM procedures. Use of Propofol or Sevoflurane is acceptable.
- Patient is positioned supine and draped to allow access to abdomen and chest for urgent needle decompression of pneumoperitoneum and pneumothorax.
- Positive pressure ventilation is recommended as it minimizes the risk for pneumomediastinum by isolating positive pressure to respiratory system via endotracheal tube
- Monitor for signs of subcutaneous emphysema and sudden increase in end tidal carbon dioxide.
- Majority of cases of subcutaneous emphysema resolve with conservative treatment
- Recommend performing in OR setting to allow for rapid surgical management of serious procedural complications outlined earlier in this chapter.

References

1. Goulson DT, Fragneto RY. Anesthesia for gatrointestinal endoscopic procedures. Anesthesiol Clin. 2009;27:71–85.
2. Wiersema MJ, Vilmann P, Giovannini M, et al. Endosonography-guided fine-needle aspiration biopsy: diagnostic accuracy and complication assessment. Gastroenterology. 1997;112:1087.
3. Gardner TB, et al. Direct endoscopic necrosectomy for the treatment of walled-off pancreatic necrosis: results from a multicenter U.S. series. Gastroinstest Endosc. 2011;73:718–26.
4. Ponsky JL, Marks JM, Pauli EM. How I do it: per-oral endoscopic myotomy (POEM). J Gastrointest Surg. 2012;16:1251–5.
5. Practice Advisory for Preanesthesia Evaluation An Updated Report by the American Society of Anesthesiologists Task Force on Preanesthesia Evaluation. Anesthesiology. 2012;116: 1–17.
6. Engelhardt T, Webster NR. Review article pulmonary aspiration of gastric contents in anaesthesia. Br J Anaesth. 1999;83:453–60.
7. Smetana Gw: Preoperative pulmonary evaluation: Identifying and reducing risks for pulmonary complications. Clev Clin J Med. 2006;73:3646.
8. Cohen LB, Wecsler JS, Gaetano JN, et al. Endoscopic sedation in the United States: results from a nationwide survey. Am J Gastroenterol. 2006;101:967–74.
9. Trummel J. Sedation for gastrointestinal endoscopy: the changing landscape. Curr Opin Anaesthesiol. 2007;20:359–64.
10. Demirarany, Korkut E, Tamer A, et al. The comparison of dexmedetomidine and midazolam used for sedation of patients during upper endoscopy: a prospective, randomized study. Can J Gastroenterol. 2007;21:25–29.
11. Litman RS. Conscious sedation with remifentanil during painful medical procedures. J Pain Symptom Manage. 2000;19:468–71.
12. Evans LT, Saberi S, Kim HM, et al. Pharyngeal anesthesia during sedated EGDs: is "the spray" beneficial? A meta-analysis and systematic review. Gastrointest Endosc. 2006;63:761–6.
13. Skoury A, Ayoub C, Abdul-Baki H, et al. Lidocaine lollipop as single-agent anesthesia in upper GI endoscopy. Gastrointest Endosc. 2007;66:786–93.
14. Chirica M, Champault A, Dray X, et al. Esophageal perforations. J Visc Surg. 2010;147, e117.
15. Inoue H, Tianle KM, Ikeda H, Hosoya T, Onimaru M, Yoshida A, Minami H, Kudo SE. Peroral endoscopic myotomy for esophageal achalasia: technique, indication, and outcomes. Thorac Surg Clin. 2011;21:519–25.
16. Donepudi S, Chavalitdhamrong D, Pu L, Draganov P. Air embolism complicating gastrointestinal endoscopy: a systematic review. World J Gastrointest Endosc. 2013;5(8):359–65.
17. Giovannini M, Binmoeller K, Seifert H. Endoscopic ultrasound-guided cystogastrostomy. Endoscopy. 2003;35:239–45.
18. Cotton PB. Outcomes of endoscopy procedures: struggling towards definitions. Gastrointest Endosc. 1994;40:514.
19. Tanaka E, Murata H, Minami H, Sumikawa K. Anesthetic management of peroral endoscopic myotomy for esophageal achalasia: a retrospective case series. J Anesth. 2013;02.

Chapter 8
Anesthesia for Colonoscopy

George A. Dumas and Gwendolyn L. Boyd

Abstract Millions of colonoscopies are performed around the world each year. Colonoscopies are associated with discomfort and pain, which can be problematic for the patient as well as the endoscopist. Most screening colonoscopies are performed on an outpatient basis where access to anesthesia providers may be limited. Interventional colonoscopies, retrograde double-balloon enteroscopies, and colonoscopies requiring deep levels of sedation are often performed with the assistance of anesthesia providers. Patients with multiple comorbidities, uncooperative patients, pediatric patients, patients with a history of difficult sedations, and patients with a history of airway related difficulties are best served by the involvement of an anesthesiologist. Sedation and patient care strategies will be reviewed in this chapter. Ultimately, the best anesthetic technique will be determined by patient factors, procedural difficulty, procedural duration, anticipated depth of sedation required, and ability to modify the chosen technique as the situation changes.

Keywords Anesthesia • Colonoscopy • Depth of sedation • Propofol sedation • Non-propofol sedation • Depth of anesthesia monitor • Moderate sedation • Aspiration during colonoscopy • Difficult mask ventilation • Awareness during colonoscopy • Deep sedation • Ketamine sedation • Difficult colonoscopy • Sedation complications

G.A. Dumas, MD (✉)
Department of Anesthesiology and Perioperative Medicine, University of Alabama at Birmingham, 619 19th ST S, JT 845, Birmingham, AL 35249-6810, USA
e-mail: gadumas@uabmc.edu

G.L. Boyd, MD
Department of Anesthesiology and Perioperative Medicine, University of Alabama at Birmingham, UAB Callahan Eye Hospital and University of Alabama Hospital, 619 S 19th Street, 945 JT, Birmingham, AL 35233, USA
e-mail: gboyd@uabmc.edu

© Springer International Publishing Switzerland 2017   101
B.G. Goudra, P.M. Singh (eds.), *Out of Operating Room Anesthesia*,
DOI 10.1007/978-3-319-39150-2_8

Introduction

Millions of colonoscopies are performed around the world each year. Colonoscopies are associated with discomfort and pain, which can be problematic for the patient as well as the endoscopist.

- Most screening colonoscopies are performed on an outpatient basis where access to anesthesia providers may be limited.
- Interventional colonoscopies, retrograde double-balloon enteroscopies, and colonoscopies requiring deep levels of sedation are often performed with the assistance of anesthesia providers.
- Patients with multiple comorbidities, uncooperative patients, pediatric patients, patients with a history of difficult sedations, and patients with a history of airway related difficulties are best served by the involvement of an anesthesiologist.

Sedation and patient care strategies will be reviewed in this chapter. Ultimately, the best anesthetic technique will be determined by patient factors, procedural difficulty, procedural duration, anticipated depth of sedation required, and ability to modify the chosen technique as the situation changes.

Defining Depth of Sedation

The common use of propofol sedation for colonoscopies has made it imperative for anesthesia providers to understand the implications of various depths of sedation. The American Society of Anesthesiologists has described the continuum of depth of sedation (Table 8.1) [1].

- Moderate sedation and analgesia is often referred to as conscious sedation. Many colonoscopies are performed under "conscious sedation."
- Anesthesia providers must be trained to rescue patients from deeper levels of sedation than were intended [1].

Pre-procedure Evaluation

Aspiration Risk

- Patients presenting for colonoscopy may be at increased risk of aspiration and aspiration pneumonia, particularly when deep sedation is used [2].
- Deep levels of anesthesia are known to obtund upper airway protective reflexes.
- In one study, aspiration occurred in 0.16% of colonoscopies [3]. Most of these patients received propofol for sedation.

Table 8.1 Depth of sedation continuum

	Minimal sedation/ anxiolysis	Moderate sedation/ analgesia	Deep sedation/ analgesia	General anesthesia
Responsiveness	Normal response to verbal stimulation	Purposeful response to tactile or verbal stimulation (reflex withdrawal to pain is not purposeful)	Purposeful response after repeated or painful stimulation (reflex withdrawal to pain is not purposeful)	Unarousable, even with painful stimulus
Airway	Unaffected	No intervention needed	Intervention may be needed	Intervention often needed
Spontaneous ventilation	Unaffected	Adequate	May be inadequate	Frequently inadequate
Cardiovascular function	Unaffected	Usually maintained	Usually maintained	May be impaired

Excerpted from Continuum of depth of sedation: definition of general anesthesia and levels of sedation/analgesia, approved by the ASA House of Delegates on October 13, 1999 and last amended on October 15, 2014, of the American Society of Anesthesiologists. A copy of the full text can be obtained from ASA, 1061 American Lane Schaumburg, IL 60173-4973 or online at www.asahq.org. With permission from the American Society of Anesthesiologists

- Swallowing impairment occurs with deeper levels of sedation. Aspiration due to swallowing impairment may occur at common infusion targets used during deep propofol sedation [4].
- The swallowing reflex completely returns about 15 min after return of consciousness when propofol is used [5].
- The swallowing reflex is depressed for 2 h after return of consciousness following midazolam use during colonoscopy [6].
- Increased patient age and high BMI are additional risk factors for swallowing impairment with propofol [4].

Split-dose bowel preparation solutions may be given before colonoscopy. Better bowel preparation is obtained with split-dose regimens as long as the "runaway time" or time since the last dose of oral bowel preparation solution does not exceed 5 h [7].

- Patients receiving split-dose bowel preparation solutions have similar residual gastric volumes to patients that were given single dose solutions the night before examination [8].
- In most patients, a 2 h fasting period should be sufficient after the second dose of bowel preparation solution.

A thorough history will reveal conditions which may predispose the patient to gastric aspiration.

- Passive regurgitation with aspiration is a proposed mechanism during colonoscopy [9].
- Initial management of aspiration in a deeply sedated or completely anesthetized patient consists of aggressive suctioning in the head down position and possible tracheal intubation with suctioning prior to initiation of ventilation [10].
- In high risk patients, in addition to strict adherence to fasting guidelines, pharmacotherapy with proton pump inhibitors, H-2 blockers, antacids, and/or prokinetic agents may be warranted.
- Endotracheal intubation for airway protection in high risk patients may be indicated.

Difficult Mask Ventilation

- As depth of sedation increases, so does the likelihood of requirement of airway and ventilatory intervention.
- Screening patients for potential difficulty of mask ventilation cannot be underestimated.
- In patients with a difficult mask ventilation, the risk of difficult intubation may be increased four times [11].

Criteria for difficult mask ventilation are listed in Box 8.1 [11–13].

Box 8.1. Difficult Mask Ventilation Predictors

Age older than 55 years
BMI >26 kg/m^2
Lack of teeth
Presence of beard
History of snoring or sleep apnea
Mallampati III or IV
Limited mandibular protrusion
Male
Airway mass or tumor
Neck irradiation
Neck circumference >40 cm

- More than one predictor should raise the level of concern even more [11].
- Neck irradiation is the most significant predictor of impossible mask ventilation [13].
- Difficult mask ventilation in a pediatric patient is especially concerning due to limited amount of time to rescue the situation [12].

Patient Expectations of Sedation

- Many patients expect to be totally unconscious during colonoscopies and are unaware that they may be aware during parts of the procedure.
- Patients who have not received pre-procedural counseling about sedation or have never had a colonoscopy in the past are the most likely to have concern about awareness [14].
- In a survey of patients prior to colonoscopy, anxiety about awareness during the procedure was more concerning than respiratory complications, vomiting, incomplete colonic examination, and post-procedural drowsiness [14].
- A discussion about awareness during colonoscopy will improve patient expectations and satisfaction [14].

Intraoperative Management

Monitors

Patients should be monitored during colonoscopies according to the standards for basic anesthetic monitoring.

- Oxygenation should be assessed continuously with pulse oximetry and exposure of the patient to assess color.
- Ventilation should be evaluated by continuous end-tidal carbon dioxide analysis and other qualitative clinical signs which may include chest excursion and auscultation of breath sounds.
- Circulation is assessed with continuous display of the electrocardiogram/heart rate and blood pressure determination at least every 5 min.
- An EEG based monitor, including the bispectral index (BIS) or patient state index (PSI) monitor, may be helpful for determining depth of sedation. Although optional, use of these monitors may be beneficial in decreasing complications associated with deeper levels of sedation.
- Placement of monitoring devices should be simple. The patient is typically in the lateral decubitus position and access to the patient's airway should not be compromised by the endoscopist.

Depth of Sedation

Several factors must be considered when choosing depth of sedation for colonoscopies. Some of these factors are listed on Box 8.2.

Box 8.2. Depth of Sedation Considerations

Recall
Patient movement
Hypotension
Airway events
Aspiration
Difficult colonoscopy
Cognitive recovery

In a recent study, depth of sedation during colonoscopy with propofol and fentanyl was examined [15]. "Light" sedation was described as a bispectral index (BIS) of 70–80 and "deep" sedation was described as BIS of <60.

- Patients receiving deep sedation had lower levels of recall, less patient movement, more hypotension, and more airway obstruction.
- Patients with light sedation were still mostly satisfied despite a higher incidence of recall (12 % versus 1 %).
- Recovery was more rapid with light sedation although, at hospital discharge, cognitive impairment was similar in both groups [15].

Typically, propofol based sedation is associated with deeper levels of sedation than non-propofol based sedation [9].

- Deep sedation, as defined by the administration of propofol, is associated with an increased risk of aspiration, splenic injury, and colon perforation [2].
- Titrating propofol administration to EEG based readings can help providers reduce the amount of time that patients are under deeper levels of anesthesia during colonoscopies. This should lessen the risks associated with deeper levels of sedation (aspiration, hypotension, respiratory depression, etc.), while still being able to utilize the clinical benefits of propofol [9].

Traditional Agents

- A rapid, short acting benzodiazepine like midazolam is typically combined with a rapid, short acting opiate such as fentanyl.
- Midazolam is known to have anxiolytic, amnestic, and sedative properties. It is also a respiratory depressant.
- Benzodiazepines have synergetic effects with opiates that result in more profound sedation, respiratory depression, and hemodynamic compromise.
- Fentanyl and other opiates offer analgesic and sedative qualities.

- Fentanyl is known to cause respiratory depression and nausea, but like midazolam, a reversal agent is available.
- Meperidine and morphine have a slower onset and longer duration than fentanyl. This makes fentanyl a more appropriate choice for colonoscopy.

Propofol

- Propofol has been increasingly used for sedation during colonoscopy.
- A major advantage of propofol is its rapid onset and rapid offset.
- Propofol provides sedation and amnesia; however, minimal analgesia is provided.
- Shorter recovery times, return of cognitive function, and antiemetic properties are very useful.
- Unfortunately, there is not a reversal agent for propofol.
- Levels of consciousness may change rapidly during administration of propofol anesthesia.
- Unintentional deep sedation or even general anesthesia, with depression in respiratory, cardiovascular, and neurologic function, may result due to rapidly changing levels of consciousness. Thus, the availability of a qualified anesthesia provider is critical.
- Compared to traditional agents (benzodiazepines and narcotics), recovery and discharge times are shorter with propofol based anesthesia. Also, patient satisfaction is higher [16, 17].

Judicious use of midazolam and or fentanyl to supplement a propofol based colonoscopy is associated with better operating conditions and shorter procedure times [18].

- Recovery time, patient satisfaction, and recall are similar to patients receiving only propofol provided that small amounts of midazolam are given.
- Administration of more than 2 mg of midazolam may be predictive of impaired cognitive function at discharge when used to supplement propofol based sedation during colonoscopy [18].

Ketamine

- Ketamine can serve as an adjunct to sedation regimens during colonoscopy.
- Ketamine is known to have anesthetic and analgesic effects.
- Airway patency is maintained while ventilatory and cardiovascular effects are minimal with low doses.
- Addition of low-dose ketamine (0.3 mg/kg) to midazolam-fentanyl-propofol sedation has been shown to improve sedation, improve hemodynamics, reduce propofol consumption, and has less adverse effects, including reduced airway support maneuvers, in patients undergoing colonoscopy [19].

Remifentanil

- Remifentanil is an ultra-short acting opioid agonist.
- Remifentanil only anesthetics for colonoscopy have been shown to result in faster recovery, good patient satisfaction, and enhanced communication between patient and endoscopist when compared to standard midazolam-meperidine combinations [20, 21].
- Lower doses of remifentanil (0.4 mcg/kg loading dose and 0.04 mcg/kg/min infusion dose) may also reduce remifentanil cardio-respiratory side effects [21].
- Patients receiving remifentanil only anesthetics may be almost fully alert suggesting that additional sedation may be optional.

Dexmedetomidine

- Dexmedetomidine is a selective alpha-2 receptor agonist.
- It has anxiolytic, sedative and analgesic effects without significant respiratory depression.
- Its use has been associated with hypotension and bradycardia.
- Complex administration, cost, and hemodynamic instability has led some to see limited utility with dexmedetomidine during colonoscopy [22]. Others believe it may have some utility [23].

Nitrous Oxide

- Benefits of nitrous oxide include its analgesic effects and its short pharmacologic half-life.
- Other benefits include minimal cardio-respiratory depression compared to large doses of many intravenous agents.
- Systematic reviews have shown that N_2O/O_2 is equal to controlling pain and discomfort compared to conventional sedation during colonoscopy [24, 25]. Patients recover more quickly and have shorter hospital stays when nitrous oxide is used compared to traditional intravenous sedation and analgesia [24, 25].
- More rapid recovery and return of psychomotor function with nitrous oxide may improve patient throughput.

Volatile Anesthetics

- Sevoflurane combined with nitrous oxide is useful in the ambulatory setting due to rapid return of psychomotor function and enhanced readiness for discharge [26].

- A sevoflurane based anesthetic compared to a propofol based anesthetic may lead to fewer airway complications (apnea, airway interventions) in geriatric colonoscopies, while providing similar procedural conditions [27].

Difficult Colonoscopy

The difficult colonoscopy may be defined as not being able to reach the cecum, time required to complete the procedure, extent of patient discomfort, or the endoscopist's level of exertion. Some of the risk factors for difficult colonoscopy are listed on Box 8.3 [28–32].

Box 8.3. Risk Factors for Difficult Colonoscopy

Colon loops and angulations
Diverticular disease
Poor bowel preparation
Body habitus
Prior surgery
Female gender
Men with history of constipation or laxative use
Young patients

- Loops and angulations, particularly in the sigmoid colon, may be the most common source of difficulty.
  - Endoscopic control becomes difficult and can cause discomfort.
  - Adequate sedation is often required.
  - Successful cecal intubation may be proportionate to sedation level [32].
- Diverticular disease may cause the colon to be more spastic causing difficulties with insufflation and bowel preparation [30, 32].
- Poor bowel preparation makes visualization difficult.
- Obese body habitus can make it difficult to apply abdominal counter-pressure to minimize looping. However, lower body mass and diminished size of the abdominal cavity with reduced visceral fat may make it more difficult to fold the colon [29].
- Prior surgery, like abdominal hysterectomy, may also increase technical difficulty [28].
- The female colon, being longer and potentially more angulated as it traverses into the pelvis, can present difficulties [32].
- Men with a history of constipation or laxative use may have redundant colon making it more difficult to reach the cecum [31].
- Young patients may experience discomfort from stretching of the mesocolon which is tight [30].

Some maneuvers may help advancement of the endoscope:

- Changing patient position from the left lateral decubitus position to supine to right lateral to prone may aid in advancement of the scope. In this situation, it is important for the patient not to be overly sedated.
- Applying abdominal counter pressure can help.
- Instructing the patient to hold a deep breath will lower the diaphragm and potentially aid in advancing the scope past a colonic flexure [32].
- Variable-stiffness scopes may help the endoscopist.
- Propofol sedation, which is often deep, has been shown to increase axial and radial forces during scope advancement and withdrawal and decrease examination time [33]. Endoscopists are able to push through loops and angulations in the colon with deep propofol sedation much more easily.

Complications

- Sedation, colon distention, and mesenteric stretching can cause hypoxia, hypoventilation, arrhythmias, hemodynamic compromise, abdominal discomfort, and vasovagal reactions.

While deeper levels of sedation more easily allow the endoscopist to complete the colonoscopy, it can lead to other complications like aspiration pnuemonitis and pneumonia.

- Splenic injury may occur more often in deeply sedated patients due to increased patient toleration to loops in the colonoscope which stress colonic to splenic attachments [2].
- Colonic perforation may occur from 0.6/1000 to 0.9/1000 colonoscopies [34, 35]. Deeper sedation may predispose to an increased incidence of perforations as patients are unable to show discomfort associated with the scope being advanced against resistance [36].

Author's Technique

A general goal of lessening the time in deep sedation will help reduce risks of aspiration, hypoxia, hypoventilation, and endoscopic trauma. Patients should be counseled about awareness during colonoscopy. A propofol based sedation plan allows rapid titration as needed to facilitate advancement of the endoscope through difficult colonic loops and angulations. This should also allow for lightening of sedation during less difficult portions and during colonoscope withdrawal. Judicious use of midazolam and fentanyl may be used to supplement propofol based sedation. Ketamine, ideally at lower doses, is a helpful adjunct for difficult to sedate patients and those with high analgesic requirements. Inhaled anesthetics and intravenous agents requiring complex administration are probably better left for rare situations.

References

1. American Society of Anesthesiologists; Quality Management and Departmental Administration. Continuum of depth of sedation: definition of general anesthesia and levels of sedation/analgesia [Internet]. 2014 [updated 2014 Oct 15; cited 2016 Jan 5]. Available from: http://www.asahq.org/~/media/Sites/ASAHQ/Files/Public/Resources/standards-guidelines/continuum-of-depth-of-sedation-definition-of-general-anesthesia-and-levels-of-sedation-analgesia.pdf.
2. Cooper GS, Kou TD, Rex DK. Complications following colonoscopy with anesthesia assistance: a population-based analysis. JAMA Int Med. 2013;173(7):551–6. doi:10.1001/jamainternmed.2013.2908.
3. Agostoni M, Fanti L, Gemma M, Pasculli N, Beretta L, Testoni PA. Adverse events during monitored anesthesia care for GI endoscopy: an 8-year experience. Gastrointest Endosc. 2011;74(2):266–75. doi:10.1016/j.gie.2011.04.028.
4. Marco G, Laura P, Alessandro O, Massimo A, Francesca P, Barbara R, et al. Swallowing impairment during propofol target-controlled infusion. Anesth Analg. 2015. doi:10.1213/ane.0000000000000796.
5. Rimaniol JM, D'Honneur G, Duvaldestin P. Recovery of the swallowing reflex after propofol anesthesia. Anesth Analg. 1994;79(5):856–9.
6. D'Honneur G, Rimaniol JM, el Sayed A, Lambert Y, Duvaldestin P. Midazolam/propofol but not propofol alone reversibly depress the swallowing reflex. Acta Anaesthesiol Scand. 1994;38(3):244–7.
7. Bucci C, Rotondano G, Hassan C, Rea M, Bianco MA, Cipolletta L, et al. Optimal bowel cleansing for colonoscopy: split the dose! A series of meta-analyses of controlled studies. Gastrointest Endosc. 2014;80(4):566–76.e2. doi:10.1016/j.gie.2014.05.320.
8. Huffman M, Unger RZ, Thatikonda C, Amstutz S, Rex DK. Split-dose bowel preparation for colonoscopy and residual gastric fluid volume: an observational study. Gastrointest Endosc. 2010;72(3):516–22. doi:10.1016/j.gie.2010.03.1125.
9. Goudra B, Singh PM, Gouda G, Borle A, Carlin A, Yadwad A. Propofol and non-propofol based sedation for outpatient colonoscopy-prospective comparison of depth of sedation using an EEG based SEDLine monitor. J Clin Monit Comput. 2015. doi:10.1007/s10877-015-9769-5.
10. Engelhardt T, Webster NR. Pulmonary aspiration of gastric contents in anaesthesia. Br J Anaesth. 1999;83(3):453–60.
11. Langeron O, Masso E, Huraux C, Guggiari M, Bianchi A, Coriat P, et al. Prediction of difficult mask ventilation. Anesthesiology. 2000;92(5):1229–36.
12. El-Orbany M, Woehlck HJ. Difficult mask ventilation. Anesth Analg. 2009;109(6):1870–80. doi:10.1213/ANE.0b013e3181b5881c.
13. Kheterpal S, Martin L, Shanks AM, Tremper KK. Prediction and outcomes of impossible mask ventilation: a review of 50,000 anesthetics. Anesthesiology. 2009;110(4):891–7. doi:10.1097/ALN.0b013e31819b5b87.
14. Chatman N, Sutherland JR, van der Zwan R, Abraham N. A survey of patient understanding and expectations of sedation/anaesthesia for colonoscopy. Anaesth Intensive Care. 2013;41(3):369–73.
15. Allen M, Leslie K, Hebbard G, Jones I, Mettho T, Maruff P. A randomized controlled trial of light versus deep propofol sedation for elective outpatient colonoscopy: recall, procedural conditions, and recovery. Can J Anaesth. 2015;62(11):1169–78. doi:10.1007/s12630-015-0463-3.
16. McQuaid KR, Laine L. A systematic review and meta-analysis of randomized, controlled trials of moderate sedation for routine endoscopic procedures. Gastrointest Endosc. 2008;67(6):910–23. doi:10.1016/j.gie.2007.12.046.
17. Singh H, Poluha W, Cheung M, Choptain N, Baron KI, Taback SP. Propofol for sedation during colonoscopy. Cochrane Database Syst Rev. 2008;(4):Cd006268. doi:10.1002/14651858.CD006268.pub2.

18. Padmanabhan U, Leslie K, Eer AS, Maruff P, Silbert BS. Early cognitive impairment after sedation for colonoscopy: the effect of adding midazolam and/or fentanyl to propofol. Anesth Analg. 2009;109(5):1448–55. doi:10.1213/ane.0b013e3181a6ad31.

19. Tuncali B, Pekcan YO, Celebi A, Zeyneloglu P. Addition of low-dose ketamine to midazolam-fentanyl-propofol-based sedation for colonoscopy: a randomized, double-blind, controlled trial. J Clin Anesth. 2015;27(4):301–6. doi:10.1016/j.jclinane.2015.03.017.

20. Manolaraki MM, Theodoropoulou A, Stroumpos C, Vardas E, Oustamanolakis P, Gritzali A, et al. Remifentanil compared with midazolam and pethidine sedation during colonoscopy: a prospective, randomized study. Dig Dis Sci. 2008;53(1):34–40. doi:10.1007/s10620-007-9818-0.

21. Hong MJ, Sung IK, Lee SP, Cheon BK, Kang H, Kim TY. Randomized comparison of recovery time after use of remifentanil alone versus midazolam and meperidine for colonoscopy anesthesia. Dig Endosc Off J Jpn Gastroenterol Endosc Soc. 2015;27(1):113–20. doi:10.1111/den.12383.

22. Jalowiecki P, Rudner R, Gonciarz M, Kawecki P, Petelenz M, Dziurdzik P. Sole use of dexmedetomidine has limited utility for conscious sedation during outpatient colonoscopy. Anesthesiology. 2005;103(2):269–73.

23. Dere K, Sucullu I, Budak ET, Yeyen S, Filiz AI, Ozkan S, et al. A comparison of dexmedetomidine versus midazolam for sedation, pain and hemodynamic control, during colonoscopy under conscious sedation. Eur J Anaesthesiol. 2010;27(7):648–52. doi:10.1097/EJA.0b013e3283347bfe.

24. Welchman S, Cochrane S, Minto G, Lewis S. Systematic review: the use of nitrous oxide gas for lower gastrointestinal endoscopy. Aliment Pharmacol Ther. 2010;32(3):324–33. doi:10.1111/j.1365-2036.2010.04359.x.

25. Aboumarzouk OM, Agarwal T, Syed Nong Chek SA, Milewski PJ, Nelson RL. Nitrous oxide for colonoscopy. Cochrane Database Syst Rev. 2011;(8):Cd008506. doi:10.1002/14651858. CD008506.pub2.

26. Theodorou T, Hales P, Gillespie P, Robertson B. Total intravenous versus inhalational anaesthesia for colonoscopy: a prospective study of clinical recovery and psychomotor function. Anaesth Intensive Care. 2001;29(2):124–36.

27. Syaed El Ahl MI. Modified sevoflurane-based sedation technique versus propofol sedation technique: a randomized-controlled study. Saudi J Anaesth. 2015;9(1):19–22. doi:10.4103/1658-354x.146265.

28. Cirocco WC, Rusin LC. Factors that predict incomplete colonoscopy. Dis Colon Rectum. 1995;38(9):964–8.

29. Anderson JC, Gonzalez JD, Messina CR, Pollack BJ. Factors that predict incomplete colonoscopy: thinner is not always better. Am J Gastroenterol. 2000;95(10):2784–7. doi:10.1111/j.1572-0241.2000.03186.x.

30. Waye JD. Completing colonoscopy. Am J Gastroenterol. 2000;95(10):2681–2. doi:10.1111/j.1572-0241.2000.03172.x.

31. Anderson JC, Messina CR, Cohn W, Gottfried E, Ingber S, Bernstein G, et al. Factors predictive of difficult colonoscopy. Gastrointest Endosc. 2001;54(5):558–62.

32. Witte TN, Enns R. The difficult colonoscopy. Can J Gastroenterol. 2007;21(8):487–90.

33. Korman LY, Haddad NG, Metz DC, Brandt LJ, Benjamin SB, Lazerow SK, et al. Effect of propofol anesthesia on force application during colonoscopy. Gastrointest Endosc. 2014;79(4):657–62. doi:10.1016/j.gie.2013.12.002.

34. Levin TR, Zhao W, Conell C, Seeff LC, Manninen DL, Shapiro JA, et al. Complications of colonoscopy in an integrated health care delivery system. Ann Intern Med. 2006;145(12): 880–6.

35. Ko CW, Riffle S, Michaels L, Morris C, Holub J, Shapiro JA, et al. Serious complications within 30 days of screening and surveillance colonoscopy are uncommon. Clin Gastroenterol Hepatol Off Clin Pract J Am Gastroenterol Assoc. 2010;8(2):166–73. doi:10.1016/j.cgh.2009.10.007.

36. Adeyemo A, Bannazadeh M, Riggs T, Shellnut J, Barkel D, Wasvary H. Does sedation type affect colonoscopy perforation rates? Dis Colon Rectum. 2014;57(1):110–4. doi:10.1097/dcr.0000000000000002.

Chapter 9
Anesthesia for ERCP

Rajiv R. Doshi and Mary Ann Vann

Abstract Anesthesia for endoscopic retrograde cholangiopancreatography (ERCP) continues to challenge even the most experienced anesthesiologist. The need for patient comfort and optimal procedural conditions has changed the anesthesia for these procedures from conscious sedation to deep sedation or even general anesthesia. The ongoing debate about deep sedation versus general anesthesia is dependent on a number of variables including severity of patient illness, availability of space and ancillary personnel, and positioning needs of the patient. A detailed discussion of the assessment and medical optimization of the patient, positioning of the patient, and utilization of anesthetic agents and airway adjuncts will aid the anesthesia provider to deliver a safe and comfortable anesthetic.

Keywords ERCP • Endoscopic retrograde cholangiopancreatography • Deep sedation • Monitored anesthesia care • General anesthesia • Capnography • Propofol • Prone position • Aspiration • Obstructive sleep apnea

Introduction

- Endoscopic retrograde cholangiopancreatography (ERCP) is a complex and invasive endoscopic procedure requiring highly specialized equipment and instrumentation combined with live fluoroscopic imaging.
- ERCP has been integral in the treatment of disorders of the pancreaticobiliary tree, sometimes supplanting to the need for surgical intervention.
- While diagnostic ERCP has primarily been replaced with better noninvasive radiologic imaging, therapeutic ERCP indications continue to increase in number. Additionally, with better training and significant advances in technology, therapeutic procedures can be offered to patients that are sicker and with more complex anatomy. Patients with biliary sepsis present for urgent therapeutic ERCP to relieve obstructions and drain infected material.

R.R. Doshi, MD (✉) • M.A. Vann, MD
Department of Anesthesia, Critical Care, and Pain Medicine, Beth Israel Deaconess
Medical Center, 330 Brookline Ave, Boston, MA 02215, USA
e-mail: mavann@earthlink.net

© Springer International Publishing Switzerland 2017   113
B.G. Goudra, P.M. Singh (eds.), *Out of Operating Room Anesthesia*,
DOI 10.1007/978-3-319-39150-2_9

- The need for patient comfort while maximizing patient safety and optimizing procedural conditions for ERCP success has made anesthetic considerations critical to the success of these complex procedures.
- Current indications for ERCP fall into three broad categories [1]:

  - Stone disease (jaundice, biliary pain, cholangitis, biliary pancreatitis, pancreatic duct stones)
  - Ampullary/papillary abnormalities (Sphincter of Oddi dysfunction (SOD), ampullary cancer)
  - Biliary and pancreatic ductal abnormalities (leaks, strictures, malignancies)

- It is important to discuss the unique space constraint issues and patient positioning issues prior to determining the suitability of delivering an anesthetic to a patient undergoing ERCP procedures.

Specific Procedural Issues Unique to ERCP Procedures

ERCP Procedure Room Layout

- Most ERCP procedures in high volume centers are performed in dedicated fluoroscopic procedure rooms with a compact layout. Anesthesia providers are positioned at the patient's head.
- ERCP procedures in low-volume centers may be performed in a radiology suite or in the operating room using a portable C-arm fluoroscopy machine.
- Rooms are compact but must accommodate the one or two endoscopists, a technician, 1–2 nurses, and an anesthesia provider. Additionally, the rooms have fixed radiographic equipment and video imaging equipment. Anesthesia personnel usually have an anesthesia machine as well as an anesthesia cart. ERCP equipment is stored in the procedure room; mobile units are rolled into procedure rooms that contain low-use equipment needed for procedures.
- Space constraints with personnel and equipment need to be taken into account prior to administration of any anesthetic as removal of additional personnel or equipment may be required for further intervention.

Positioning for ERCP

- ERCP can be performed in three positions: prone (most common), supine, and left lateral decubitus.

ERCP: Prone Position

- This is the most common position for ERCP since it allows the endoscopist optimal visualization and access to anatomical structures.

- Contraindications for prone position for ERCP include significant aspiration risk, advanced pregnancy, tense ascites, severe immobilizing cervical spine disease, and critically ill patients who cannot be turned prone due to lines/infusions/ongoing treatments. Patients who have marginal cardiopulmonary status are also not appropriate candidates for the prone position.
- Prone positioning in conscious patients requires a cooperative patient who can lie on their abdomen for at least 5–10 min until adequate sedation is achieved.
- Frail, elderly patients may have limited mobility and may require significant assistance to achieve the correct position. Additionally, arthritic changes in the cervical spine may make turning of the head difficult to facilitate passage of the endoscope. Pressure and skin injuries are also more common in frail elderly patients, so extra care must be taken in moving and positioning.
- Post-cholecystectomy patients or patients with any intervention of the anterior abdomen (e.g. percutaneous transhepatic biliary drain) may require analgesia prior to positioning.
- Anesthesia providers should ensure IV lines are not inadvertently displaced during movement and positioning. If analgesia or sedation is administered prior to movement, monitoring should be initiated prior to transfer. There should be minimal interruption of monitoring after assuming the prone position.

ERCP: Supine Position

- Reserved for patients who are critically ill where position changes may lead to unacceptable changes in ventilation or cardiovascular status. Patients who are actively vomiting, known gastric outlet obstruction (physical or functional), and patients at high aspiration risk have their procedure performed in the supine position (e.g. active severe pancreatitis).
- Patients with cervical spine disorders, altered airway anatomy, or patients at high risk for airway obstruction may benefit from the supine position.
- Facilities performing general anesthesia for ERCP will often maintain their patients in the supine position to secure the airway.
- Advanced pregnancy and patients with increased intra-abdominal pressure due to pathology (tumor, ascites) may benefit from the supine with left lateral tilt position to prevent aortocaval compression.

ERCP: Left Lateral Decubitus Position

- This position is only possible in rooms where the fluoroscope can be rotated to obtain anterior-posterior views.
- This is a potential alternative position for patients who cannot or will not assume the prone position.
- Endoscopists may find this position less favorable in terms of visualizing the ampulla and cannulating the bile ducts. The literature does not seem to support this finding in deeply sedated patients [2].

Focused History and Physical Findings in Patients Presenting for ERCP

Introduction

- Prior to anesthesia consultation, the endoscopist has evaluated the patient and has deemed the patient a candidate for ERCP. The endoscopist needs to determine the case urgency based in patient's clinical condition (semi-elective, urgent, emergent).
- A complete and uninterrupted assessment of the patient should occur prior to administration of anesthesia by an appropriate anesthesia provider. Ideally, the person performing the anesthetic should perform the preanesthetic assessment.
- The patient's height and weight and body mass index should be obtained. Morbid obesity presents a multitude of management difficulties for both the anesthesia provider and the endoscopist.
- Previous medication allergy history and specifically iodinated contrast allergy should be obtained.
- A current list of medications should be obtained prior to initiation of the procedure. If patient is an inpatient, a current home medication list is also important. Many patients are on antiplatelet agents, direct thrombin inhibitors, or oral or intravenous anticoagulants that can lead to excessive bleeding with specific ERCP procedures.
- Previous procedural/surgical history and issues with anesthesia should be obtained. Any history of difficult mask airway or intubation should be clarified and previous records should be obtained. This is especially true for patients with history of sleep apnea.
- Patients with family members with anesthetic histories suggestive of malignant hyperthermia or prolonged neuromuscular blockade with succinylcholine should be identified.
- The patient's current cardiopulmonary status and current medical conditions should be obtained and documented.
- Organ system dysfunction related to the hepatic or pancreaticobiliary systems should be fully characterized with imaging and appropriate laboratory values.
- Patients with serious organ system dysfunction may have concomitant bleeding disorders. Patients on anticoagulants/antiplatelet drugs should be identified. If sphincterotomy or biopsy is planned, timely assessment of coagulation or platelet function should be conducted prior to such intervention.
- Family history, social history and review of systems should be obtained. Patients with chronic opioid abuse or significant opioid use secondary to pain management should be identified, as there can be difficulty in sedating these patients appropriately.

Pathophysiologic Considerations (by Organ System) Prior to ERCP

Gastrointestinal

- A previous history of intestinal diversion surgery (e.g. Roux-en-Y gastric bypass or gastrojejunostomy) can potentially prolong an otherwise routine ERCP and necessitate alterations in the anesthetic plan. Tumor burden, especially if extending to the gastric outlet or within the abdomen increasing intra-abdominal pressure may place the patient at high risk for aspiration.
- Significant liver dysfunction may increase the risk of variceal bleeding on insertion of the ERCP scope. Additionally, large-volume ascites without paracentesis significantly increases risk of aspiration due to increased intra-abdominal pressure.

Cardiac

- Patients with uncontrolled hypertension or unexplained hypotension should be evaluated and treated prior to ERCP if possible. Adjustments to chronic cardiac medications may need to occur due to malabsorption and/or hypoalbuminemia from the current disease process.
- Older patients undergoing ERCP may have a history of myocardial infarction with cardiac stents requiring potent antiplatelet agents that can cause significant bleeding during ERCP, particularly sphincterotomy. The most commonly used agents are clopidogrel, prasugrel, and ticagrelor. These agents should be discontinued only after direct interaction with a cardiology specialist; ERCP procedures can be performed without discontinuation but must be discussed in advanced with all team members.
- Congestive heart failure can present acutely or as an acute exacerbation of a chronic condition. Acute decompensated heart failure should be treated aggressively prior to ERCP. Patients with significant oxygen requirements from chronic CHF may require general and mechanical ventilation.
- Cardiac arrhythmias, particularly atrial fibrillation, usually require systemic anticoagulation. Discontinuation of anticoagulation must be done under the direction of the prescribing physician (outpatient) or medical service (inpatient). Bridging anticoagulation should be performed by the prescribing physician in consultation with the patient's cardiologist. Laboratory values to ensure no residual anticoagulation should be performed prior to ERCP.
- Anesthetic management of patients with implantable cardiac devices such as permanent pacemakers, automated implantable cardiac defibrillators, and cardiac resynchronization therapy devices should be managed per local, national, and international guidelines [3]. Patients with left ventricular assist devices

(LVAD) that require ERCP intervention should be managed by cardiac anesthesiologists or anesthesiologists familiar with these devices in consultation with cardiac anesthesia. If cardiac anesthesiologists are not available, these patients should be transferred to facilities where cardiac anesthesiologists or heart failure support can be obtained.

Pulmonary

- Patients on supplemental oxygen at home may require higher oxygen supplementation during sedation for ERCP. Additionally, they may also be candidates for intubation and general anesthesia in order to maintain proper oxygenation.
- A history of obstructive sleep apnea can make deep sedation more difficult in patients in the prone position. Risk scoring scales such as STOP-BANG scoring system can identify patients at higher risk of adverse events during ERCP procedures [4]. Risk factors include age >50 years, body mass Index >35 kg/m^2, male gender, neck circumference >40 cm, hypertension, and history of snoring, tiredness/sleepiness, and observed apneas [5].

Hematologic/Oncologic

- Severe liver dysfunction can impair coagulation factor synthesis and increase bleeding risk during ERCP. Moderate pancreatitis that has required fluid resuscitation may cause mild to moderate derangements in coagulation. Pancreatitis patients or patients with cholangitis may develop renal dysfunction which may lead to acute uremia and qualitative platelet dysfunction, further impairing coagulation.
- Dosage and administration of oral or intravenous anticoagulants, antiplatelet agents, and direct thrombin inhibitors need to be confirmed prior to proceeding with ERCP.

Neurologic

- A history of dementia or delirium related to the patient's current medical conditions might make informed consent difficult or even impossible. Depressed or altered sensorium may place the patient at higher risk for aspiration and may necessitate utilization of general anesthesia

Orthopedic

- Frail, elderly patients are at higher risk for injury due to degenerative arthritis and osteoporosis. Patients may not be able to move themselves and moving them inappropriately may lead to injury. Arthritis of the neck may make oral cannulation difficult or even impossible in the prone position due to limited neck mobility.
- Identification of hardware/scarring of the lower extremity is important for avoidance of placement of the dispersive pad for the electrosurgical unit required for sphincterotomy.

Endocrine

- Patients with diabetes are at higher risk for cardiovascular complications. Hyperglycemia can occur in patients with pancreatic disorders due to injury to beta cells and decreased insulin production.
- Non-diabetic patients who are bacteremic or septic may have glucose dysregulation and may be hyper- or hypoglycemic.

Gynecologic

- If patient suspects pregnancy, this should be investigated promptly prior to procedure initiation.

Physical Examination

- An assessment of baseline neurologic function and level of consciousness is mandatory prior to proceeding with anesthesia for ERCP.
- Vitals signs should be checked and recorded including measurements of blood pressure, heart rate, respiratory rate, and oxygen saturation in the presence and absence (if possible) of supplemental oxygen. Blood glucose should also be checked.
- A directed physical examination based on the patient's known active medical issues should be performed before the procedure.

  - Physical examination of the heart and lungs

    - Bronchospasm should be treated with beta-agonists prior to the procedure
    - The cause of rales on examination should be aggressively pursued prior to procedure (e.g. cardiac or non-cardiac causes)

- Evidence of a consolidative process (pneumonia) warrants a discussion of risk/benefit of proceeding versus delaying procedure after initiating treatment for the consolidative process.
- Significant cardiac abnormalities on exam such as the presence of a new systolic or diastolic murmur require further investigation.

- A complete airway examination should be performed with documentation of the patient's Mallampati score. This should be performed in conjunction with assessment for risk factors for obstructive sleep apnea. Additionally, patency of the nares is important in case placement of a nasopharyngeal airway is necessary.

  - Airway examination

    - High Mallampati scores may be associated with difficult mask ventilation as well as difficult intubation if general anesthesia is required.
    - If neck movement is limited or restricted secondary to other disease processes or arthritis, consideration of other positions should be entertained.
    - It is important to identify oral abnormalities (e.g. macroglossia, high arched palate), dysmorphic facial features, and jaw abnormalities (e.g. micrognathia) that may contribute to ventilation difficulties during sedation or difficult securing the airway for general anesthesia.

- All patients should have a physical inspection for stigmata of liver dysfunction (e.g., icteric sclera, asterixis) and presence of significant or occult bruising.
- The abdomen should be inspected for dressings (from recent surgeries), drains, stomas, and the presence of tense ascites.

Is the Patient in an Optimum State to Proceed with Anesthesia?

- Minimum required fasting times should be strictly adhered to prior to ERCP. Current American Society of Anesthesiologists recommendations for preoperative fasting are a minimum of 6 hours after a light meal in healthy patients [6]. Patients may benefit from appropriate intravenous repletion of fluids lost while fasting.
- Preoperative tests should only be ordered to for "(1) discovery or identification of a disease or disorder that may affect perioperative anesthetic care; (2) verification or assessment of an already known disease, disorder, medical or alternative therapy that may affect perioperative anesthetic care; and (3) formulation of specific plans and alternatives for perioperative anesthetic care." [7]

  - Patients undergoing ERCP will have complete blood counts including platelet count, coagulation studies, and pancreas and liver function tests prior to arrival to the procedural area (if not, they should be obtained prior to the procedure).

- Pregnancy tests should be obtained in high-risk patients of childbearing age or if there is any question of pregnancy.
- Electrocardiograms (ECG) are not mandatory in patients undergoing low-risk cardiac procedures such as ERCP. However, ECG and other studies may be warranted based on the patient's previous cardiac history and should be obtained prior to the procedure.
- Chest radiographs should be reviewed for occult lung pathology that may affect anesthetic management, such as consolidation, excessive atelectasis, fluid overload, or cardiomegaly.
- If the patient is pregnant, specialists in maternal fetal medicine should be involved prior to ERCP initiation to determine best plan of care as well as need for preprocedure, intraprocedure, and/or postprocedure fetal monitoring.
- Preprocedural administration of antibiotics is usually required prior to instrumentation or cannulation of the common bile duct. Fluoroquinolones are commonly used but determination of the appropriate prophylactic antibiotic regimen should be made by the endoscopist and checked against the patient's allergies prior to administration.
- All patients should have an American Society of Anesthesiologist Physical Status classification assigned prior to anesthetic administration. Sedation related complications are higher in patients with an ASA physical status classification of 3 or higher [8].

Commonly Used Anesthesia Techniques

General Anesthesia Versus Monitored Anesthesia Care

- While conscious sedation can be performed on select patients undergoing ERCP, a recent study shows that 1/3 to 1/2 of patients experience discomfort and pain during and after the ERCP procedure [9]. Risk factors for pain during and after the procedure included age <45, suboptimal quality of life scores, and the need for therapeutic ERCP [9]. A Cochrane systematic review of conscious sedation versus deep sedation/general anesthesia reported no significant differences in cardiac or respiratory complications with an overall better recovery profile with propofol (deep sedation) [10].
- There is ongoing debate regarding the utilization of general anesthesia versus the administration of deep sedation/monitored anesthesia care for ERCP.
- High volume academic centers that perform ERCPs safely utilize monitored anesthesia care for these procedures, especially for healthy, non-obese patients. In a retrospective observation study from a high-volume ERCP center, 89.7% patients had ERCPs performed with monitored anesthesia care with only 3.7% of cases being converted to a general anesthetic [11]. No serious (irreversible) complications occurred during the study period. Other groups have reported even better success without need to convert to general anesthesia and endotracheal intubation [12].

- General anesthesia for ERCP procedures is most commonly described with endotracheal intubation. However, there are reports in the literature of placement of laryngeal mask airway without airway complications and without significant difficultly in performing the ERCP procedure [13].
- Data from ERCPs performed at three community hospitals (n = 650) suggested a tendency toward general anesthesia with a statistically lower risk of cardiopulmonary complications in the general anesthesia group [14]. Complications included hypoxia (requiring either non-invasive positive pressure ventilation or intubation) and arrhythmias.
- The decision to perform monitored anesthesia care versus general anesthesia is based on number of factors including:
  - Preference of the anesthesia group to perform general anesthesia versus sedation. Factors such as shared airway, increased risk of aspiration, and duration of procedure are active considerations.
  - Skill level of individual endoscopist and total number of ERCPs performed in the institution
  - Space/layout constraints in the event of cardiac or pulmonary complications necessitating further intervention (e.g. intubation or advanced cardiac life support). Some procedure rooms are too small to move patient on the ERCP bed and need to be flipped supine to another bed.

Monitoring

- Standard American Society of Anesthesiologists standards for monitoring include: non-invasive blood pressure at least every 5 min, continuous oxygen saturation, electrocardiogram, quantitative capnography, and available temperature monitoring for patients undergoing monitored anesthesia care or general anesthesia.
- Supplemental oxygen is administered with nasal prongs or specialized oxygen delivery devices designed for ERCP. There are various masks and bite blocks that have built-in ports for supplemental oxygen delivery and end-tidal carbon dioxide monitoring while allowing for passage of the endoscope. Additionally, wall oxygen can be attached via small suction catheters and bent in a fishhook shape and placed between the labial commissure and the oral bite block.
- For monitored anesthesia care, capnography sampling ports are built into the nasal cannula allowing for real-time monitoring.
- A recent study with healthy patients in the supine position suggests that nasal cannula where oxygen delivery is through one prong and capnography is via the other prong may be the best at delivery of high concentrations of oxygen and sampling of carbon dioxide [15]. This has not been validated in patients undergoing procedures in the prone position or patients undergoing ERCP.

- Many anesthesia providers have noted that there is significant sampling difficulty of end-tidal carbon dioxide during ERCP that may require multiple adjustments of the nasal cannula. Additionally, the accuracy of end tidal capnography monitoring is diminished in GI locations that utilize carbon dioxide as the insufflating gas. There may be excessively high levels of exhaled carbon dioxide detected due to passive efflux from the GI tract and inadvertent rebreathing.
- Level of consciousness should be documented during the administration of monitored anesthesia care. Depth of anesthesia monitors may be useful in the management of patients that may have a history of difficulty with sedation in the past.

Single Drug Regimens Versus Combination Drug Regimens

- Propofol is the single most commonly used drug in the performance of monitored anesthesia care for ERCP.
- Propofol has a rapid onset of action for sedation (30–60 s), short duration of effect (4–8 min), and relative stable pharmacokinetics in patients with renal dysfunction or moderate liver dysfunction [16].
- Propofol monotherapy appeared to be no different in terms of sedation safety, procedural outcomes, and complications as compared with balanced propofol sedation (propofol with midazolam and fentanyl administered at the beginning of the anesthetic) [17]. There was a slight decrease in recovery time in the propofol monotherapy group.
- At least 2 studies with propofol monotherapy as their primary anesthetic demonstrated more procedural and postprocedural pain [16, 18].
- Some groups have utilized non-opioid adjuncts to improve analgesia without utilizing opioids. Ketamine in low doses (10–30 mg) decreases the total amount of propofol required for maintenance and provides supplemental analgesia without additional respiratory depression. Addition of ketamine to propofol/remifentanil combinations avoided deep sedation, found improved analgesia and decreased nausea and vomiting postprocedure [19].
- Dexmedetomidine, an intravenous selective alpha2-adrenergic agonist, provides sedation without respiratory depression. The utility of dexmedetomidine for ERCP is has shown mixed results. One study has shown it to be inferior in terms of sedation quality to propofol or propofol/adjunct medication regimens [20] while another study finds it to be superior to propofol/ketamine in terms of recovery time and hemodynamic stability [21]. Addition of dexmedetomidine to various sedation regimens may prolong recovery times [22].
- The use of antisialogogues to minimize secretions in the mouth particularly in the prone/semi-prone position may be useful during management of the oropharynx during these procedures.
- Many groups utilize topical anesthetics to decrease the discomfort and stimulation of endoscope placement. This is usual and routine practice for upper endoscopic procedures under conscious sedation in the United States. Lidocaine

gargle and sprays as well as benzocaine topical spray have been used. There is a risk of methemoglobinemia with benzocaine spray.

Anticipated Adverse Events

- ERCP-related adverse events can be defined as either procedure specific complications related to therapeutic maneuvers performed during the ERCP and general complications.
- Procedure specific complications include pancreatitis, bleeding, perforation, and cholangitis/infection and are classified as mild, moderate, or severe based on the degree of physiologic perturbation or degree of intervention required to restore normal physiologic function [23]. Anesthesia providers should be in constant communication with the endoscopist and prepare for physiologic perturbations due to these issues, which may even require abrupt cessation of the procedure to treat.
- General complications related to anesthesia encompass sedation related issues such as airway obstruction with oxygen desaturation and oversedation.
- Patients undergoing upper endoscopy procedures including ERCP are at risk of aspiration and laryngospasm.
- Pulmonary complications are primarily sedation related and include respiratory depression, airway obstruction, hypoxia, and pulmonary aspiration. Cardiovascular complications may include hypertension and hypotension, cardiac arrhythmias, and myocardial ischemia/infarction [24].
- Data from the American Society of Anesthesiologists Closed Claims Database from 1990 and later identified respiratory events and specifically inadequate oxygenation and ventilation as the most common remote location malpractice claim [24]. Note that 15 % of claims had capnography and 15 % had no documented respiratory monitoring; additional respiratory events included esophageal intubation, difficult intubation and aspiration of gastric contents [24]. This data was obtained prior to routine use of capnography.
- Contributing factors to the risk of complications are ASA physical status >3, obesity, and age greater than 70 years [8, 25].
- Retrospective database analysis of 11,497 ERCPs over 12 years found severe or fatal complications associated with the following variables: severe and incapacitating systemic disease, obesity, known or suspected bile-duct stones, pancreatic manometry, and complex (grade 3) procedures [23].
- Sedation related adverse events in a cohort of 799 patients undergoing advanced upper endoscopic procedures revealed hypoxemia as the most common adverse event, with 14.4 % requiring an airway maneuver (chin lift, modified mask, or nasal airway) [26]. No patients required endotracheal intubation. Other issues included hypotension and oversedation.

Prevention and Management of Adverse Events

Management

- Timing of emergent interventions is crucial. Proper training of all procedural and periprocedural staff is necessary prior to emergency events so that roles and responsibilities are well defined. Additionally, simulated emergencies also identify deficiencies in crisis management, such as the location of emergency equipment and drugs.
- Management of sedation related complications is about preempting the most common problems before they become concerning or critical.

Respiratory Depression

- Respiratory depression due to sedation medications is the most common event. Propofol has a narrow therapeutic window and can lead to airway obstruction relatively quickly. Use of opioids during ERCP depresses frequency of respirations and is synergistic with propofol and benzodiazepines.
- Deep sedation mandates the use of quantitative capnography; progressive increases in the value of exhaled end-tidal carbon dioxide may suggest hypoventilation. Ensure that carbon dioxide is not the insufflating gas prior to this determination, as carbon dioxide from the upper GI tract can contaminate the carbon dioxide sampling port of the nasal cannula.
- Supplemental oxygen is almost always required for cases involving deep sedation. Patients who receive supplemental oxygen and subsequently hypoventilate will have delayed oxygen desaturation; any drop in oxygen saturation during deep sedation should be addressed quickly. Airway maneuvers such as chin lift or jaw thrust may be required to "stimulate" the patient; occasionally, mask ventilation or airway instrumentation may be needed.

Airway Obstruction

- Identification of patients at high risk for airway obstruction should be identified prior to the procedure, and backup airway plans and equipment for a response should be available.
- Hypoventilation due to airway obstruction is difficult to detect in the presence of supplemental oxygen. Quantitative capnography is useful and recommended in this setting. Abrupt decreases in amplitude or absence of end-tidal carbon dioxide waveform is highly suggestive of airway obstruction.

- Most airway obstruction occurs due to the tongue, and can be relieved with chin lift or jaw thrust maneuvers. Many endoscopy bite blocks cause the tongue to be pushed back obstructing the airway. New endoscopic bite blocks resembling an oral airway have been designed to alleviate this problem.
- For patients at higher risk for obstruction (obesity, OSA, high ASA physical status classification), continuous positive airway pressure can be performed. An anesthesia group at a tertiary academic medical center utilizes nasopharyngeal trumpets attached via an endotracheal tube connector to the anesthesia circuit to provide continuous positive pressure to patients at high risk for upper airway obstruction. This can also be utilized in patients where an abrupt decrease in oxygen or ventilation may have disastrous consequences [27]
- Laryngospasm, or acute glottis closure, can happen for a multitude of reasons during ERCP [28]. It can occur during placement of endoscope, particularly if the vocal cords are irritated or if secretions reach the vocal cords. Additionally, patient specific factors, such as asthma, reflux, and Parkinson's places the patient at higher risk. Treatment is by prompt recognition of obstruction by capnography, discontinuation of the procedure, and supportive airway management usually requiring jaw thrust and bag-mask ventilation. Concomitant administration of propofol (30–50 mg) and if necessary, low dose succinylcholine (10–20 mg) during airway maneuvers is useful to break the laryngospasm. Endotracheal intubation can be performed if necessary.

Pulmonary Aspiration

- The most common risk factors for aspiration identified in upper endoscopy include [29]:
  - Increased risk of vomiting (gastric outlet obstruction, gastric stasis, fluids/chyme incidentally found after placement of endoscope)
  - Elderly patients
  - Patients receiving topical anesthetic for ease of endoscopic cannulation
  - Outpatients or inpatients who violated established preprocedure fasting (NPO) guidelines

- Procedures that may release proteinaceous material into the intestinal lumen and potentially become aspirated should be considered for endotracheal intubation outright, such as draining of pancreatic pseudocysts [28].
- Subclinical aspiration may be considered when patient coughs and retches continuously. This usually occurs within the initial few minutes of the procedure during the cannulation attempts (which may as a result of or exacerbated by light anesthesia). Deepening sedation can occasionally resolve this issue but may require conversion to general anesthesia. Other methods include using opioids (fentanyl 25 µg) or ketamine (10–20 mg) 3–5 min prior to blunt stimulation from endoscope cannulation and decrease subsequent airway

secretions. Some anesthesia providers also pretreat patients with an antisialo-gogue (glycopyrrolate 0.2–0.4 mg given slowly at least 5–15 min prior to the procedure).

Cardiac Complications

- Hypotension during ERCP is most commonly caused by the vasodilating effects of anesthetic agents coupled with volume depletion, either from oral intake restriction or from intercurrent illness such as sepsis. Appropriate hydration based on the patient's acute and chronic medical needs is appropriate. Additionally, small doses of vasopressors [phenylephrine (50–100 μg) or ephedrine (5–10 mg)]. Alternatively, combination anesthetics (propofol with opioid or ketamine) may reduce the overall hypotensive effect of any one anesthetic agent.
- Hypertension during ERCP may be from light anesthesia, pain, and stimulation during portions of the procedure. Using adjunctive analgesics (fentanyl, ketamine) either as needed (PRN) or as an infusion in combination with propofol (remifentanil infusion 0.1 mcg/kg/min or less) may attenuate the stress response and control hypertensive episodes.
- Cardiac arrhythmias should be monitored closely. Non-malignant cardiac arrhythmias should not be treated if they do not result in hypotension.
- If hemodynamically unstable arrhythmias occur in the middle of a complicated ERCP, vasopressor support may be indicated until such time the procedure can be completed or aborted. Patients with new onset arrhythmias should have electrolytes checked and should also be monitored for developing bacteremia/septicemia.
- Bradycardia can occur during esophageal endoscopic intubation and may be treated by removal of the scope and pre-emptive treatment with glycopyrrolate 0.2 mg IV.
- Tachycardia should be aggressively treated in patients with pre-existent cardiac disease or valvular abnormalities where fast heart rates are detrimental (e.g. aortic stenosis).
- Individuals with history of angina pectoris or at-risk myocardium as determined by nuclear/pharmacologic stress testing should be identified prior to ERCP. Avoidance of hypoxemia and maintenance of blood pressure is key to optimal management. New ST segment elevations/depressions or T-wave inversions should be reason to terminate the procedure as soon as possible.

Other Adverse Events

- Allergic reactions can occur with antibiotic administration and with administration of intraluminal contrast media. There is a low incidence of reactions to contrast media used during ERCP. Treatment of contrast reactions (anaphylactoid)

should be similar to recommendations for anaphylactic reactions (airway, epinephrine, fluids) as per the American College of Radiology [30].
- Symptomatic treatment for nausea and vomiting may be treated with a serotonin 5-HT$_3$ receptor antagonists in the recovery period.

Preferred Technique

- Identify risk factors for hypoxemia and airway obstruction, and identify relevant organ dysfunction that may impact care (cardiac, pulmonary disease, active vomiting) or response to sedative drugs.
- Obtain relevant physical exam including full airway examination and auscultation of heart and lung fields.
- Obtain informed consent from patient (ideally) or patient's power of attorney.
- Younger patients (age <40), ASA I or II patients, patients with chronic anxiety or psychiatric disorders, patients with current substance abuse, and patients on chronic opioid therapy may benefit from preoperative anxiolysis with an intravenous benzodiazepine (midazolam 1–2 mg IV) prior to initiation of the procedure. After prone positioning, procedural sedation would consist of moderate dose intravenous propofol infusion 100–150 mcg/kg/min. Rate of sedation can be increased with cautious low dose boluses of propofol (20–30 mg every 1–2 min) until no response to oral suctioning. Adjuncts to enhance propofol sedation include administration of lidocaine 40–100 mg, ketamine 10–30 mg or fentanyl 25–50 µg.
- Frail, elderly patients sedation regimens would consist of lower dose intravenous propofol infusion 80–100 mcg/kg/min with or without bolus administration. These patients may require significant assistance and attention to pressure or skin injury during positioning prior to sedation. They may also benefit from topical oropharyngeal anesthesia (benzocaine spray or lidocaine spray/gargle) to prevent stimulation and tachycardia/hypertension that may occur from passage of the endoscope.
- Well-lubricated nasopharyngeal trumpets are especially useful when placed early in patients at high risk for airway compromise, such as obstructive sleep apnea patients and morbidly obese patients.
- Even in centers that usually provide monitored anesthesia care for ERCP, it is common to intubate morbidly obese patients or those with recent abdominal surgery, for optimal patient safety and comfort.
- Given the high volume of ERCPs performed at our institution and frequent use of monitored anesthesia care, we do not routinely use depth of anesthesia monitors. However, for other centers undertaking a new practice of monitored anesthesia care for ERCP procedures, depth of anesthesia monitors may allow for better overall titration of medications.
- General anesthesia with endotracheal intubation is reserved for patients with airway anomalies, a high risk of aspiration, or need for deeper anesthesia for

comfort during the procedure (e.g. recent abdominal surgery). Airway adjuncts (aforementioned nasopharyngeal airway connected to anesthesia circuit, nasopharyngeal airway alone) may be used in patients with higher Mallampati scores, severe sleep apnea, or morbid obesity.

References

1. Kim JK, Carr-Locke DL. Indications for ERCP. In: ERCP and EUS. New York: Springer; 2015. p. 19–35.
2. Mashal B, Edwyn Harrison M, Ananya D, Rodney E, Michael C. Optimal positioning for ERCP: efficacy and safety of ERCP in prone versus left lateral decubitus position. ISRN Endoscopy. 2013;2013, Article ID 810269:6. doi:10.5402/2013/810269.
3. Crossley GH, Poole JE, Rozner MA, Asirvatham SJ, Cheng A, Chung MK, et al. The Heart Rhythm Society (HRS)/American Society of Anesthesiologists (ASA) Expert Consensus Statement on the perioperative management of patients with implantable defibrillators, pacemakers and arrhythmia monitors: facilities and patient management this document was developed as a joint project with the American Society of Anesthesiologists (ASA), and in collaboration with the American Heart Association (AHA), and the Society of Thoracic Surgeons (STS). Heart Rhythm. Elsevier. 2011;8(7):1114–54.
4. Coté GA, Hovis CE, Hovis RM, Waldbaum L, Early DS, Edmundowicz SA, et al. A screening instrument for sleep apnea predicts airway maneuvers in patients undergoing advanced endoscopic procedures. Clin Gastroenterol Hepatol. 2010;8(8):660–1. Elsevier.
5. Chung F, Yegneswaran B, Liao P, Chung SA, Vairavanathan S, Islam S, et al. STOP questionnaire: a tool to screen patients for obstructive sleep apnea. Anesthesiology: Am Soc Anesthesiol. 2008;108(5):812–21.
6. Apfelbaum JL, et al. Practice guidelines for preoperative fasting and the use of pharmacologic agents to reduce the risk of pulmonary aspiration: application to healthy patients undergoing elective procedures. Anesthesiology. 2011;114(3):495–511.
7. Apfelbaum JL, Connis RT, Nickinovich DG, Pasternak LR, Arens JF, Caplan RA, et al. Practice advisory for preanesthesia evaluation: an updated report by the American Society of Anesthesiologists Task Force on Preanesthesia Evaluation. Anesthesiology. 2012;116(3):522–38.
8. Frieling T, Heise J, Kreysel C, Kuhlen R, Schepke M. Sedation-associated complications in endoscopy – prospective multicentre survey of 191142 patients. Z Gastroenterol. 2013;51(6): 568–72.
9. Jeurnink SM, Steyerberg EW, Kuipers EJ, Siersema PD. The burden of endoscopic retrograde cholangiopancreatography (ERCP) performed with the patient under conscious sedation. Surg Endosc. 2012;26(8):2213–9.
10. Garewal D, Powell S, Milan SJ, Nordmeyer J, Waikar P. Sedative techniques for endoscopic retrograde cholangiopancreatography. Cochrane Database Syst Rev. 2012;(6):CD007274.
11. Barnett SR, Berzin T, Sanaka S, Pleskow D, Sawhney M, Chuttani R. Deep sedation without intubation for ERCP is appropriate in healthier, non-obese patients. Dig Dis Sci. 2013;58(11): 3287–92.
12. Goudra B, Singh P, Sinha A. Outpatient endoscopic retrograde cholangiopancreatography: safety and efficacy of anesthetic management with a natural airway in 653 consecutive procedures. Saudi J Anaesth. 2013;7(3):259–65.
13. Osborn IP, Cohen J, Soper RJ, Roth LA. Laryngeal mask airway--a novel method of airway protection during ERCP: comparison with endotracheal intubation. Gastrointest Endosc. 2002;56(1):122–8.
14. Sorser S, Fan D, Tommolino E, Gamara R, Cox K, Chortkoff B, et al. Complications of ERCP in patients undergoing general anesthesia versus MAC. Dig Dis Sci. 2014;59(3):696–7. Springer US.

15. Ebert TJ, Novalija J, Uhrich TD, Barney JA. The effectiveness of oxygen delivery and reliability of carbon dioxide waveforms: a crossover comparison of 4 nasal cannulae. Anesth Analg. 2015;120(2):342–8.

16. Lichtenstein DR, Jagannath S, Baron TH, Anderson MA, Banerjee S, Dominitz JA, et al. Sedation and anesthesia in GI endoscopy. Gastrointest Endosc. 2008;68(2):205–16.

17. Lee TH, Lee CK, Park S-H, Lee S-H, Chung I-K, Choi HJ, et al. Balanced propofol sedation versus propofol monosedation in therapeutic pancreaticobiliary endoscopic procedures. Dig Dis Sci. 2012;57(8):2113–21. Springer US.

18. Haytural C, Aydinli B, Demir B, Bozkurt E, Parlak E, Dişibeyaz S, et al. Comparison of propofol, propofol-remifentanil, and propofol-fentanyl administrations with each other used for the sedation of patients to undergo ERCP. BioMed Res Int. 2015;2015:465.

19. Fabbri LP, Nucera M, Marsili M, Malyan Al M, Becchi C. Ketamine, propofol and low dose remifentanil versus propofol and remifentanil for ERCP outside the operating room: is ketamine not only a "rescue drug'? Med Sci Monit. 2012;18(9):CR575–80.

20. Muller S, Borowics SM, Fortis EAF, Stefani LC, Soares G, Maguilnik I, et al. Clinical efficacy of dexmedetomidine alone is less than propofol for conscious sedation during ERCP. Gastrointest Endosc. 2008;67(4):651–9.

21. Abdalla MW, El Shal SM, El Sombaty AI, Abdalla NM, Zeedan RB. Propofol dexmedetomidine versus propofol ketamine for anesthesia of endoscopic retrograde cholangiopancreatography (ERCP) (A randomized comparative study). Egypt J Anaesth. 2015;31(2):97–105.

22. Goyal R, Hasnain S, Mittal S, Shreevastava S. A randomized, controlled trial to compare the efficacy and safety profile of a dexmedetomidine-ketamine combination with a propofol-fentanyl combination for ERCP. Gastrointest Endosc. 2016;83(5):928–33.

23. Cotton PB, Lehman G, Vennes J, et al. Endoscopic sphincterotomy complications and their management: an attempt at consensus. Gastrointest Endosc. 1991;37:383–93.

24. Metzner J, Domino KB. Risks of anesthesia care in remote locations. Anesthesia Patient Safety Foundation Newsletter [Internet]. 2011 Spring-Summer [cited 2015 Nov 24]. Available from: http://www.apsf.org/newsletters/html/2011/spring/06_remotelocation.htm.

25. Metzner J, Posner KL, Domino KB. The risk and safety of anesthesia at remote locations: the US closed claims analysis. Curr Opin Anaesthesiol. 2009;22(4):502–8.

26. Coté GA, Hovis RM, Ansstas MA, Waldbaum L, Azar RR, Early DS, et al. Incidence of sedation-related complications with propofol use during advanced endoscopic procedures. Clin Gastroenterol Hepatol. 2010;8(2):137–42.

27. Goudra B, Singh PM. ERCP: the unresolved question of endotracheal intubation. Dig Dis Sci. 2013;59(3):513–9.

28. Gavel G, Walker RW. Laryngospasm in anaesthesia. Continuing education in anaesthesia, critical care & pain. Oxford University Press. 2013;14(2):mkt031–51.

29. Green J. Guidelines on complications of gastrointestinal endoscopy. British Society of Gastroenterology [Internet]. British Society of Gastroenterology; Guidelines Index 2006 [accessed 02 Dec 2015]. Available from: http://www.bsg.org.uk/images/stories/docs/clinical/guidelines/endoscopy/complications.pdf.

30. ACR manual on contrast media. Version 9, 2013 [Internet] Reston, VA: American College of Radiology, ACR Committee on Drugs and Contrast Media; c2015. [cited 2015 Dec 1]. Available from: http://www.acr.org/~/media/37D84428BF1D4E1B9A3A2918DA9E27A3.pdf.

Chapter 10
Anesthesia for Bronchoscopy

Mona Sarkiss

Abstract

- Diagnostic flexible bronchoscopic procedures, such as airway exam, bronchoalveolar lavage, and Transbronchial biopsies (TBBX), are commonly performed under moderate sedation (Wahidi et al., Chest 140(5):1342–1350, 2011).
- Advanced diagnostic bronchoscopic procedure, namely Endobronchial ultrasound fine needle aspiration (EBUS-FNA), can be performed under moderate sedation or general anesthesia. The choice of anesthesia technique is based on the patient's tolerance, co-morbidities, expected duration of the procedure, and the skills of bronchoscopist (Casal et al., Am J Respir Crit Care Med 191(7):796–803, 2015).
- Therapeutic bronchoscopic procedures such as debulking of central airway tumors, management of hemoptysis, and stenting of the central airway are generally performed through the rigid bronchoscope under general anesthesia. Minor therapeutic procedures can be performed through the flexible bronchoscope under moderate sedation (Sarkiss, Curr Opin Pulm Med 17(4):274–278, 2011).

Keywords Flexible bronchoscopy • Rigid bronchoscopy • Endobronchial ultrasound • Jet ventilation • Total intravenous anesthesia • Laryngeal mask airway

Introduction

- Diagnostic flexible bronchoscopic procedures, such as airway exam, bronchoalveolar lavage, and Transbronchial biopsies (TBBX), are commonly performed under moderate sedation [1].
- Advanced diagnostic bronchoscopic procedure, namely Endobronchial ultrasound fine needle aspiration (EBUS-FNA), can be performed under moderate sedation or general anesthesia. The choice of anesthesia technique is based on

M. Sarkiss, MD, PhD
Department of Anesthesiology and Perioperative Medicine, University of Texas MD Anderson Cancer Center, 1400 Holcombe Blvd. Unit 409, Houston, TX 77030, USA
e-mail: msarkiss@mdanderson.org

© Springer International Publishing Switzerland 2017
B.G. Goudra, P.M. Singh (eds.), *Out of Operating Room Anesthesia*,
DOI 10.1007/978-3-319-39150-2_10

the patient's tolerance, co-morbidities, expected duration of the procedure, and the skills of bronchoscopist [2].

- Therapeutic bronchoscopic procedures such as debulking of central airway tumors, management of hemoptysis, and stenting of the central airway are generally performed through the rigid bronchoscope under general anesthesia. Minor therapeutic procedures can be performed through the flexible bronchoscope under moderate sedation [3].

Focused History and Physical Findings in Patients Presenting for the Procedure

Upper Airway Assessment

Irrespective of the anesthesia technique planned for the bronchoscopic procedure a thorough examination of the upper airway is essential for the determination of

- The ability of the patient to maintain an adequate airway while under moderate or deep sedation
- The ease of endotracheal intubation and similarly the insertion of the rigid bronchoscope if need
- The ease of insertion of Laryngeal Mask Airway (LMA) and the likelihood of achieving an adequate seal around the glottic opening and ventilation.

Factors that should alert the anesthesiologist and the bronchoscopist to possible difficulties with airway adequacy and control during the procedure are

- History of obstructive sleep apnea
- High mallampati airway class
- Short thyromental distance and small chin indicating anterior larynx view with direct laryngoscopy
- Upper airway changes secondary to external beam irradiation

  - Edema
  - Fibrosis
  - Poor laryngeal mobility and/or loss of laryngeal click
  - Limited mouth opening
  - Known glottic, supraglottic or infraglottic tumor.

Pulmonary Co-morbidities

Reviewing and understanding the location and ventilatory effects of the airway pathology at hand, is essential for both the anesthesiologist and the bronchoscopist. Computed Tomography (CT) images, Pulmonary function testing and flow volume loops are fundamental for planning the most suitable type of anesthesia, airway device and mode of ventilation to utilize during a particular airway procedure e.g.,

- Patients with high FiO$_2$ requirement necessitating the use of supplemental oxygen
- Patients with reactive, obstructive or restrictive airway disease
- Upper airway pathology e.g. edema and/or space occupying lesions
- Upper and mid tracheal pathology
- Tumors with ball valve effect
- Tumors and/or infections known to cause airway bleeding

Cardiac Co-morbidities

Cardiac and circulatory co-morbidities can be related or unrelated to the pulmonary pathology.

- Pulmonary and/or mediastinal tumors abutting the heart and major vessels may cause direct mechanical effect or secondary effects on the patient's hemodynamics due to hypoxemia and hypercarbia.
- Cardiac arrhythmias such as atrial fibrillation, premature atrial beats, premature ventricular beats, supraventricular tachycardia and malignant ventricular tachycardia has been reported in patients with various pulmonary pathology.
- Compressive and obstructive effect of the mediastinal pathology on the inflow and outflow of the cardiac chambers e.g., SVC syndrome, pulmonary veins occlusion, pulmonary artery thrombi and emboli, pericardial effusion, and pericardial tamponade.
- Pulmonary hypertension and core pulmonale related to restrictive and obstructive pulmonary disease respectively
- Appropriate choice of anesthesia technique, monitoring devices, and medications to support the circulatory system during the procedure is essential.

Laboratory Testing

Baseline laboratory testing can reflect the effects of the underlying pulmonary pathology as well as guide the anesthesiologist in formulation of the anesthesia plan.

CBC

- Elevated white cell count could reflect and underlying pulmonary infection or the concurrent intake of steroids for the management of COPD or autoimmune pulmonary diseases.
- Acute anemia can be due to hemoptysis and reflects the amount of blood lost.

- Thrombocytopenia especially in the setting of hemoptysis and/or lung biopsies should alert the anesthesiologist to order a type and screen and have packed RBCs and/or platelet available for transfusion in case of emergency bleeding during a bronchoscopic procedure

Electrolytes

- Hyponatremia can be associated with para- malignant syndrome encountered in patients with lung cancer
- Hyperkalemia should alert the anesthesiologist to avoid the use of succinylcholine as a muscle relaxant.
- Elevated bicarbonate levels may be related to carbon dioxide retention secondary to obstructive sleep apnea or other ventilator pathology.

Coagulation Studies

- Simple bronchoscopic procedures such as flexible bronchoscopy for airway exam and broncho-alveolar lavage can be safely performed in patients with coagulopathy.
- Procedures involving biopsy of airway pathology, mediastinal lymphadenopathy and lung parenchymal lesions or rigid bronchoscopy for management of central airway tumor and hemoptysis might necessitate a baseline coagulation studies and correction of the coagulopathy in order to perform the procedure safely.

Renal and Hepatic Function

Baseline renal and liver function testing can be beneficial in the selection of anesthesia medications based on the drug metabolism and clearance

Type and Screen

Although massive bleeding is rarely encountered in patients undergoing bronchoscopic procedures, a type and screen is considered judicious in patients undergoing rigid bronchoscopy for central airway tumor debulking and/or hemoptysis management.

Is the Patient in an Optimum State to Proceed with Anesthesia?

Bronchoscopic procedures are generally considered an urgent procedure to diagnose and/or manage airway or lung pathology.

- The common indications for diagnostic flexible bronchoscopy are
  - Airway exam for detection of airway pathology such as space occupying lesions, infections and source of hemoptysis.
  - Broncho-alveolar Lavage (BAL) to obtain washings from the distal airway to detect bacterial and viral infections and obtain samples for microbiology cultures
  - Transbronchial Biopsies (TBBx) is a blind technique where a needle is inserted through the wall of the tracheobronchial tree to obtain a fine needle aspirate from the lung parenchyma. TBBx is commonly used to diagnose infectious, malignant or autoimmune pathologies of the lung.
- Advanced diagnostic bronchoscopy or Endobronchial Ultrasound Guided fine needle aspiration of mediastinal lymph nodes (EBUS-FNA) can also be considered an urgent procedure where the staging of the mediastinum is essential to formulate the patient's treatment plan. Additionally, EBUS-FNA is used for diagnosis of mediastinal lymphadenopathy of unknown etiology
- Rigid bronchoscopic procedures are frequently emergent and urgent procedures to manage airway obstruction and/or hemoptysis.

Due to the urgent or emergent nature of bronchoscopic procedures patient optimization might not be considered a first priority. However an in depth understanding of the patient's airway pathology is necessary for safe anesthetic management.

Commonly Used Anesthesia Techniques Including Monitoring with References

In a consensus statement published by the American College of Chest Physicians in 2011, the use of topical anesthesia, analgesia and sedation was suggested in all patients undergoing bronchoscopic procedures. This statement was based on the current literature that advocates the safety of topical anesthesia, analgesia and sedation when the appropriate agent for the appropriate patient has been selected.

Topical Anesthesia

- Topical anesthesia is used to reduce coughing and discomfort during bronchoscopy.
- Lidocaine is the most commonly used agent. The maximum dose of Lidocaine when sprayed in the airway is 8.2 mg/Kg. Dose reduction is recommended in patients with impaired liver function and old age [4].
- The use of other agents such as cocaine, Benzocaine or tetracaine is discouraged due to known side effects of addiction in the case of cocaine and higher incidence of methemoglobinemia with tetracaine and benzocaine.

- Topical anesthetics can be sprayed or applied directly in the airway before and during bronchoscopy. Additionally, transcricoid, transtracheal injections or laryngeal nerve blocks can be used [1].

Moderate Sedation

A single agent or different drug combinations have been studied and proved to be both safe and effective in reducing discomfort, anxiety and coughing during bronchoscopic procedures [1, 3]. The most commonly used agents are benzodiazepines, opioids, propofol, antihistamine and anti-cholinergic drugs

- *Midazolam* is the most commonly used benzodiazepine due to its rapid onset of action, rapid peak effect short duration. Midazolam has been associated with prolonged recovery time but without an increase in complication rates. Adverse effects of Benzodiazepine are easily reversed with Flumazenil.
- *Fentanyl* similar to Midazolam is a preferred drug for sedation during bronchoscopy due to its rapid onset of action, rapid peak effect and short duration. Fentanyl is commonly used in combination with Midazolam due to their synergistic effect and the additional cough suppressant effect of Fentanyl [5]. Respiratory depression associated with the use of opioids can be easily reversed with Naloxone.
- *Propofol* has the same mechanism of action as benzodiazepine with the added advantage of ultra-short onset time, rapid peak and rapid elimination and recovery time [6]. Propofol can be used alone or in combination with other sedative agents.
- *Anticholinergic agents* such as Atropine and glycopyrrolate have the theoretical advantage of reducing airway secretions but were proven to confer no advantage of improved lung functions or decreased secretions during bronchoscopy. The AACP consensus statement has advised against their routine use during bronchoscopy [1].

General Anesthesia

Indications

- General anesthesia is the technique of choice for rigid bronchoscopy and for prolonged procedure or when patient intolerance to the procedure is expected.
- Patient intolerance to the procedure performed under sedation can be due to anxiety, high oxygen requirement, severe airway pathology with high grade airway obstruction and/or hemoptysis

Techniques

Total intravenous anesthesia with ultra-short acting medications is the technique of choice [7].

- Commonly used medications are propofol, ketamine, remifentanil and dexmedetomidine.
- Care should be taken with the use of muscle relaxants. Muscle weakness and paralysis reduce coughing and motion and thus facilitating the accuracy and ease of airway manipulation during the procedure [3].
- Muscle paralysis should be avoided in patients with airway fistulas to the mediastinum or its structures and when positive pressure ventilation is not feasible due to central airway obstruction [3].

Airway Devices

- Moderate sedation can be performed while oxygen is delivered via nasal cannula and high flow oxygen as needed. Face mask e.g., POM face mask with a modification to allow for the insertion of the bronchoscope can be used for patients with higher FiO2 requirement. Additionally, non-invasive positive pressure NIPP nasal or face mask with special adaptor for the insertion of the bronchoscope can be used in patients with sleep apnea [8].
- General anesthesia necessitates the presence of an airway devise such as LMA or endotracheal tube (ETT). The LMA has the advantage of being placed above the central airway allowing for complete airway inspection and free mobility of the bronchoscope in the central airway
- The rigid bronchoscope is the most suitable airway device for therapeutic bronchoscopy where airway obstruction, bleeding and/or compression can be safely managed.

Modes of Ventilation Under General Anesthesia

- Spontaneous Ventilation as described before is necessary in patients with airway fistula where positive pressure ventilation can lead to air leak causing pneumo-mediastinum, pneumothorax and pneumo-peritonium. Spontaneous ventilation can be achieved through LMA, ETT or rigid bronchoscope. For the rigid bronchoscopy supplemental 100% oxygen can be administered passively thorough the side port of the rigid bronchoscope to allow for delivery of a higher FiO_2
- Controlled ventilation whether volume cycled or pressure cycled can be used based on the underlying lung pathology. When LMA is utilized, care should be taken to set airway pressure limit between 20 and 25 Cm H_2O in order to avoid leak around the device. Controlled ventilation through the rigid bronchoscope requires packing of the mouth and occlusion of the nostril to reduce leak.

- Jet Ventilation is the ideal mode of ventilation during rigid bronchoscopy [9, 10]. Care should be taken to keep the side ports of the rigid bronchoscope open to air in order to avoid barotrauma secondary to air trapping.

Monitoring

- Standard monitors such as electrocardiogram, pulse oximeter and blood pressure monitoring is mandatory for all cases.
- Additional monitoring are available such as Bispectral index monitoring to titrate the depth of anesthesia especially with the TIVA technique [11]. Non-invasive and invasive arterial and hemodynamic monitoring can be vital when the airway pathology is affecting the circulatory system e.g., massive hemoptysis, SVC syndrome.

Anticipated Adverse Events

Airway Reactivity

Causes

Airway reactivity or bronchospasm can be encountered in patients with predisposing factors undergoing any bronchoscopic procedure e.g.

- History of bronchial asthma or reactive airway disease
- Respiratory infections
- COPD exacerbation
- Airway irritation secondary to bleeding manipulation of the airway by the bronchoscope or other instruments.

Management

- Intra-procedural nebulization or inhalation of β- agonists e.g., Albuterol
- Utilization of inhalation agents e.g., Sevoflurane

Airway Bleeding

Causes

- Preexisting bleeding source such as central or distal airway tumor, infection or bronchiectasis

- Iatrogenic bleeding related to
  - Biopsy of central airway lesions,
  - Transbronchial lung biopsy (TBBx),
  - Biopsy of mediastinal lymph nodes either blind or ultrasound guided
  - Tumor debulking during rigid bronchoscopy.

Management

Airway bleeding should be managed promptly and its management is based on the location and the severity of the bleeding.

- Superficial or mild to moderate bleeding can be managed with topical instillation of cold saline, diluted epinephrine, tranexamic acid or thrombin in the airway
- Anticipated larger volume of bleeding threating to cause flooding of the airway and hypoxemia is best managed with the rigid bronchoscopy inserted in the airway. Different techniques can be used
  - Direct compression and tamponade by the rigid bronchoscopy
  - Argon Plasma Coagulation (APC), LASER or electrocautery

Additionally, tools for lung isolation such as bronchial blockers and double lumen tubes should be readily available and appropriately utilized as a temporizing measure while surgical management is arranged.

Hypoxemia

Hypoxemia during bronchoscopic procedures can be defined as oxygen saturation <90% for more than 1 min. However, other definitions have been quoted in research articles. Even though hypoxemia is considered an infrequent encounter during bronchoscopy, its cause should be sought and managed appropriately.

Causes

Common causes of hypoxemia during bronchoscopy are

- Baseline oxygen dependence
- Frequent suctioning
- Low FiO_2 needed during APC, electrocautery and LASER
- Airway bleeding
- Bronchospasm
- Airway obstruction by tumor, bleeding or instruments used for the procedure.

Management

- Treat the cause
- Increase oxygen flow through nasal cannula
- Increase FiO_2 delivered by using face mask, non-rebreather, non-invasive BIPAP or CPAP mask.
- Persistent hypoxemia unresponsive to increasing oxygen flow and FiO_2 delivered warrants intubation with LMA or ETT where 100% FiO_2 can be reliably delivered to the patient.

Hypercapnia

Hypercarbia and Hypercapnia are not reliably detected during bronchoscopy unless the patient has an airway device with CO_2 monitoring in place e.g., ETT, LMA. The effect of hypercapnia can be noted in increased somnolence, tachycardia and hypertension.

Causes

- Baseline due pulmonary pathology such as COPD, PE, or airway obstruction
- Deep sedation with respiratory depressant medications
- Hypoventilation
- Airway obstruction during the procedure with large bronchoscope (EBUS bronchoscope external diameter of 6.2 mm) and/or other instruments.

Management

- Pre-procedure optimization of the patient's pulmonary co-morbidities e.g. inhaled bronchodilator therapy, steroids.
- Utilizing ultra-short acting anesthetics and sedative in order to have minimal to no residual respiratory depression post procedure e.g., propofol, reminfentanil.
- Most patients with an airway device in place can tolerate hypercapnia during bronchoscopy. However care must be taken to reverse the hypercapnia pharmacologically or by hyperventilation before the patient is discharged.
- Hypercapnia in patients without airway device in place may be due to airway obstruction and/or apnea. In such instance pharmacologic reversal of the sedatives and/or insertion of an airway device such as LMA or ETT is necessary to treat the hypercarbia.

Airway Obstruction

Causes

- External compression by benign or malignant space occupying lesions e.g., anterior mediastinal mass
- Internal growth in the central airway
- Blood clots, mucous plugs, fungal infection

Management

Airway obstruction is managed by the interventional bronchoscopists but it imposes several challenges to the anesthesiologists.

- Selections of the airway device: LMA is preferred for airway examination for upper and mid tracheal lesions in order to avoid obscuring and/or traumatizing the lesion.
- The rigid bronchoscope is an ideal device when the central airway is compressed by external mass as it is able to stent the central airway lumen open facilitating ventilation.
- Large obstructing lesions of the trachea and main bronchi pose a risk of air trapping behind the mass due to ball-valve effect. If the air trapping is disregarded or went unnoticed, hemodynamic instability can ensue due to increased intrathoracic pressure and impediment of the venous return. Increasing the I:E ratio in patients managed with positive pressure ventilation can reduce the risk of air trapping as it allows longer time for the passive exhalation.

Authors Preferred Technique and the Justification

The authors preferred anesthesia technique for bronchoscopic procedures is the use of Total Intravenous Anesthesia (TIVA) (Table 10.1). Compared to inhalation anesthesia, TIVA guarantees an adequate delivery of the anesthetic irrespective of the changes in the upper and lower airway occurring during the procedure e.g.

- Frequent suctioning of airway secretion, blood and saline washes can alter the concentration of inhalation anesthetic dose delivered to the patient.
- Frequent changes in airway devices used during a procedure, e.g., LMA, rigid bronchoscopy, endotracheal tube (ETT), can lead to interruption in the delivery of inhalation anesthetic and varying depth of anesthesia while the airway device is being exchanged.
- Multiple insertion and removal of the bronchoscope through an airway device during a procedure can lead to leak of the inhalation agent to the environment of the bronchoscopy suite and exposure of the healthcare worker to anesthetic agents.

Table 10.1 A table to summarize the important aspects of anesthetic management

Medication	Short acting or ultra-short acting anesthetics in order to avoid post procedure depression of respiratory function e.g., Propofol, Remifentanil
Anesthesia technique	TIVA in most cases. Inhalation anesthesia in patients with reactive airway
Ventilation	High FiO_2 to maintain adequate saturation, expect and manage Hypercabnia, FiO_2 reduction during LASER and cautery in the airway
Monitoring	Standard. BIS monitor for the depth of TIVA. Consider invasive or non-invasive hemodynamic monitoring for rigid bronchoscopy cases
Airway devices	LMA, rigid bronchoscope and less frequently ETT
Recovery	30–45 min with the use of ultra-short acting anesthetic medications

However, it is important to note that in the event of bronchospasm during bronchoscopic procedures, inhalation agents are considered a potent bronchodilator and the benefits of its use might outweigh the risks.

The authors preferred airway device for bronchoscopic procedures is the LMA and the rigid bronchoscopy.

- The LMA allows for a complete inspection of the central airway as compared to the ETT. An appropriately placed ETT obscures the upper airway down to the mid-trachea.
- LMA insertion avoid trauma to upper and mid tracheal lesions that can occur with ETT insertion.
- Endotracheal intubation can be performed easily through the LMA if needed
- The large barrel of the rigid bronchoscope allows the bronchoscopist to use a wider variety of instrument to manage the airway pathology.
- The rigid bronchoscope can be used to manage complications that are anticipated during bronchoscopic procedures e.g., tamponade tracheal and bronchial bleeding and coring of tumors obstruction the central airways.

References

1. Wahidi MM, et al. American College of Chest Physicians consensus statement on the use of topical anesthesia, analgesia, and sedation during flexible bronchoscopy in adult patients. Chest. 2011;140(5):1342–50.
2. Casal RF, et al. Randomized trial of endobronchial ultrasound-guided transbronchial needle aspiration under general anesthesia versus moderate sedation. Am J Respir Crit Care Med. 2015;191(7):796–803.
3. Sarkiss M. Anesthesia for bronchoscopy and interventional pulmonology: from moderate sedation to jet ventilation. Curr Opin Pulm Med. 2011;17(4):274–8.
4. British Thoracic Society Bronchoscopy Guidelines Committee, a.S.o.S.o.C.C.o.B.T.S. British Thoracic Society guidelines on diagnostic flexible bronchoscopy. Thorax. 2001;56(Suppl 1): i1–21.
5. Fox BD, et al. Benzodiazepine and opioid sedation attenuate the sympathetic response to fiberoptic bronchoscopy. Prophylactic labetalol gave no additional benefit. Results of a randomized double-blind placebo-controlled study. Respir Med. 2008;102(7):978–83.

6. Clark G, et al. Titrated sedation with propofol or midazolam for flexible bronchoscopy: a randomised trial. Eur Respir J. 2009;34(6):1277–83.
7. Purugganan RV. Intravenous anesthesia for thoracic procedures. Curr Opin Anaesthesiol. 2008;21(1):1–7.
8. Clouzeau B, et al. Fiberoptic bronchoscopy under noninvasive ventilation and propofol target-controlled infusion in hypoxemic patients. Intensive Care Med. 2011;37(12):1969–75.
9. Kraincuk P, et al. A new prototype of an electronic jet-ventilator and its humidification system. Crit Care. 1999;3(4):101–10.
10. Fernandez-Bustamante A, et al. High-frequency jet ventilation in interventional bronchoscopy: factors with predictive value on high-frequency jet ventilation complications. J Clin Anesth. 2006;18(5):349–56.
11. Bruhn J, et al. Depth of anaesthesia monitoring: what's available, what's validated and what's next? Br J Anaesth. 2006;97(1):85–94.

Chapter 11
Airway Devices in GI Endoscopy

Basavana Goudra and Preet Mohinder Singh

Abstract This chapter discusses the currently available airway management options in the management of patients undergoing upper gastrointestinal (GI) under deep sedation. Some of the devices are approved by the Food and Drug Administration (FDA), while others are waiting for the approval. While prospective randomized controlled trials studying the safety and efficacy of the methods discussed are not available, sufficient retrospective data is published. It is hoped that adaptation of some of the methods described will increase the safety during GI endoscopy.

Keywords Propofol • Endoscopy • ERCP • Bite Block • Airway • Sedation

Importance of Airway Management in Out of OR Anesthesia

The challenges faced by an anesthesiologist involved in GI endoscopy are unique and different from those faced by an operating room anesthesiologist. Studies have repeatedly demonstrated that hypoxemia is the commonest and most serious adverse event during the procedures performed out of the operating room. GI endoscopic procedures contribute to majority of these adverse events.

Metzner et al. was one of the first to report the risks of providing anesthesia in out of OR locations [1–3]. They concluded that "closed Claims database suggest that anesthesia at remote locations poses a significant risk for the patient, specifically in relation to oversedation and inadequate oxygenation/ventilation during monitored anesthesia care". The proportion of respiratory events for remote location

B. Goudra, MD, FRCA, FCARCSI (✉)
Department of Anesthesiology and Critical Care Medicine,
Hospital of the University of Pennsylvania, 3400 Spruce Street,
5042 Silverstein Building, Philadelphia, PA 19104, USA
e-mail: goudrab@uphs.upenn.edu

P.M. Singh, MD, DNB, MNAMS
Department of Anesthesiology, Critical Care and Pain Medicine,
All India Institute of Medical Sciences, New Delhi, India

© Springer International Publishing Switzerland 2017
B.G. Goudra, P.M. Singh (eds.), *Out of Operating Room Anesthesia*,
DOI 10.1007/978-3-319-39150-2_11

claims was double compared to that of operating room claims (44 vs. 20%, P<0.001), with issues related to oxygenation and (or) ventilation being the most common. These events occurred approximately seven times more frequently in remote locations than in operating rooms (21 vs. 3%, P<0.001). However, these are likely to be a small proportion of the total number of such adverse events in these locations. It should be noted that all adverse events are not reported to the American Society of Anesthesiologists (ASA) and as a result are unavailable for an analysis. Additionally, many near misses are never reported.

Two recent single center publications further strengthen these conclusions. Goudra et al. published their experience of nearly 5 years in providing mild-moderate and deep sedation/general anesthesia to patients undergoing both routine and diagnostic gastrointestinal endoscopic procedures [4, 5]. Although the data was analyzed retrospectively, the documentation of all events was made on the day of occurrence. The overall incidence of cardiac arrest and death (all causes, until discharge) was 6.07 and 4.28 per 10,000 in patients sedated with propofol, compared with 0.67 and 0.44 in patients receiving non–propofol-based sedation. The incidences were per 10,000 procedures performed. The incidence of cardiac arrest during and immediately after the procedure (recovery area) for all endoscopies was 3.92; of which, 72% were airway related. About 90.0% of all peri-procedural cardiac arrests occurred in patients who received propofol and many were hypoxemia related. Although other factors might have played a part either in the occurrence or the ultimate outcome of these adverse events, it is beyond doubt that hypoxemia played a significant role. The role of deep sedation in the occurrence of hypoxemia is further highlighted in a recent meta-analysis. In this study, the rates of sedation related complications were lower in patients undergoing advanced endoscopic procedures and receiving propofol from non-anesthesia providers [6]. However, both the patient and the endoscopist satisfaction were also lower in the non-anesthesia administered propofol group. This was possibly related to lighter degrees of sedation, as evidenced by lower doses of propofol administered. The most recent study to validate these findings is of Wernli et al. [7]. Once again, propofol sedation in patients undergoing colonoscopy was associated with a 13% increase in the incidence of all complications, including those related to airway.

In view of these findings, it is sensible that those involved in administering anesthesia/deep sedation in GI endoscopy are familiar with existing devices, device modifications and the devices in the pipeline. However, until the new devices become widely available.

Old Devices-New Adaptations

Existing Mapleson breathing systems can be modified to suit the requirements of patients undergoing GI endoscopy.

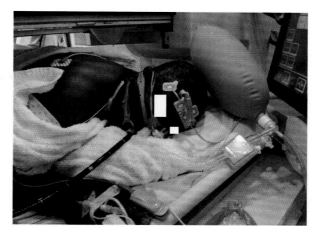

Fig. 11.1 A nasal airway connected to a Mapleson C breathing system. Also seen in the picture is the sensor for SEDLine depth if sedation monitor

Nasal Airway Connected to a Portable Mapleson Breathing System

As illustrated in the Fig. 11.1, a nasal airway (popularly referred to as a nasal trumpet in the USA), is inserted into the nostril on the floor of the nose, underneath the inferior turbinate [8]. The patent needs to be adequately sedated before an attempt is made at insertion. It is advised to let the patient breath 100% oxygen via a tight fitting face mask, while the initial slow bolus administration of propofol is in progress. On disappearance of the eyelash reflex, face mask is removed and sufficient lubricant is instilled into the appropriate side of the nose. Any contraindication (high INR, polyps, bleeding diathesis) should be documented at the time of pre-procedural evaluation and should caution or exclude such insertion. Irrespective of any contraindications, force should never be used during insertion. Cases of catastrophic bleeding are reported. Any tear into the mucosa might force the airway into the retropharyngeal space. Blood supply to the conchae is from the ophthalmic artery which is a branch of internal carotid artery. Controlling such bleeding might require intervention from an otorhinolaryngologist. If resistance is encountered, an attempt is made to insert into the other nostril. Additional doses of propofol might be needed during the process.

Before the nasal airway is inserted, it is also important to prepare the airway itself, so that it can be secured. There are multiple ways of achieving this. Although tape can be used, it might not be stable. The way practiced at the hospital of the university of Pennsylvania is demonstrated in Fig. 11.2. An endotracheal tube connector is obtained. They can be either purchased on their own or removed from a new endotracheal tube. Using the steps in the figure, the endotracheal tube connector and the nasal airway are held together. Typically, a 32 fr size is used for adult

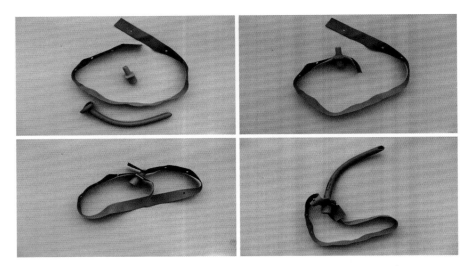

Fig. 11.2 Various steps to prepare a nasal airway before insertion and thereafter connection to a Mapelson C breathing system

females and 34 fr for an adult male. Smaller airway might be appropriate for smaller size adults of both gender.

After insertion of the nasal airway, it is connected to a pre-prepared Mapleson breathing system, which was used during pre-oxygenation. An oxygen flow of 6–8 l is typically used, however it can be increased to allow for the leaks in the event of attempted ventilation. It is important to maintain a sedation depth that would allow spontaneous ventilation. Such a degree of sedation would allow scope insertion including maneuvering required for advanced endoscopic procedures. Although no prospective controlled studies exist on the safety and efficacy of this technique during gastrointestinal endoscopy under deep propofol sedation, sufficient body of retrospective data is available [9–11].

In addition to providing high concentration of oxygen at the laryngeal inlet, the nasal airway might provide a degree of positive pressure ventilation by occluding the second nostril and mouth around the endoscope. However, it is by no means guaranteed to provide a good seal or allow consistent intermittent positive pressure ventilation (IPPV). In the event of desaturation due to apnea, if the initial efforts at IPPV fail, it is very important to request the endoscopist to withdraw the endoscope and initiate positive pressure ventilation.

As a result of propofol deep sedation, muscles of the jaw become relaxed and the tongue falls back to obstruct the oropharynx. This might be associated with obstruction of the nasopharyngeal air passage brought about by the soft palate falling back onto the posterior nasopharynx. Chin lift, jaw thrust and suctioning of the oropharynx are often forgotten and needs implementation early on. Any laryngospasm needs to be identified on time and appropriate measures including administration of succinylcholine instituted.

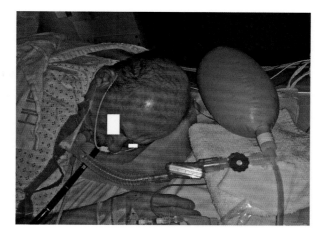

Fig. 11.3 A nasal airway in the mouth which is connected to a Mapleson C breathing system

Oral Airway Connected to a Portable Mapleson Breathing System

Figure 11.3 illustrates the nasal airway inserted on the side of the month to achieve similar objectives as nasal airway. Securing the trumpet is similar to the nasal airway. Once again, no randomized studies are available to confirm its safety and efficacy.

Using either of the above techniques would limit the ability to sample the end tidal gas for a reliable display of end tidal carbon dioxide graph or number. This limitation was studied and reported [12]. It might be sensible to use alternate means of respiration like impedance pneumogram or acoustic respiratory monitoring. The limitation of the former is its inability to detect breathing against a closed glottis, while the latter is expensive and insufficiently studied.

Nasal Airway Connected to a Jet Ventilator

Supraglottic jet ventilation is occasionally employed in upper GI endoscopy. As displayed in the Fig. 11.4, the nasal airway is connected to the luer connector of jet ventilator tubing.

High frequency Jet ventilation (HFJV) uses a high-pressure gas source which is applied to an open airway in short bursts. This can be achieved with a hand held device (manual jet ventilation originally described by sanders), where rate and duration of the breath are set by the user depending on the chest expansion and the saturation. An automated system that delivers oxygen or air-oxygen mixture, at respiratory rates substantially higher than physiologic (between 60 and 300 breaths/min, often termed HFJV) is another option. This allows for a nearly motionless

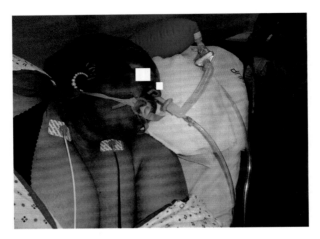

Fig. 11.4 A nasal airway connected to a C Mapleson breathing system. The Luer fitting on the elbow of the breathing system is connected to a hand held jet ventilator

operative field as well as frees the anesthesiologist from ventilation responsibilities during the procedure. Patients with restrictive lung disease, poor chest wall compliance, and significant obesity are poor candidates for automated jet ventilator. They can develop atelectasis during prolonged procedures due to low VTs (small tidal volume) and low mean airway pressure. Development of excessive airway pressures and pneumothorax is a limitation of manual jet ventilation.

Unlike in rigid bronchoscopy where jet ventilation is popular, its use is limited to few enthusiasts in the area of GI endoscopy. A case can be made for its use in patients undergoing Endoscopic Retrograde Cholangiopancreatography (ERCP). However, it is important to align the tip of the nasal airway with the laryngeal opening. It is also essential that the tip of the nasal airway is not obstructed as this can lead to potential air entry into the soft tissues (as pharyngeal trauma cannot be excluded either during nasal airway or endoscope insertion) with catastrophic airway occlusion. Morbidly obese is another potential group who can benefit from jet ventilation [13, 14]. There are no studies conforming its safety and efficacy in the setting of GI endoscopy.

New Devices

Goudra Bite Block Goudra Mask Airway

Goudra Bite block (GBB) combines the features of a standard bit block and a face mask, while Goudra mask airway (GMA) combines the features of a standard bit block, face mask and an airway [15, 16]. As can be deciphered from Figs. 11.5 and 11.6, the endoscope is inserted through the stretchable opening of an airtight diaphragm. The bite block itself has an extended flange with an inflatable seal. When the bite block is appropriately inserted, secured and inflated, it will provide an airtight seal. However, to facilitate positive pressure ventilation, it would be important

Fig. 11.5 Goudra Bite
Block (GBB) with a scope
insertion port in the middle
(More details at goudra.
com)

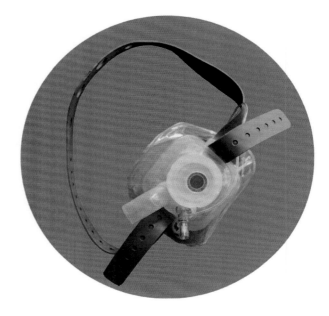

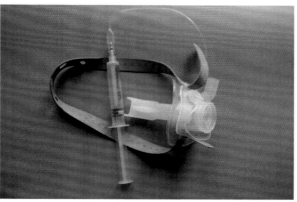

Fig. 11.6 Goudra Mask Airway (GMA) (More details at goudra.com)

to occlude both nostrils and occasionally press the flange to the face. The 15 mm connector is attached to a portable or standard anesthesia breathing system. The device is waiting for FDA clearance.

Wei's Nasal Airway

WEI Nasal Jet (WNJ) is an adaptation of an existing standard nasopharyngeal airway with a dedicated channel for providing jet ventilation [17]. Additionally, it allows to sample the end tidal gas with another dedicated channel. The details are

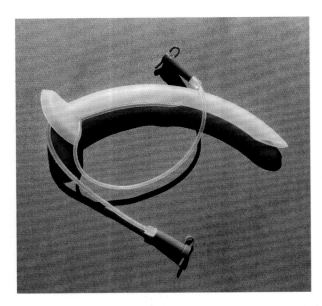

Fig. 11.7 We nasal jet tube. The narrow tube emanating from the proximal end of the tube is for connecting to a jet ventilator, while the other narrow tube is for End tidal Carbon dioxide monitoring

explained in Fig. 11.7. It will present the same challenges as those posed by the standard nasal airway.

Conclusions

Although, providing anesthesia/deep sedation poses unique challenges, by intelligent adaptation of existing devices, the risks can be reduced significantly. The newer devices should help to standardize the care and improve safety.

References

1. Metzner J, Domino KB. Risks of anesthesia or sedation outside the operating room: the role of the anesthesia care provider. Curr Opin Anaesthesiol. 2010;23(4):523–31.
2. Metzner J, Posner KL, Domino KB. The risk and safety of anesthesia at remote locations: the US closed claims analysis. Curr Opin Anaesthesiol. 2009;22(4):502–8.
3. Metzner J, Posner KL, Lam MS, Domino KB. Closed claims' analysis. Best Pract Res Clin Anaesthesiol. 2011;25(2):263–76.
4. Goudra B, Nuzat A, Sngh PM, Borle A, Carlin A, Gouda G. Association between type of sedation and the adverse events associated with gastrointestinal endoscopy: an analysis of 5 years' data from a tertiary center in the USA. Clin Endosc. 2016. doi: 10.5946/ce.2016.019.

5. Goudra B, Nuzat A, Singh PM, Gouda GB, Carlin A, Manjunath AK. Cardiac arrests in patients undergoing gastrointestinal endoscopy: a retrospective analysis of 73,029 procedures. Saudi J Gastroenterol Off J Saudi Gastroenterol Assoc. 2015;21(6):400–11.
6. Goudra BG, Singh PM, Gouda G, Borle A, Gouda D, Dravida A, et al. Safety of Non-anesthesia Provider-Administered Propofol (NAAP) sedation in advanced gastrointestinal endoscopic procedures: comparative meta-analysis of pooled results. Dig Dis Sci. 2015;60(9):2612–27.
7. Wernli KJ, Brenner AT, Rutter CM, Inadomi JM. Risks associated with anesthesia services during colonoscopy. Gastroenterology [Internet]. [cited 2016 Jan 3]. Available from: http://www.sciencedirect.com/science/article/pii/S0016508515018132.
8. Ellis H, Lawson A. Anatomy for anaesthetists. 9th ed. Chichester: Wiley-Blackwell; 2013. 360 p.
9. Goudra B, Singh P, Sinha A. Outpatient endoscopic retrograde cholangiopancreatography: safety and efficacy of anesthetic management with a natural airway in 653 consecutive procedures. Saudi J Anaesth. 2013;7(3):259.
10. Goudra B, Singh PM. ERCP: the unresolved question of endotracheal intubation. Dig Dis Sci. 2014;59(3):513–9.
11. Goudra BG, Singh PM, Penugonda LC, Speck RM, Sinha AC. Significantly reduced hypoxemic events in morbidly obese patients undergoing gastrointestinal endoscopy: predictors and practice effect. J Anaesthesiol Clin Pharmacol. 2014;30(1):71–7.
12. Goudra BG. Comparison of acoustic respiration rate, impedance pneumography and capnometry monitors for respiration rate accuracy and apnea detection during GI endoscopy anesthesia. Open J Anesthesiol. 2013;03(02):74–9.
13. Levitt C, Wei H. Supraglotic pulsatile jet oxygenation and ventilation during deep propofol sedation for upper gastrointestinal endoscopy in a morbidly obese patient. J Clin Anesth. 2014;26(2):157–9.
14. Goudra BG, Penugonda LC, Sinha A. A novel way of anesthetizing and maintaining airway/ventilation in an ultra-morbidly obese patient presenting for upper GI endoscopy. J Clin Anesth. 2012;24(7):604–5.
15. Goudra B, Chandramouli M, Singh P, Sandur V. Goudra ventilating bite block to reduce hypoxemia during endoscopic retrograde cholangiopancreatography. Saudi J Anaesth. 2014;8(2):299.
16. Goudra bite block for upper gastrointestinal endoscopy. PubMed – NCBI [Internet]. [cited 2016 Mar 21]. Available from: http://www.ncbi.nlm.nih.gov/pubmed/25657763.
17. Testing the efficacy and safety of the WEI Nasal Jet – full text view. ClinicalTrials.gov [Internet]. [cited 2016 Mar 21]. Available from: https://clinicaltrials.gov/ct2/show/NCT02005406.

Part IV
Anesthesia for Cardiac Procedures

Chapter 12
Anesthesia and Sedation Strategies in Electrophysiology: General Concepts

Anjan Trikha, Bharathram Vasudevan, and Anuradha Borle

Abstract Numerous procedures are carried out in the cardiac electrophysiology laboratory including catheter ablation for various arrhythmias and implantation of devices such as pacemakers and implantable cardioverter-defibrillators (ICD). Patients undergoing these procedures pose unique challenges to the anesthetist as they have serious cardiovascular conditions like unstable arrhythmias, coronary artery disease and poor cardiac function, often with left ventricular ejection fraction less than 35 %. Many of these procedures can be carried out under local anesthesia with conscious sedation administered by a trained nurse. However, monitored anesthesia care with varying levels of sedation provided by trained anesthesia personnel is preferable in patients with multiple comorbidities and severe cardiac conditions. General anesthesia is needed for patient populations such as pediatric patients, those with poor functional status who cannot lie on their back and for complex catheter ablation procedures which require minimal patient movement for prolonged durations. Midazolam and fentanyl are the commonly used agents for conscious sedation. Propofol, etomidate or ketamine are commonly used for deeper sedation or general anesthesia. The effects of anesthetic drugs on the cardiac conduction system should be kept in mind as they can interfere with identifying arrhythmias during electrophysiological studies.

Keywords Anesthesia • Sedation • Monitored anesthesia care • Cardiac electrophysiology • Catheter ablation • Atrial fibrillation • Pacemaker • Implantable cardioverter-defibrillator • Cardiac resynchronization therapy • Midazolam • Fentanyl • Propofol • Ketamine • Etomidate • High frequency jet ventilation

A. Trikha, MD, DA, FICA, MNAMS (✉) • B. Vasudevan, MBBS • A. Borle
Department of Anaesthesiology, Pain Medicine and Critical Care,
All India Institute of Medical Sciences, Ansari Nagar, New Delhi, Delhi, India
e-mail: anjantrikha@hotmail.com; drbharathram@yahoo.in; andromeda85@gmail.com

© Springer International Publishing Switzerland 2017
B.G. Goudra, P.M. Singh (eds.), *Out of Operating Room Anesthesia*,
DOI 10.1007/978-3-319-39150-2_12

Introduction

The number of procedures being carried out in the cardiac electrophysiology laboratory (EP lab) has increased tremendously in the past few decades. They have grown from simple diagnostic electrophysiology studies for cardiac conduction abnormalities to complex therapeutic procedures offering treatment for a variety of cardiac conditions. For instance, more than 12,500 implantable cardioverter-defibrillators (ICD) are implanted every month in the United States of America [1]. Many of the procedures in the EP lab can be done under local infiltration anesthesia with minimal sedation that is usually administered by non-anesthesia personnel. Certain complex procedures and patient populations require deep sedation or general anesthesia and the expertise of an anesthesiologist. The focus of this chapter is to provide a general overview of anesthesia and sedation strategies employed in the EP laboratory.

Arrhythmias and EP Lab Procedures

An in-depth knowledge of the mechanisms of arrhythmias and various procedures done in the EP laboratory are crucial for safe and effective anesthetic management for the procedure. The types of interventions done in any EP lab can be divided into two –

1. Device based interventions and
2. Catheter based interventions

Device Based Interventions

Device based interventions include implantation of pacemakers, implantable cardioverter-defibrillators and lately biventricular pacing gadgets for cardiac resynchronization therapy (CRT) with or without implantable cardioverter-defibrillator. Permanent pacemakers are indicated for symptomatic bradycardia in patients with sick sinus syndrome, atrioventricular block, bifascicular or trifascicular blocks, carotid sinus hypersensitivity and neurally mediated bradycardia [2]. ICD is indicated for both primary prevention and secondary prevention of sudden cardiac death. Patients with previous history of cardiac arrest due to ventricular fibrillation or sustained ventricular tachycardia require an ICD as a secondary prevention measure. ICD implantation for primary prevention is indicated in patients at risk for sudden cardiac death and sustained ventricular tachyarrhythmias (e.g. – patients with previous myocardial infarction and ischemic cardiomyopathy with left ventricular ejection fraction (LVEF) less than 35 %). CRT involves biventricular pacing to improve coordination and increase ejection fraction in patients with poor left ventricular function (LVEF less than 35%) and QRS duration more than 0.12 s. CRT can also be combined with an ICD to prevent sudden cardiac death in such patients. Readers are referred to the 'appropriate use' criteria published by the American College of Cardiology Foundation in association with other related societies for knowing the exact indications for placement of these devices [3]. Implantation of these devices is done by transvenous route (usually subclavian vein) and the generator is placed in a subcutaneous pocket in the infra-clavicular region.

Catheter Based Interventions

These include the diagnostic electrophysiological studies and catheter ablations done for various tachyarrhythmias. The arrhythmias amenable to catheter ablation include atrioventricular reentrant tachycardia (AVRT), atrioventricular nodal reentrant tachycardia (AVNRT), Wolff-Parkinson-White syndrome, atrial tachycardia, atrial flutter, atrial fibrillation (AF) and ventricular tachycardia (VT). Catheter ablation is offered for patients with symptomatic and recurrent tachyarrhythmias not responding to medical treatment or recurrent VT requiring multiple ICD generated shocks if the same has been implanted earlier [4–6]. It may also be indicated as the first-line of treatment in some arrhythmias with high cure rates after ablation. Catheter ablations have been associated with better outcomes and improved quality of life [6].

Cardiac electrophysiologic mapping refers to the determination of spatial and temporal distribution of electrical activity of heart to find the specific mechanism of arrhythmias and to identify the target location for ablation. EP testing involves placement of electrode catheters at multiple predetermined positions inside the heart and programmed pacing is done to obtain intra-cardiac localized electrograms. Classical locations for placement of catheters are in the right atrium, near the bundle of His, in the right ventricle and the coronary sinus. The sequence of activation at these different positions and time delay between the recorded electrograms help in the exact diagnosis and localization of the target area. Various strategies of mapping are employed that include activation mapping, entrainment mapping, pace mapping and substrate mapping. During such procedures, arrhythmias may be induced by programmed electrical stimulation, burst pacing or pharmacological methods (catecholamine infusion). Conventional mapping techniques uses fluoroscopy to position the electrode catheters. Newer non-fluoroscopic catheter navigational systems (such as CARTO and Ensite NAVx) provide three-dimensional electroanatomical mapping of the heart chambers and help in catheter localization and navigation by using electromagnetic and impedance based technologies respectively. They provide the advantage of three dimensional modeling and also a decrease in fluoroscopy times [7].

Catheter ablation at the identified site is performed usually using radiofrequency energy delivered by a catheter tip to the endocardial surface which causes a burn by resistive heating. Some arrhythmias have a known anatomical cause and the ablation energy is directed to this site – e.g. atrial flutter arises from a reentrant mechanism at the cavo-tricuspid isthmus between the inferior vena cava and tricuspid valve.

To avoid excessive tissue damage with radiofrequency ablation, saline irrigation to cool the catheter tip has been used but this can lead to fluid overload in susceptible patients [8]. Cryothermal energy to produce cryo-ablation has also been used, although less frequently. The advantage of cryo-ablation is the ability to produce reversible test lesions by controlling the temperature and a reduced risk of thromboembolism [9].

Anesthetic Drugs and Cardiac Electrophysiology

The ideal anesthetic agent for cardiac electrophysiology procedures should not interfere with the ability to identify arrhythmias during an electrophysiological procedure. While all anesthetic agents can affect the cardiac conduction system, a balanced anesthesia technique has been shown not to interfere in the ability to identify aberrant pathways during open surgical ablation [10]. The anesthetic agents commonly used in the EP laboratory with their relevant pharmacokinetic and pharmacodynamic properties are discussed below.

- **Propofol** is an alkyl phenol exerting its hypnotic effects through GABA and NMDA receptors. It is commonly used for sedation as well as induction and maintenance of general anesthesia. Propofol is a profound cardiovascular depressant. It causes hypotension after an induction dose due to reduction in systemic vascular resistance and also associated myocardial depression. However, it is not accompanied by an increase in heart rate due to probable inhibition of baroreceptor reflex. The effects may lead to hemodynamic instability especially in patients with poor LV function (candidates for CRT) and in elderly population. Small titrated doses of propofol have been found to be safe in these patients. The onset time is prolonged in patients with heart failure due to longer circulation times and the administration of a repeat bolus should be delayed. Though various studies have shown that propofol does not affect conduction at sinus node, AV node or through accessory pathways, it has been reported to interfere with the induction of supraventricular tachycardia especially in children, which should be kept in mind during electrophysiological studies [11–14].
- **Etomidate** is an imidazole derivative acting on the GABA receptor. It is cardiovascular stable drug and is an attractive choice for induction of anesthesia in patients with cardiovascular instability. It causes lesser depression of respiratory drive than propofol and may be advantageous in situations requiring short GA with minimal airway manipulation. Two main disadvantages of etomidate include the high incidence of myoclonus and prolonged adrenal suppression after long term infusions. Myoclonus can interfere with the ECG recording which is undesirable in cardiac electrophysiological studies [15, 16]. Pretreatment with midazolam has been shown to reduce the incidence of myoclonus [17, 18].

- **Ketamine**, a NMDA receptor antagonist is an indirectly acting sympathomimetic leading to an increase in blood pressure, heart rate and cardiac output. This leads to increased myocardial oxygen demand which may have deleterious effects in cardiac patients with coronary artery disease or pulmonary hypertension. Ketamine also causes psychomimetic effects leading to emergence phenomenon postoperatively. These hemodynamic and psychomimetic effects of ketamine can be attenuated with prior administration of midazolam or dexmedetomidine [19]. It should also be noted that in critically ill patients with catecholamine depletion, ketamine can lead to myocardial depression by its direct effect on the heart. The advantages of using ketamine for sedation include profound analgesia and its minimal effects on respiratory drive. Wutzler et al. found that the hemodynamic effects of ketamine were beneficial compared to propofol in patients undergoing radiofrequency ablation for supraventricular tachycardia with pre-existing bradycardia and hypotension [20].
- **Benzodiazepenes** are commonly used for sedation and anxiolysis. Midazolam is especially suited for intravenous procedural sedation because of its faster onset and shorter duration of action. It does not cause significant cardiovascular instability though it can decrease peripheral vascular resistance and cardiac output more than other benzodiazepenes. It has no effect on cardiac conduction system. Exaggerated sedation and cardiovascular responses can be seen in the elderly and requires appropriate titration [7]. Midazolam can sometimes cause paradoxical agitation which can be treated with flumazenil or propofol [21, 22].

Short acting opioids such as fentanyl, alfentanil, sufentanil and remifentanil are also used for sedation and analgesia in these groups of patients. Fentanyl and midazolam combination is one of the most commonly used sedation technique in procedures carried out in EP labs. They have a synergistic effect when used along with other sedatives or induction agents. High dose opioid based anaesthesia has been associated with hemodynamically stable intraoperative period when compared to other intravenous or inhalational anesthetics. Opioids can cause bradycardia at high doses due to a direct membrane action or via opioid receptors [23]. They have also been associated with QTc prolongation and remifentanil has been reported to cause slowing of conduction in sino-atrial and AV node during electrophysiological studies in children [24].

Dexmedetomidine is a highly selective alpha-2 agonist and is often used for sedation and monitored anesthesia care with minimal effects on respiration. During cardiac electrophysiologic procedures, it has been shown to produce slowing in both sino-atrial and AV node function which can be deleterious in patients at risk for AV nodal block and bradycardia [25, 26]. Also it can lead to sympatholysis which can interfere with the induction of arrhythmias during the electrophysiological study thereby hampering diagnosis and treatment.

Neuromuscular blocking agents are rarely used in the EP lab as most procedures are done under sedation and muscle relaxants might interfere with the ability to test the phrenic nerve which may be injured during catheter ablation procedures. They also affect the cardiac conduction system. Succinylcholine can lead to both brady and rarely tachyarrhythmias. It can also lead to elevation of serum potassium which may alter the electrophysiological responses. Pancuronium can lead to tachycardia due to its vagolytic properties. Atracurium and mivacurium can cause hypotension and reflex tachycardia by histamine release. Vecuronium can cause bradycardia when combined with potent opioids while rocuronium is relatively cardiovascular stable [7, 23].

All inhalational anaesthetics can affect the conduction system of heart. Volatile agents, especially halothane sensitize the myocardium to the arrhythmogenic action of catecholamines thereby leading to abnormal automaticity and this can cause premature contractions and arrhythmias [23]. All volatile agents also lead to prolongation of QTc which may lead to induction of torsades de pointes [27]. A study comparing isoflurane and propofol in children undergoing ablation procedure for supraventricular tachycardia found no clinically significant interference by either of the agents, while another report found significant prolongation of accessory pathway refractory period with sevofurane when compared with propofol in children [13, 28].

Finally, the context-sensitive half-life of propofol and opioids after prolonged infusions should be kept in mind and the dose should be titrated accordingly. Context-sensitive half-life is the time taken for the plasma drug concentration to decrease by 50 % after discontinuation of an infusion. It depends on the duration of infusion ('context' = duration) and the half-life of the drug increases with an increase in duration of the infusion except for drugs with very short elimination half times (e.g. Remifentanil).

Most procedures in EP lab are done under local infiltration anesthesia and therefore a thorough understanding of the relevant local anesthetic pharmacology is essential. Local anesthetics are either amioesters or aminoamides that act on the voltage gated sodium channels in the axons and reversibly block nerve conduction. Lidocaine, bupivacaine, levobupivacaine and ropivacaine are the commonly used drugs. Local anesthetics also block the sodium channels in the cardiac tissue and cause a dose dependent prolongation in cardiac conduction and a decrease in myocardial contractility. The prolongation of cardiac conduction is seen as an increase in the duration of PR interval and QRS complex. However, there are significant differences in the action of different local anesthetics on the cardiac tissue. The maximal rate of depolarization in the purkinje fibers and ventricular muscle is depressed by local anesthetics, more so by bupivacaine than lidocaine [29]. Bupivacaine has higher affinity and dissociates slower from the sodium channels leading to incomplete recovery between action potentials. These differences are responsible for bupivacaine being the most cardiotoxic local anesthetic, while lidocaine is used as an antiarrhythmic agent. Ropivacaine and levobupivacaine are relatively lesser cardiotoxic than bupivacaine [30]. Systemic toxicity after local infiltration or peripheral nerve block can occur due to overdose or inadvertent intravascular injection and manifests with central nervous system toxicity at lower blood levels and cardiovascular toxicity at higher blood levels. To prevent systemic toxicity, it is important to adhere to the maximum recommended dosages of 5 mg/kg for lidocaine, 7 mg/kg for lidocaine with epinephrine and 3 mg/kg for bupivacaine, levobupivacaine and ropivacaine [23].

Thus all anesthetic agents have their own merits and demerits and careful consideration of these properties has to done while selecting an agent depending upon the individual needs of the patient and the specific procedure.

Anesthetic Management

Personnel Providing Anesthesia or Sedation in EP Lab

Anesthesia for various procedures in the electrophysiology lab can vary from local anesthesia with minimal sedation administered by a trained nurse to monitored anesthesia care and general anesthesia provided by an anesthesiologist [31]. Many procedures in the EP lab can be carried out under local anesthesia combined with conscious sedation administered by a trained nurse under the supervision of the cardiologist. The safety of nurse administered sedation has been well established in some studies [32, 33]. On the other hand, the advantages and benefits of having trained anesthesia personnel have also been shown in some studies especially in complex procedures and biventricular implants [34, 35]. The cardiologist can concentrate on the procedure exclusively and general anesthesia has been shown to improve outcomes in certain procedures such as ablation for atrial fibrillation [36, 37]. The decision of opting for trained anesthesia personnel (an anesthesiologist or a certified registered nurse anesthetist) is based on the procedure and patient characteristics.

Pre-anesthetic Considerations

All patients scheduled to undergo a device or catheter based intervention should be screened by the cardiac electro physiologist to determine the need for a preprocedure anesthesia consultation. Situations demanding a proper anesthesia care include – procedures requiring an immobile patient for prolonged periods like complex ablation procedures, complicated lead extractions, hemodynamically unstable patients, patients with an anticipated difficult airway, patients with congestive heart failure who have poor LV function and are unable to lie down flat, those with obstructive sleep apnea syndrome, severe respiratory disease, other comorbidities, those on drug therapy which could complicate usage of sedation, patients for biventricular pacing and any patient who is scheduled for a general anesthesia [38].

Patient scheduled for such procedures can be very different from that seen in a routine surgical population. Patients with severe systolic dysfunction (ejection fraction less than 30%), recent myocardial infarction, arrhythmias with unstable hemodynamics and failed interventions often present for procedures in the electro-physiological laboratory. Assessment of the patient should include a thorough eval-uation of patient's cardiovascular history and drug therapy, current clinical and functional status which may require an EKG, echocardiography and a complete airway examination [39].

Electrophysiology Lab Environment

The EP lab environment is different from a routine operating room environment with many large gadgets like the fluoroscopy machine and screen which may hinder access to the patient during the procedure. Long connections for anesthesia circuit, intravenous lines and monitoring lines are therefore needed. The patient table in a radiological suite is also different from a routine operating table and the head end cannot be elevated separately which may be a limitation for the airway manage-ment. Electrophysiology suites are usually located far away from the main operat-ing theatre complex making it necessary to stock adequate anesthetic supplies including drugs and devices for emergency management. One another concern for persons working in these suites is the exposure to radiation and therefore protective equipment like lead aprons, thyroid shields and eye-glasses should be used [38].

Technique of Anesthesia

As mentioned earlier, the anesthetic or sedation technique may range from local infiltration anesthesia with mild or moderate sedation to deep sedation or general anesthesia. Mild to moderate conscious sedation can be administered by trained nurses in most patients while monitored anesthesia care may be required in some specific patient populations as listed above. Deep sedation or general anesthesia requires the presence of an anesthesiologist or anesthesia care team.

Mild to moderate sedation is most commonly achieved with a combination of midazolam and fentanyl [40]. Titrated doses should be used in elderly patients and in patients with poor cardiac reserve. Low dose ketamine can be added to provide analgesia with no respiratory depression in suitable patients [41]. Dexmedetomidine has a limited role when patients are prone to bradycardia and conduction blocks. Most diagnostic electrophysiologic studies, catheter ablations and device implanta-tions (pacemakers, ICD, CRT) can be done under local infiltration combined with mild to moderate sedation [31]. Device implantation requires a properly adminis-tered effective local infiltration for creation of a subcutaneous pocket. Intraoperative cardioversion or defibrillation threshold testing of ICD needs a short period of deep sedation which can be achieved by a titrated bolus of propofol or thiopental or etomidate [42]. Small titrated doses of propofol have been found to be safe even in patients with poor cardiac function. Spontaneous ventilation is usually maintained, but patients might need assisted ventilation with deeper levels of sedation using propofol. Assisted ventilation using mask with or without adjuncts like oropharyngeal or nasopharyngeal airway is done till the patient regains spontaneous ventilation [7].

General anesthesia is needed for patients with congestive heart failure and associated valvular heart disease or pulmonary hypertension who cannot lie on their back, pediatric patients, patients prone for airway obstruction or apnea on sedation and anxious uncooperative patients. Also GA is needed for some procedures like complex catheter ablation of destabilizing arrhythmias (VT with ischemic heart disease), catheter ablation for AF which may require prolonged immobility and for complicated lead extractions which are prone for complications or hemodynamic instability. Pulmonary vein isolation for AF under GA has been reported to be associated with better outcomes. General anesthesia is commonly induced with titrated doses of propofol or etomidate and muscle relaxation can be achieved with a faster onset non-depolarizing agent like rocuronium. Muscle relaxant is avoided intraoperatively in catheter ablation procedures where phrenic nerve integrity testing may be needed. Maintenance of anesthesia can be done with total intravenous (TIVA) or inhalational techniques depending on the patient's hemodynamic condition and the need for novel methods of ventilation like high frequency jet ventilation [7, 39, 41].

Sometimes a combination of anesthetic techniques is employed with the patient under conscious sedation during diagnostic electro physiologic study followed by deep sedation or GA for ablation. Induction of GA at the very beginning is desirable especially in patients with difficult airway as airway management is difficult intraoperatively due to positioning.

Regional anesthesiais rarely used as an anesthetic technique in the EP lab. Thoracic paravertebral block combined with sedation has been used for a case of ICD and laser lead extraction [43]. On the contrary, thoracic epidural anesthesia and stellate ganglion blockade are being increasingly used as therapeutic modalities for sympatholysis in refractory ventricular arrhythmias [44–46]. The discussion of these autonomic modulation techniques for treatment of sympathetically mediated arrhythmias is beyond the scope of this chapter.

Airway Management

Patients who are under mild sedation and breathing spontaneously may develop airway obstruction when additional doses of sedatives or opioids are used to deepen the sedation levels. Such patients may require assisted bag and mask ventilation that may be difficult due to the gadgets at the head end. Therefore such incremental doses should be titrated carefully and all airway equipment should be readily available. Coughing, sneezing or vigorous respiratory movements can cause excessive movement of the inter-atrial septa which can lead to inadvertent complications during procedures requiring trans-septal puncture such as pulmonary vein isolation procedure for AF. GA with controlled ventilation has been shown to decrease these complications. Recently, high frequency jet ventilation has been employed to decrease respiratory movements during pulmonary vein isolation and is associated with better catheter stability and outcomes. During HFJV, the ventilator rate is set at more than 100 cycles/min using a special ventilator. The potential disadvantages include hypercapnia, barotrauma and atelectasis. Inhalation anesthetic delivery is poor during HFJV, thereby necessitating the use of total intravenous anesthesia [7, 47–49].

Intraoperative Monitoring and Management

Intraoperative monitoring consists of ECG, heart rate, blood pressure and oxygen saturation in all patients. A 12-lead ECG setup is used in all electrophysiological interventions. All patients should have defibrillation pads attached prior to the procedure for emergency cardioversion/defibrillation during the procedure. End tidal carbon dioxide ($ETCO_2$) monitoring should be standard during GA and is desirable under sedation also as it gives valuable information regarding respiratory rate and occurrence of apnea. Face masks with an integrated sample line for $ETCO_2$ monitoring are available and can be used in patients under sedation to provide supplemental oxygen as well as to monitor $ETCO_2$. Invasive arterial pressures are monitored in patients and procedures at risk for hemodynamic instability. Induction of arrhythmias and use of vasoactive drugs through the catheter by the cardiologist can lead to sudden changes in the hemodynamic status of the patient. It should also be kept in mind that saline irrigated catheters can lead to significant volume overload in patients with poor systolic function. Activated clotting time monitoring is done in patients who receive heparin for trans-arterial or trans-septal left heart catheterization and is maintained at more than 300 s during the procedure. Esophageal temperature monitoring can be beneficial to detect hypothermia as well as excessive tissue injury and esophageal burns during pulmonary vein isolation procedure for AF. The use of transesophageal echocardiography can give valuable information regarding the cardiac function and also guide the electrophysiologist regarding catheter position and for diagnosing thrombus in the left atrial appendage or complications such as cardiac tamponade.

Postoperative Care and Complications

Recovery from anesthesia should be smooth and timed after complete hemostasis of the vascular access site is confirmed in order to prevent unwanted movement of limbs which may lead to disruption of hemostasis. Patients who received general anesthesia are ideally monitored in a post-anesthesia care unit. Vascular access related complications such as bleeding, hematoma, pseudoaneurysm, AV fistula and infection are the most frequent complications after any EP lab procedure. Other complications that can occur are listed in Box 12.1 [50]. Systemic embolization can lead to stroke but the risk remains low (<1 %) [51]. Patients who develop life threatening complications require immediate interventions and post-operative ICU care. Some procedures such as complicated lead extractions can have a higher risk of vascular injury and based on the individualized case needs they may be carried out in a hybrid operating room where access to cardiopulmonary bypass (CPB) is readily available [38].

Box 12.1: Complications of EP Lab Procedures
Vascular access site complications (hematoma, pseudoaneurysm, AV fistula)
Pericardial effusion and cardiac tamponade
Cardiac conduction blocks including complete AV nodal block
New arrhythmias
Stroke
Phrenic nerve injury
Esophageal injury and atrial-esophageal fistula
Pneumothorax
Radiation burn
Subcutaneous generator pocket hematoma or infection

Conclusion

Anesthesia outside the operating room provides unique challenges to the anesthesia care team. Those specific to cardiac electrophysiology are the need for minimal interference by anesthetic drugs on the cardiac conduction system, caring for patients with significant cardiac morbidity and the possibility of many life threatening complications and hemodynamic instability during the procedure. With newer technologies and complex procedures, there is increasing need for an anesthesiologist in the electrophysiology lab.

References

1. Kremers MS, Hammill SC, Berul CI, Koutras C, Curtis JS, Wang Y, et al. The National ICD Registry Report: version 2.1 including leads and pediatrics for years 2010 and 2011. Heart Rhythm Off J Heart Rhythm Soc. 2013;10(4):e59–65.
2. Epstein AE, DiMarco JP, Ellenbogen KA, Mark Estes INA, Freedman RA, Gettes LS, et al. ACC/AHA/HRS 2008 Guidelines for Device-Based Therapy of Cardiac Rhythm Abnormalities: Executive SummaryA Report of the American College of Cardiology/American Heart Association Task Force on Practice Guidelines (Writing Committee to Revise the ACC/AHA/NASPE 2002 Guideline Update for Implantation of Cardiac Pacemakers and Antiarrhythmia Devices) Developed in Collaboration With the American Association for Thoracic Surgery and Society of Thoracic Surgeons. J Am Coll Cardiol. 2008;51(21): 2085–105.

3. Russo AM, Stainback RF, Bailey SR, Epstein AE, Heidenreich PA, Jessup M, et al. ACCF/ HRS/AHA/ASE/HFSA/SCAI/SCCT/SCMR 2013 appropriate use criteria for implantable cardioverter-defibrillators and cardiac resynchronization therapy: a report of the American College of Cardiology Foundation appropriate use criteria task force, Heart Rhythm Society, American Heart Association, American Society of Echocardiography, Heart Failure Society of America, Society for Cardiovascular Angiography and Interventions, Society of Cardiovascular Computed Tomography, and Society for Cardiovascular Magnetic Resonance. J Am Coll Cardiol. 2013;61(12):1318–68.

4. Blomström-Lundqvist C, Scheinman MM, Aliot EM, Alpert JS, Calkins H, Camm AJ, et al. ACC/AHA/ESC guidelines for the management of patients with supraventricular arrhythmias--executive summary: a report of the American College of Cardiology/American Heart Association Task Force on Practice Guidelines and the European Society of Cardiology Committee for Practice Guidelines (Writing Committee to Develop Guidelines for the Management of Patients With Supraventricular Arrhythmias). Circulation. 2003;108(15):1871–909.

5. Aliot EM, Stevenson WG, Almendral-Garrote JM, Bogun F, Calkins CH, Delacretaz E, et al. EHRA/HRS Expert Consensus on Catheter Ablation of Ventricular Arrhythmias: developed in a partnership with the European Heart Rhythm Association (EHRA), a Registered Branch of the European Society of Cardiology (ESC), and the Heart Rhythm Society (HRS); in collaboration with the American College of Cardiology (ACC) and the American Heart Association (AHA). Heart Rhythm Off J Heart Rhythm Soc. 2009;6(6):886–933.

6. Calkins H, Kuck KH, Cappato R, Brugada J, Camm AJ, Chen S-A, et al. 2012 HRS/EHRA/ ECAS Expert Consensus Statement on Catheter and Surgical Ablation of Atrial Fibrillation: recommendations for patient selection, procedural techniques, patient management and follow-up, definitions, endpoints, and research trial design. Eur Eur Pacing Arrhythm Card Electrophysiol J Work Groups Card Pacing Arrhythm Card Cell Electrophysiol Eur Soc Cardiol. 2012;14(4):528–606.

7. Saksena S, editor. Interventional cardiac electrophysiology: a multidisciplinary approach. Minneapolis: Cardiotext Publishing; 2015.

8. Seiler J, Steven D, Roberts-Thomson KC, Inada K, Tedrow UB, Michaud GF, et al. The effect of open-irrigated radiofrequency catheter ablation of atrial fibrillation on left atrial pressure and B-type natriuretic peptide. Pacing Clin Electrophysiol PACE. 2014;37(5):616–23.

9. Piccini JP, Daubert JP. Cryoablation of atrial fibrillation. J Interv Card Electrophysiol Int J Arrhythm Pacing. 2011;32(3):233–42.

10. Irish CL, Murkin JM, Guiraudon GM. Anaesthetic management for surgical cryoablation of accessory conducting pathways: a review and report of 181 cases. Can J Anaesth J Can Anesth. 1988;35(6):634–40.

11. Warpechowski P, Lima GG, Medeiros CM, Santos ATL, Kruse M, Migloransa MH, et al. Randomized study of propofol effect on electrophysiological properties of the atrioventricular node in patients with nodal reentrant tachycardia. Pacing Clin Electrophysiol PACE. 2006;29(12):1375–82.

12. Warpechowski P, dos Santos ATL, Pereira PJI, de Lima GG. Effects of propofol on the cardiac conduction system. Rev Bras Anestesiol. 2010;60(4):438–44.

13. Erb TO, Kanter RJ, Hall JM, Gan TJ, Kern FH, Schulman SR. Comparison of electrophysiologic effects of propofol and isoflurane-based anesthetics in children undergoing radiofrequency catheter ablation for supraventricular tachycardia. Anesthesiology. 2002;96(6): 1386–94.

14. Owczuk R, Wujtewicz MA, Zienciuk-Krajka A, Lasińska-Kowara M, Piankowski A, Wujtewicz M. The influence of anesthesia on cardiac repolarization. Minerva Anestesiol. 2012;78(4): 483–95.

15. Hullander RM, Leivers D, Wingler K. A comparison of propofol and etomidate for cardioversion. Anesth Analg. 1993;77(4):690–4.

16. Doenicke AW, Roizen MF, Kugler J, Kroll H, Foss J, Ostwald P. Reducing myoclonus after etomidate. J Am Soc Anesthesiol. 1999;90(1):113–9.

17. Schwarzkopf KRG, Hueter L, Simon M, Fritz HG. Midazolam pretreatment reduces etomidate-induced myoclonic movements. Anaesth Intensive Care. 2003;31(1):18–20.
18. Hwang J-Y, Kim J-H, Oh A-Y, Do S-H, Jeon Y-T, Han S-H. A comparison of midazolam with remifentanil for the prevention of myoclonic movements following etomidate injection. J Int Med Res. 2008;36(1):17–22.
19. Levänen J, Mäkelä ML, Scheinin H. Dexmedetomidine premedication attenuates ketamine-induced cardiostimulatory effects and postanesthetic delirium. Anesthesiology. 1995;82(5): 1117–25.
20. Wutzler A, Huemer M, Boldt L-H, Parwani AS, Attanasio P, Tscholl V, et al. Effects of deep sedation on cardiac electrophysiology in patients undergoing radiofrequency ablation of supraventricular tachycardia: impact of propofol and ketamine. Eur Eur Pacing Arrhythm Card Electrophysiol J Work Groups Card Pacing Arrhythm Card Cell Electrophysiol Eur Soc Cardiol. 2013;15(7):1019–24.
21. Tae CH, Kang KJ, Min B-H, Ahn JH, Kim S, Lee JH, et al. Paradoxical reaction to midazolam in patients undergoing endoscopy under sedation: Incidence, risk factors and the effect of flumazenil. Dig Liver Dis Off J Ital Soc Gastroenterol Ital Assoc Study Liver. 2014;46(8): 710–5.
22. Weinbroum AA, Szold O, Ogorek D, Flaishon R. The midazolam-induced paradox phenomenon is reversible by flumazenil. Epidemiology, patient characteristics and review of the literature. Eur J Anaesthesiol. 2001;18(12):789–97.
23. Miller RD, Eriksson LI, Fleisher LA, Wiener-Kronish JP, Cohen NH, Young WL, editors. Miller's anesthesia. 8th ed. Philadelphia: Elsevier; 2015.
24. Niksch A, Liberman L, Clapcich A, Schwarzenberger JC, Silver ES, Pass RH. Effects of remifentanil anesthesia on cardiac electrophysiologic properties in children undergoing catheter ablation of supraventricular tachycardia. Pediatr Cardiol. 2010;31(7):1079–82.
25. Ergul Y, Unsal S, Ozyilmaz I, Ozturk E, Carus H, Guzeltas A. Electrocardiographic and electrophysiologic effects of dexmedetomidine on children. Pacing Clin Electrophysiol PACE. 2015;38(6):682–7.
26. Hammer GB, Drover DR, Cao H, Jackson E, Williams GD, Ramamoorthy C, et al. The effects of dexmedetomidine on cardiac electrophysiology in children. Anesth Analg. 2008;106(1):79–83, table of contents.
27. Staikou C, Stamelos M, Stavroulakis E. Impact of anaesthetic drugs and adjuvants on ECG markers of torsadogenicity. Br J Anaesth. 2014;112(2):217–30.
28. Caldwell JC, Fong C, Muhyaldeen SA. Should sevoflurane be used in the electrophysiology assessment of accessory pathways? Europace. 2010;12(9):1332–5.
29. Moller R, Covino BG. Cardiac electrophysiologic properties of bupivacaine and lidocaine compared with those of ropivacaine, a new amide local anesthetic. Anesthesiology. 1990;72(2): 322–9.
30. Groban L, Dolinski SY. Differences in cardiac toxicity among ropivacaine, levobupivacaine, bupivacaine, and lidocaine. Tech Reg Anesth Pain Manag. 2001;5(2):48–55.
31. Furniss SS, Sneyd JR. Safe sedation in modern cardiological practice. Heart Br Card Soc. 2015;101(19):1526–30.
32. Al Fagih A, Al Shurafa H, Al Ghamdi S, Dagriri K, Al Khadra A. Safe and effective use of conscious sedation for defibrillation threshold testing during ICD implantation. J Saudi Heart Assoc. 2010;22(4):209–13.
33. Ichihara N, Miyazaki S, Taniguchi H, Usui E, Takagi T, Iwasawa J, et al. Simple minimal sedation for catheter ablation of atrial fibrillation. Circ J Off J Jpn Circ Soc. 2015;79(2):346–50.
34. Trouvé-Buisson T, Arvieux L, Bedague D, Casez-Brasseur M, Defaye P, Payen J-F, et al. Anaesthesiological support in a cardiac electrophysiology laboratory: a single-centre prospective observational study. Eur J Anaesthesiol. 2013;30(11):658–63.
35. Sayfo S, Vakil KP, Alqaqa'a A, Flippin H, Bhakta D, Yadav AV, et al. A retrospective analysis of proceduralist-directed, nurse-administered propofol sedation for implantable cardioverter-defibrillator procedures. Heart Rhythm Off J Heart Rhythm Soc. 2012;9(3):342–6.

36. Malcolme-Lawes LC, Lim PB, Koa-Wing M, Whinnett ZI, Jamil-Copley S, Hayat S, et al. Robotic assistance and general anaesthesia improve catheter stability and increase signal attenuation during atrial fibrillation ablation. Eur Eur Pacing Arrhythm Card Electrophysiol J Work Groups Card Pacing Arrhythm Card Cell Electrophysiol Eur Soc Cardiol. 2013;15(1):41–7.
37. Di Biase L, Conti S, Mohanty P, Bai R, Sanchez J, Walton D, et al. General anesthesia reduces the prevalence of pulmonary vein reconnection during repeat ablation when compared with conscious sedation: results from a randomized study. Heart Rhythm Off J Heart Rhythm Soc. 2011;8(3):368–72.
38. Roberts JD. Ambulatory anesthesia for the cardiac catheterization and electrophysiology laboratories. Anesthesiol Clin. 2014;32(2):381–6.
39. Shook DC, Savage RM. Anesthesia in the cardiac catheterization laboratory and electrophysiology laboratory. Anesthesiol Clin. 2009;27(1):47–56.
40. Pachulski RT, Adkins DC, Mirza H. Conscious sedation with intermittent midazolam and fentanyl in electrophysiology procedures. J Intervent Cardiol. 2001;14(2):143–6.
41. Kwak J. Anesthesia for electrophysiology studies and catheter ablations. Semin Cardiothorac Vasc Anesth. 2013;17(3):195–202.
42. Camci E, Koltka K, Sungur Z, Karadeniz M, Yavru A, Pembeci K, et al. Implantable cardioverter-defibrillator placement in patients with mild-to- moderate left ventricular dysfunction: hemodynamics and recovery profile with two different anesthetics used during deep sedation. J Cardiothorac Vasc Anesth. 2003;17(5):613–6.
43. Tsai T, Rodriguez-Diaz C, Deschner B, Thomas K, Wasnick JD. Thoracic paravertebral block for implantable cardioverter-defibrillator and laser lead extraction. J Clin Anesth. 2008;20(5):379–82.
44. Hayase J, Patel J, Narayan SM, Krummen DE. Percutaneous stellate ganglion block suppressing VT and VF in a patient refractory to VT ablation. J Cardiovasc Electrophysiol. 2013;24(8):926–8.
45. Tan AY, Abdi S, Buxton AE, Anter E. Percutaneous stellate ganglia block for acute control of refractory ventricular tachycardia. Heart Rhythm. 2012;9(12):2063–7.
46. Bourke T, Vaseghi M, Michowitz Y, Sankhla V, Shah M, Swapna N, et al. Neuraxial modulation for refractory ventricular arrhythmias: value of thoracic epidural anesthesia and surgical left cardiac sympathetic denervation. Circulation. 2010;121(21):2255–62.
47. Goode JS, Taylor RL, Buffington CW, Klain MM, Schwartzman D. High-frequency jet ventilation: utility in posterior left atrial catheter ablation. Heart Rhythm Off J Heart Rhythm Soc. 2006;3(1):13–9.
48. Hutchinson MD, Garcia FC, Mandel JE, Elkassabany N, Zado ES, Riley MP, et al. Efforts to enhance catheter stability improve atrial fibrillation ablation outcome. Heart Rhythm Off J Heart Rhythm Soc. 2013;10(3):347–53.
49. Raiten J, Elkassabany N, Mandel JE. The use of high-frequency jet ventilation for out of operating room anesthesia. Curr Opin Anaesthesiol. 2012;25(4):482–5.
50. Haines DE, Beheiry S, Akar JG, Baker JL, Beinborn D, Beshai JF, et al. Heart Rhythm Society expert consensus statement on electrophysiology laboratory standards: process, protocols, equipment, personnel, and safety. Heart Rhythm Off J Heart Rhythm Soc. 2014;11(8):e9–51.
51. Haeusler KG, Kirchhof P, Endres M. Left atrial catheter ablation and ischemic stroke. Stroke J Cereb Circ. 2012;43(1):265–70.

Chapter 13
Anesthesia for Cardioversion

Michele L. Sumler and McKenzie Hollon

Abstract Elective cardioversion is a procedure often requiring an off-site anesthetic. Cardioversion is a brief but painful procedure which utilizes electrical current for the treatment of cardiac dysrhythmias. The anesthetic management can vary widely, however general anesthesia, with out without airway control, is often indicated. Preoperative assessment, optimization, and preparation of an anesthetic plan for cardioversion presents several unique anesthetic considerations. Additionally, knowledge of the procedure and the underlying physiology and pathology assists the anesthesiologist in preparing for management of adverse events.

Keywords Synchronized Cardioversion • Atrial Fibrillation • Arrythmias • Off-site anesthetic

Introduction

Cardioversion is a brief but painful procedure utilizing electrical current for the treatment of cardiac dysrhythmias. Direct current cardioversion can be used to normalize abnormal cardiac rhythms, stable or unstable, except ventricular fibrillation. Indications for electrical cardioversion include supraventricular tachycardias, atrial fibrillation, atrial flutter, ventricular tachycardia with pulse and any reentrant tachycardia with narrow or wide QRS (with hemodynamic instability). Cardioversion is most commonly used to treat atrial fibrillation [1].

The circumstances for the procedure can vary widely, from an elective, off site anesthetic to an emergent procedure in a hemodynamically tenuous patient. In most cases, it is an outpatient procedure very rarely requiring an overnight hospital stay [2]. Beyond typical anesthetic considerations, the essential components of anesthetic management include understanding of the physiologic consequences of the underlying arrhythmia and the cardioversion. Familiarity with the defibrillation

M.L. Sumler, MD (✉) • M. Hollon, MD
Department of Anesthesiology, Emory University Hospital,
1364 Clifton Road, Atlanta, GA 30322, USA
e-mail: msumler@emory.edu; mmayo2@emory.edu

Table 13.1 Comparison of monophasic and biphasic waveforms

	Monophasic	Biphasic
Current direction	Unidirectional	Bidirectional
Waveform	Positive Sinusoidal	Rectilinear
Typical energy level	200–300 Joules	100–200 Joules
Median successful energy for cardioversion of AF	200 Joules	100 Joules

equipment and procedure, as well as knowledge of potential complications associated with cardioversions, are essential components of anesthetic management unique to this procedure.

Direct current cardioversion is preformed by sensing the intrinsic activity of the heart to synchronize the delivery of an electrical shock with the R wave of the QRS complex. The goal of synchronization is to ensure the electrical stimulation does not coincide with a vulnerable period of ventricular function. Synchronizing with the early portion of the QRS avoids the delivery of the shock during the terminal portion of the refractory state when adjacent myocardial fibers are in differing states of repolarization and chances of inducing ventricular fibrillation exists. Success of the cardioversion depends on multiple factors, including the patient's underlying disease as well as the effective delivery of electrical current to the atrial myocardium. Current may be delivered transcutaneously through chest electrodes, or more rarely through internal cardiac electrodes. Density of current delivered is influenced by the defibrillator's capacitor voltage, the output waveform, the size and position of the electrodes, and the impedance to flow between electrodes and the target myocardium [3]. The output waveform influences the energy delivery, and there are two types, monophasic and biphasic Table 13.1.

Biphasic shocks have been shown to require the use of less energy than monophasic delivery and to have higher success rates of cardioversion. Currently biphasic shocks represent the present standard for cardioversion of atrial fibrillation [4]. Other independent factors predicting successful cardioversion are thoracic impedance and duration of dysrhythmia [5]. The American Heart Association provides guidelines on the energy requirements based on which arrhythmia is being treated, with 120–200 joules being the current initial requirement for biphasic cardioversion of atrial fibrillation [6]. To avoid myocardial damage, some have suggested that the interval between consecutive shocks should be at least 1 min [7].

Cardioversion is contraindicated in dysrhythmias due to enhanced automaticity, such as digitalis toxicity and catecholamine-induced arrhythmias. Not only is cardioversion ineffective in these enhanced automaticity states, it is also associated with a higher incidence of post shock ventricular tachycardia and fibrillation. Additionally, cardioversion is contraindicated in multifocal atrial tachycardia as it does not address the underlying cause of dysrhythmia.

Focused History and Physical Findings in Patients Presenting for Elective Cardioversion

Patient assessment should begin with traditional pre-operative anesthetic evaluation, with particular attention paid to the cardiovascular system. The patient's history should be carefully reviewed for the presence of syncope, near-syncope, dizziness, chest pain, palpitations, and history of known bradycardias or tachycardias. Evaluation should include assessment of the electrocardiogram (EKG) to characterize the patient's current rhythm as well history of any known dysrhythmia triggers. It is important to be aware of prior pharmacologic and non-pharmacologic treatments of arrhythmias, as well as the details of any prior attempts at electrical conversion.

In the case of atrial fibrillation, the duration since onset may be unknown depending on the absence or presence of symptoms, and particular attention must be paid to the guidelines for evaluation of thrombus and appropriateness of anticoagulation. Further, the presence of implantable rhythm devices, pacemakers, ICDs, or dual devices, should be investigated. Improperly performed cardioversion in patients with these devices can damage the device or lead system and lead to malfunction or loss of capture. To ensure appropriate function, the device should be interrogated before and after cardioversion [8].

Is the Patient in an Optimum State to Proceed with Anesthesia

Preoperative management of known cardiac conditions, including arrhythmias, congestive heart failure, ischemia, and hypertension should be assessed. Review of the medication history should pay particular attention to use of beta blockers, antihypertensives, antiarrythmics, and statins. If the patient is on digoxin, the level should be checked and the patient should be assessed for signs of toxicity, however it is not necessary to routinely discontinue it prior to the cardioversion. Many patients undergoing cardioversion are on anticoagulation to prevent systemic embolization of thrombus, it is important to ensure that anticoagulation is adequate prior to proceeding with the procedure. An electrolyte panel is necessary for all patients undergoing cardioversion. Evaluation of labs and familiarity with patient's history is essential as DC cardioversion is contraindicated in patients with digitalis toxicity or with hypokalemia [1].

Further testing, including echocardiogram for evaluation of the presence of thrombus, catheterization, and stress testing may be indicated based on the patient's presentation in accordance with current guidelines. In all elective cases, NPO guidelines should be followed. In the event that cardioverion is being performed emergently, full stomach measures should be taken. These measures include preoxygenation and tracheal intubation. Succinylcholine is not contraindicated in this setting but bradyarrythmias may be precipitated and hyperkalemia may be worsened with its use. Occasionally, pregnant patients may present for cardioversion. Cardioversion has been found to be safe in this patient population, although it has been associated with fetal arrhythmias [9]. In cases when the fetus is viable, it is prudent to monitor the fetal heart rate throughout the procedure.

Preparation and Commonly Used Anesthetic Technique

It is common for these procedures to be done in off-site, or non-OR locations. Off site anesthetic challenges include unfamiliar equipment, personnel unfamiliar with anesthetic aspects of care and remoteness from additional anesthetic support. Preparing for an off-site anesthetic it is essential to ensure immediate availability of emergency drugs and airway equipment. American Society of Anesthesiologists (ASA) guidelines for standard monitors apply, and the minimum for cardioversion should include continuous EKG, pulse oximetry, BP monitoring, and likely continuous capnography [10]. An oxygen source, suction capability and a means to provide positive pressure ventilation should also be readily available.

A variety of anesthetics have been used successfully for cardioversion. Though external cardioversion is brief, the electrical stimulus can equal the intensity to that of surgical incision. An ideal anesthetic would provide analgesia, sedation, minimal hemodynamic compromise, and rapid recovery. The level of sedation required may depend on the setting and the patient, with adequate sedation allowing avoidance of recall of an unpleasant experience. Preventing or attenuating the effects of a catecholamine mediated stress response which could precipitate myocardial ischemia in this high risk population is paramount. The minimum appropriate anesthetic depth for elective cardioversion is likely deep sedation and often general anesthesia is required [1].

Volatile anesthetics are not often used for multiple reasons, including setting of the procedure often being offsite and very rarely requiring an endotracheal tube. There is no perfect IV drug however there are several small studies which have compared the efficacy of various IV agents including etomidate, propofol, fentanyl and benzodiazepines. Benzodiazepines have been shown to have a longer duration of effect and greater patient variability [11]. Propofol is associated with hypotension and a higher incidence of apnea than other IV anesthetics, but in comparison recovery time is more rapid. Etomidate produces myoclonus and pain on injection, however it's use is associated with less decrease in arterial blood pressure which may make it a better choice in patients with significant cardiac disease [12]. Comparison has been made between the combinations of etomidate and fentanyl, and propofol and fentanyl, with the etomidate and fentanyl combination having a shorter induction time and greater degree of hemodynamic stability [13]. A 2015 Cochrane database review looked at all the available literature and concluded that the evidence did not support superiority of any agent nor argue for the efficacy of additional analgesic medication to improve any metrics [14]. No matter which agent is most appropriate for the individual patient, careful titration to avoid hemodynamic compromise in a high risk population is prudent.

There are instances in which a transesophageal echocardiogram (TEE) is performed immediately prior to cardioversion to rule out the presence of thrombus. In these cases, the procedure may take up to 30 min. A nasal cannula will usually suffice, however further airway management may be required to keep a patient comfortable during the procedure. A study found that deep sedation with intravenous propofol and the use of a laryngeal mask airway (LMA), provided excellent conditions without the need to remove the TEE probe [15]. This provides a reasonable option in patients in which appropriate procedural sedation and airway maintenance become problematic.

Anticipated Adverse Events

As with all procedures, the possibility of adverse events is always present. Prevention and management of adverse events should begin with pre-operative planning, including obtaining adequate IV access for resuscitation, the use of monitors for early detection of adverse events, and the development of a plan for most likely adverse events.

Depending on the depth of anesthetic required, airway may become a particular concern in cases where deep sedation without a secured airway is employed. Airway management should include proper monitors, including ETCO2, and preparation of plan of action for intervention in the case of airway compromise. It may be appropriate to bag valve mask ventilate the patient for such a brief procedure if there is no underlying pulmonary disease, the patient has been appropriately NPO, and there are no concerning findings on the airway exam. In patients with hemodynamic disturbances or concern for aspiration it may be wise to intubate the trachea for airway control.

The most common complications are arrhythmias, such as atrial, ventricular, and junctional premature beats. Other arrhythmias can also been seen transiently, including bradycardia and short periods of sinus arrest, and these commonly subside spontaneously [14]. Animal experiments have demonstrated a wide margin of safety between the energy required for cardioversion of atrial fibrillation and that associated with myocardial depression. Even without apparent myocardial damage, transient ST-segment elevation may appear on the EKG after cardioversion, and the anesthesia team should be aware of this potentially normal variant [16]. Rarely, high energy shocks can lead to myocardial necrosis which should manifest as immediate ST segment elevation which lasts for 1–2 min. EKG changes which last longer than 2 min typically indicate myocardial injury unrelated to the shock. However, more serious dysrhythmias, including ventricular fibrillation can result in cases of severe heart disease, improper synchronization, high amounts of electrical energy conduction, electrolyte abnormalities or digitalis toxicity. In some patients with longstanding atrial fibrillation, there may be underlying sinus node dysfunction or intrinsic conduction defects which are unmasked by cardioversion. These patients should be evaluated thoroughly by cardiology prior to cardioversion so that a transvenous or transcutaneous pacemaker can be used prophylactically if deemed appropriate [17].

Hemodynamic disturbances often occur and can lead to myocardial dysfunction. The population undergoing cardioversion is typically high risk, often with underlying cardiac disease and the absence of coronary perfusion during even a brief arrest may result in ischemia. Patients may experience a phenomenon called myocardial stunning which is myocardial dysfunction which is reversible within the first 24–48 h. To avoid inaccurate assessments, evaluation of cardiac function should be delayed until at least 48 h after the cardioversion [18]. Rarely, in patients with valvular heart disease or poor left ventricular systolic function, transient pulmonary edema may be seen.

Embolic and ischemic stroke are possible complications, and make this procedure contraindicated in patients with a known presence of thrombus. Thromboembolization is not uncommon, and has been associated with cardioversion in 1–7 % of patients not give prophylactic anticoagulation before cardioversion of atrial fibrillation [19]. For this reason, evaluation of coagulopathy and assurance of adequate anti-coagulation must be completed prior to the procedure. For elective cardioversions, patients who have been in atrial fibrillation for greater than 48 h, an echocardiogram should be performed to rule out the presence of an intracardiac (left atrial) thrombus. American College of Cardiology and American Heart Association guidelines recommend anticoagulation for 3–4 weeks before and after cardioversion. After completion of cardioversion, a neurologic exam for focal deficits should be assessed [1].

Painful skin burns can occur after cardioversion, and are most likely due to improper placement of the electrodes. Skin burns are less common with biphasic defibrillators and with the use of gel based pads. Some advocate prophylactic use of steroid cream and or topical ibuprofen to reduce pain and inflammation.

References

1. American College of Cardiology/American Heart Association Task Force on Practice Guidelines; European Society of Cardiology Committee for Practice Guidelines (Writing Committee to Revise the 2001 Guidelines for Management of Patients With Atrial Fibrillation); European Heart Rhythm Association; Heart Rhythm Society. Circulation. 2006;114: e257–354.
2. Lesser MF. Safety and efficacy of in-office cardioversion for treatment of supraventricular arrhythmias. Am J Cardiol. 1990;66:1267–8.
3. Ewy GA. The optimal technique for electrical cardioversion of atrial fibrillation. Clin Cardiol. 1994;17:79–84.
4. Page RL, Kerber RE, Russell JK, et al. Biphasic versus monophasic shock waveform for conversion of atrial fibrillation: the results of an international randomized, double-blind multicenter trial. J Am Coll Cardiol. 2002;39:1956–63.
5. Mittal S, Ayati S, Stein KM, et al. Transthoracic cardioversion of atrial fibrillation: comparison of rectilinear biphasic versus damped sine wave monophasic shocks. Circulation. 2000;101: 1282–7.

6. Atkins DL, Passman RS, Halperin HR, Samson RA, White RD, et al. Part 6: electrical therapies: automated external defibrillators, defibrillation, cardioversion, and pacing: 2010 American Heart Association Guidelines for Cardiopulmonary Resuscitation and Emergency Cardiovascular Care. Circulation. 2010;122(18 Suppl 3):S706–19.
7. Dahl CF, Ewy GA, Warner ED, et al. Myocardial necrosis from direct current countershock. Effect of paddle electrode size and time interval between discharges. Circulation. 1974;50:956–61.
8. Gould L, Patel S, Gomes GI, Chokshi AB. Pacemaker failure following external defibrillation. Pacing Clin Electrophysiol. 1981;4(5):575–7.
9. Schroeder JS, Harrison DC. Repeated cardioversion during pregnancy. Am J Cardiol. 1971;27:445–6.
10. Statement on nonoperating room anesthetizing locations committee of origin: standards and practice parameters (Approved by the ASA House of Delegates on October 19, 1994, and last amended on October 16, 2013).
11. Canessa R. Anesthesia for elective cardioversion: a comparison of four anesthetic agents. J Cardiothorac Vasc Anesth. 1991;5(6):566–8.
12. Desai PM, Kane D, Sarkar MS. Cardioversion: what to choose? Etomidate or propofol. Ann Card Anaesth. 2015;18(3):306–11.
13. Kalogridaki M. Anaesthesia for cardioversion: a prospective randomised comparison of propofol and etomidate combined with fentanyl. Hellenic J Cardiol. 2011;52(6):483–8.
14. Rabbino MD, Likoff W, Dreifus LS. Complications and limitations of direct current countershock. JAMA. 1964;190;417–20.
15. Ferson D, Thakar D, Swafford J, Sinha A, Sapire K, Arens J. Use of deep intravenous sedation with propofol and the laryngeal mask airway during transesophageal echocardiography. J Cardiovasc Vasc Anesth. 2003;17:443–6.
16. Lewis SR, Nicholson A, Reed SS, Kenth JJ, Alderson P, Smith AF. Anaesthetic and sedative agents used for electrical cardioversion. Cochrane Database Syst Rev. 2015;(3):CD01082.
17. Mancini GB, Goldberger AL. Cardioversion of atrial fibrillation: consideration of embolization, anticoagulation, prophylactic pacemaker, and long-term success. Am Heart J. 1982;104:617–21.
18. Kern KB, Hilwig RW, Rhee KH, Berg RA. Myocardial dysfunction after resuscitation from cardiac arrest: an example of global myocardial stunning. J Am Coll Cardiol. 1996;28(1):232–40.
19. Bjerkelund CJ, Orning OM. The efficacy of anticoagulant therapy in preventing embolism related to D.C. electrical conversion of atrial fibrillation. Am J Cardiol. 1969;23:208–16.

Chapter 14
Anesthesia for Cardiac Ablation Procedures

Igor O. Zhukov and Yuriy O. Zhukov

Abstract Ablations in the electrophysiology (EP) laboratory provide unique challenges to an anesthesiologist. The patient's underlying pathology can be confounded by the periods of induced arrhythmias, total immobility is necessary due to sensitivity of electrophysiological mapping equipment, the access to patient's airway and vasculature may be complicated; these nuances differentiate EP laboratory from the operating room environment. Routine anesthetic techniques can be applied to the ablation procedures if these caveats are discussed with proceduralist to ensure optimal patient safety and procedure success, allowing for extra monitoring modalities, anticipation of potential complications, and vigilant perioperative care.

Keywords General anesthesia • Sedation • Monitored Anesthesia Care • Electrophysiology • Ablation • Arrhythmia • Atrial Fibrillation • Ventricular Tachycardia • Pulmonary Vein • Atrio-esophageal fistula • Transesophageal echocardiography • TEE • LVAD • Impella

Introduction

A large number of procedures are performed in the EP laboratory either as an alternative to a more invasive surgical intervention or as a unique solution to patient's particular disorder. The majority of these procedures are performed without anesthesia personnel and may involve local anesthesia only, or minimal, moderate, and even deep sedation by the EP staff. However, anesthesiologist's presence is

I.O. Zhukov, MD (✉)
Division of Cardiothoracic Anesthesiology, Emory University,
1364 Clifton Rd NE, Atlanta, GA 30322, USA
e-mail: izhukov@emory.edu

Y.O. Zhukov, MD
Department of Cardiothoracic Surgery, University Hospitals Elyria Medical Center,
Elyria, OH, USA
e-mail: Yuriy.Zhukov@UHHospitals.org

© Springer International Publishing Switzerland 2017
B.G. Goudra, P.M. Singh (eds.), *Out of Operating Room Anesthesia*,
DOI 10.1007/978-3-319-39150-2_14

179

sometimes requested for the ablation procedures when the procedure or the patient are complex enough to preclude successful accomplishment of the ablation with minimal or moderate sedation only.

Sedation and Anesthesia

The American Society of Anesthesiologists (ASA) provides clear definitions for minimal, moderate, and deep sedation. The sedation is differentiated from general anesthesia based on patient's responsiveness, the need for an airway intervention, presence of spontaneous ventilation, and cardiovascular status (Table 14.1) [1].

The anesthesiologist's presence is often requested if deep sedation and/or anesthesia are required; the guidelines set by the ASA indicate that the practitioner providing a specific level of sedation must be able to rescue the patient who inadvertently entered a deeper plane of sedation. For example, a practitioner administering moderate sedation must be able to recover the patient from deep sedation, while provider prescribing deep sedation must possess the skill level necessary for reversal of general anesthetic [1]. Bubien, et.al, published a consensus of North American Society of Pacing and Electrophysiology (NASPE) endorsing the need for anesthesia service during deep sedation and general anesthesia [2]. Additional guidelines related to provider's qualification such as Advanced Cardiac Life Support training, certifications, scope of practice limitations, and the list of sedation drugs permissible for use by non-anesthesiologist staff are often generated within each institution.

Table 14.1 Distinguishing features of various sedation levels

	Minimal sedation/ anxiolysis	Moderate sedation/ analgesia ("conscious sedation")	Deep sedation/ analgesia	General anesthesia
Responsiveness	Normal response to verbal stimulation	Purposeful** response to verbal or tactile stimulation	Purposeful** response following repeated or painful stimulation	Unarousable even with painful stimulus
Airway	Unaffected	No intervention required	Intervention may be required	Intervention often required
Spontaneous ventilation	Unaffected	Adequate	May be inadequate	Frequently inadequate
Cardiovascular function	Unaffected	Usually maintained	Usually maintained	May be impaired

** Withdrawal from painful stimulus does not constitute a purposeful movement
With permission: Ref. [1]

Benefits and Tradeoffs of General Anesthesia

It has been recognized that scheduling ablation procedures with anesthesiology service providing the sedation or general anesthesia may result in the increased total cost of the procedure [3, 4]; this is likely the result of the direct anesthesiology service cost as well as the requirement for post-anesthesia recovery period in a specialized unit, potential scheduling delays while anesthesia turnover occurs, etc. These difficulties associated with anesthesia involvement have been contrasted with the great success of managing these cases with minimal and moderate sedation provided by a non-anesthesiologist [3, 4]; additionally, deep sedation with Propofol by a non-anesthesia provider is commonplace in Europe and has a great safety record [5]. Therefore, involvement of the anesthesia service is only warranted if the demonstrable patient benefit exists, the procedure carries an elevated complication risk, or the patient is not able to tolerate sedation due to physical or psychosocial reasons. On the other hand, it was observed that during Atrial fibrillation (Afib) ablation employing general anesthesia, both the time of fluoroscopy and total procedure duration were significantly shorter while resulting in a higher cure rate of atrial fibrillation, thus potentially offsetting the implied cost of general anesthesia [6].

To further complicate the decision to proceed with general anesthesia, it was observed that patients undergoing ablation under general anesthesia had higher rate of thermal esophageal injury [7]. However, in this particular study both sedation and general anesthesia groups exhibited zero incidence of atrioesophageal fistula formation and the injuries resolved spontaneously without any sequellae

Equipment and Monitoring

The American Society of Anesthesiologists extensively described the minimum monitoring requirements of the patients undergoing general anesthesia for a surgical procedure; this is applicable to ablation procedures performed under general anesthesia, as well as deep sedation and Monitored Anesthesia Care (MAC) [8].

Pulse oximetry is a rapid, quantitative, and reliable method of assessing patient's oxygenation status. It employs transillumination of tissue, usually at the fingertip, earlobe, or nare with a minimum of two wavelengths of light, thus allowing resolution of oxyhemoglobin and deoxyhemoglobin concentrations. When coupled with a variable pitch audio output this monitor provides a continuous background information about both patient's heart rate and blood oxygen concentration, and thus it is one of the essential monitors recommended by ASA during general anesthesia and deep sedation [8].

Ventilation monitoring during mechanical ventilation routinely consists of automatic tidal volumes, circuit integrity, and airway pressure monitoring by the circuitry of the anesthesia machine. Additionally, inhaled and exhaled gas spectroscopy reports fractions of inspired gases and volatile anesthetics in addition to producing a continuous capnography waveform [9]. In the absence of invasive ventilation capnography remains a valuable tool for monitoring spontaneous ventilation as it allows for apnea detection much earlier than pulse oximetry alone.

Circulation is probably the most redundantly monitored vital sign as continuous EKG (electrocardiogram) and pulse oximetry provide information about patient's heart rate. Additionally, multiple-lead EKG tracing is a valuable tool for detecting cardiac ischemia. Leads II and V5 are most commonly monitored and provide at least 80% sensitivity for myocardial ischemia, while modern telemetry machines are capable of automatically monitoring five or more leads and will alert the provider should ST morphology change.

Non-invasive blood pressure (NIBP) is recommended by the ASA to be cycled at least every 5 min and is recommended even for patients in whom invasive blood pressure assessment is employed. NIBP is reliable and is not prone to calibration errors associated with pressure transducers. Also, arterial blood pressure is sometimes transduced via the shared sheath introducers which can be subject to thrombosis, malposition, or occlusion by the ablation device. Additionally, at the time of hemodynamic instability when dedicated BP reading is vital, these sheaths may need to be exchanged for an intraaortic balloon pump (IABP) or a peripheral arterial cardiopulmonary bypass (CPB) cannula.

Body temperature monitoring is required during ablations under general anesthesia, as these procedures routinely last greater than 30 min, and often exceed 3–6 h. Both passive and active rewarming measures should be employed pre-induction and should continue throughout the procedure; these include warm blankets, socks and head covers, forced air warming, fluid warmers, conservation of airway moisture, and other site-specific means to maintain normothermia.

Radiofrequency (RF) ablation of the posterior surface of the heart exposes the patient to the risk of thermal injury to the esophagus, which is implicated in the development of an atrio-esophageal fistula, a dreaded and serious complication of left atrial ablation. The esophageal temperature can be monitored using either a standard esophageal temperature probe, or a purpose-designed unit with multiple thermistors that measures esophageal temperature along the length of the left atrium. Usually these monitors are placed with fluoroscopic guidance to ensure optimal sensitivity [10]. Once a pre-determined esophageal temperature is reached the ablation is paused or power to the ablation probe is reduced to mitigate the risk of injury. It is also worth mentioning that there is a unique potential for interference of radiofrequency used for ablation and esophageal monitoring probe. Deneke, et.al. hypothesized that thermal esophageal injury may occur in patients with esophageal temperature probes due to the probe acting as a receiver of the RF energy, which is then converted to heat; this pattern of esophageal ulceration was not seen in the unmonitored control cohort [11].

Transesophageal echocardiography (TEE), while not recommended as a routine monitoring modality in the operating room nor in the EP laboratory, has a unique application in the setting of atrial fibrillation. Given the prevalence of left atrial thrombus in approximately 10–15% of patients with atrial fibrillation [12], and an estimated 3.5 fold increase in thromboembolic complications, TEE screening is commonly, though not universally [13] performed before ablation procedures or cardioversion. Patients who are treated with long-term anticoagulation are not completely protected from forming left atrial thrombi (LAT). In a very recent meta-analysis Di Minno, et al. demonstrated LAT incidence of 3.5 % in cohorts that were reported to be 100 % anticoagulated for atrial fibrillation. The overall safety of TEE needs a separate discussion with the patient, especially those with relative or absolute contraindications including esophageal or GI pathology, history of chest irradiation, or a risk of GI bleeding from varices [14]. While the overall risk of esophageal perforation is reported to be 1:1000 or less [14], and while only a handful of reports have been generated on esophageal injury during ablation procedures [15], combined risk of esophageal damage from radiofrequency ablation and TEE probe manipulation have to be weighed carefully in a patient who is frail or otherwise predisposed to this complication.

Anesthetic Considerations: Preoperative Evaluation

As eluded above, general anesthesia is reserved for ablation procedures in which procedural challenges or patient-specific comorbidities may preclude successful completion of ablation with non-anesthetist administered sedation. Usually, this referral is initiated by the primary EP physician and thereafter is achieved through scheduling a pre-anesthesia assessment. Anesthesiologist who is performing the procedure is tasked with risk-stratifying the patient according to cardiac and pulmonary comorbidities, obesity and potential for obstructive sleep apnea (OSA), renal dysfunction, hematologic derangements, anticoagulation status, history of anesthetic problems in the past, allergies, and pertinent chronic medications.

Many ablation procedures require mapping of arrhythmogenic foci which is accomplished by inciting arrhythmias either chemically or electrically. These bouts of increased heart rate place additional strain on myocardial supply and demand balance, possibly exacerbating pre-existent coronary artery disease symptoms. Therefore, a thorough cardiac history and physical examination should be the center of pre-anesthesia evaluation.

Most recent guidelines published jointly by the ASA, AHA and ACC have simplified the risk stratification into 2 instead of 3 groups: Low risk of major adverse cardiac event (MACE) and intermediate or high risk of MACE. Procedures that require general anesthesia would commonly fall into latter category, and thus a reasonable functional status (>4 METs) must be documented, or a cardiovascular evaluation must be performed [16].

Anesthetic Considerations: Intraoperative Management

Selection of sedation strategy between monitored anesthesia care (MAC) or general anesthesia requires a discussion and agreement between the cardiologist and the anesthesiologist. Patient-specific comorbidities as described above and procedural factors such as the need for prolonged immobility, hybrid intracardial/epicardial ablation, and the need for invasive monitoring or TEE assessment will influence the decision to proceed with general anesthesia. The need for muscle relaxation to achieve absolute immobility will require placing an endotracheal tube, as opposed to maintaining the patient spontaneously ventilating with or without a Laryngeal Mask Airway (LMA). If a decision is made to secure the airway with an LMA, one must consider the difficulty reaching the patient's airway once X-ray unit is moved into position and the undesirable loss of arrhythmia mapping if a patient is shifted during intubation in the middle of the procedure.

Patients with known difficult airway and patients with unfavorable airway exam may be better served with intubation at the beginning of the procedure using a combination of video laryngoscopy, fiberoptic bronchoscope, and optimal intubation positioning, etc. Fluoroscopy tables also lack familiar mobility and it may be difficult to elevate and flex the patient, or use reverse Trendelenburg positioning; an induction and intubation while patient is lying on a more flexible transport gurney may be a better option.

Induction drug selection is generally driven more by the patient-specific factors and comorbidities rather than the type of ablation procedure. The majority of drugs used to induce general anesthesia have a very short duration of action and are not consequential to the success of arrhythmia mapping. In selecting drugs for deep sedation Wutzler and colleagues demonstrated a predictable sympathomimetic effect of Ketamine, as compared to Propofol, which has not influenced the inducibility of arrhythmia or the efficacy of ablation, but increased the heart rate and blood pressure in a predictable manner [17]. This effect can be exploited for patients in whom cardiac depressant effects of Propofol are undesirable. Etomidate is another excellent drug for induction of anesthesia in a patient with cardiovascular disease, due to minimal change in contractility and the systemic vascular resistance (SVR).

Maintenance of anesthesia is a debated topic with very little data to provide evidence for or against inhalational vs intravenous technique: Sharpe et.al. demonstrated no significant effect of common intravenous and inhalational anesthetics on sinoatrial node, atrioventricular conduction or accessory pathways implicated in Wolf-Parkinson-White syndrome [18–21]. Similarly, there was no difference in effectiveness of ablation of supraventricular tachycardia in children anesthetized with either propofol or isoflurane [22]. Therefore, factors other than arrhythmia inducibility are important when selecting intravenous versus inhalational anesthetic. The need for High Frequency Jet Ventilation (HFJV), risk of post-operative nausea and vomiting (PONV), or susceptibility to malignant hyperthermia (MH) make total intravenous anesthetic (TIVA) most desirable.

During arrhythmia mapping, the proceduralist may request a provocative maneuver for induction of arrhythmia; these are often discussed during the pre-procedure time out and may include administration of Adenosine, Isoproterenol, or rapid pacing. These periods will require increased vigilance both by the anesthesiologist and the cardiologist performing the ablation to ensure that patient is hemodynamically stable, the cerebral perfusion is maintained, and myocardial oxygen delivery is not compromised.

Complications of the Ablation Procedure

Arrhythmia ablation is estimated to carry a mortality risk of 0.1 % with tamponade, stroke, and atrio-esophageal fistula accounting for 25 %, 16 %, and 16 % of these mortalities respectively [13]. Complication rates vary depending on the ablation modality employed (radiofrequency vs. cryoablation), the experience of the provider, and the patient's comorbidities. Commonly cited complication rates, though vary from source-to-source, are summarized in the Table 14.2 below: [13, 23].

Tamponade is the most common serious complication with the incidence estimated at 1.5 %. Rapidly diagnosed by measurement of cardiac filling pressures, transesophageal or transthoracic echocardiography, or fluoroscopy this is usually managed via subxyphoid drainage using Seldinger technique and reversal of anticoagulation [13]. Concomitantly, the anesthesiologist can temporize the symptoms of cardiac tamponade by administration of intravenous fluids, blood products, and initiating or increasing administration of Epinephrine, Norepinephrine, or Vasopressin. In extreme cases, conversion to surgical drainage is indicated and the presence of cardiac anesthesiologist capable of managing multiple vasopressors, assessing TEE data, and leading resuscitative efforts is desirable.

Stroke is a second leading cause of mortality with multiple implicated etiologies. Commonly the anti-arrhythmic medications are witheld prior to the ablation which may elevate the risk of cerebrovascular accident (CVA). Also, if left atrium or ventricle are instrumented during the ablation, the injured endothelium can serve as a source of CVA-causing thrombi during the procedure. Additionally, patients remain at risk for delayed thrombotic CVA for several weeks post-procedure. Air embolism is prevented by meticulous de-airing of the catheters, while thrombotic complications stemming from thrombus formation on the ablation device are mitigated by systemic anticoagulation during procedure. Heparin is the most common anticoagulant of choice with goal Activated Clotting Time (ACT) of 300–400 s; the anticoagulation strategy is usually discussed during the preoperative time-out [13].

Phrenic nerve injury is relatively common non-life threatening complication, particularly when cryoablation of the right superior pulmonary vein is performed. It is currently recommended to use superior vena cava (SVC) pacing and diaphragmatic

Table 14.2 Incidence of complications during cardiac ablation procedures

Any serious complication	6 %
Tamponade	1.5 %
Stroke	0–7 %
Atrioesophageal fistula	0.1–0.25 %
Esophageal injury	0–17 %
Vascular injury	0–13 %
Phrenic nerve injury	1–6.5 %
Pulmonary vein stenosis	1.3–3.4 %
Pericardial effusion	2.9 %
Vagus nerve injury	1 %

monitoring for prevention of phrenic injury. In this case the use of muscle relaxants needs to be discussed with the proceduralist, and careful monitoring of airway pressure waveform should be done by the anesthesiologist during SVC pacing to detect diaphragmatic motion [13].

Unstable Ventricular Tachycardia Ablation

Unlike ablation of supraventricular arrhythmias, which can largely be managed with combination of judicious anesthetic delivery and correction of hemodynamic instability through vasopressor administration alone, recalcitrant ventricular tachycardia mapping may require longer periods of heart rhythms that are not well tolerated, especially by the patient with previous myocardial injury.

These cases realize a greater benefit from cardiac anesthesiologist's presence for placement of invasive monitors, careful titration of multiple vasopressors, transesophageal echocardiography, and in some cases placement and management of a percutaneous Left Ventricular Assist Device (LVAD). Pre-emptive placement of an Impella™ LVAD may allow for longer periods of ventricular tachycardia without significant loss of cerebral or coronary perfusion, which in turn may allow for a higher success of ablation or even permitting an ablation in a patient otherwise unfit for such procedure [24, 25]. The device is usually inserted percutaneously into femoral artery and advanced into the left ventricle (LV) so that is traverses the aortic valve. Positioning across the aortic valve is confirmed by pressure differential sensors at the inlet and the outflow of the device, fluoroscopy, and TEE. These miniature (9Fr) axial-flow LVAD units are capable of flowing up to 5 litres per minute and providing support for up to 6 h and are indicated for salvage of unstable patients or performance of procedures that otherwise could require cardiopulmonary bypass [26].

Post Anesthesia Recovery

Recovery of patients after ablation procedures poses its own challenge. The pre/post procedure unit which handles routine ablations and catheterization procedures is well-equipped to resolve issues arising from placement of percutaneous access, potential for occasional arrhythmia, fluid overload due to excess cooling fluid administration through the ablation system or flush lines, etc. However, patients recovering from general anesthesia have added requirements for monitoring of ventilation and oxygenation, potential for residual neuromuscular blockade, and post-operative nausea and vomiting (PONV); these patients historically have recovered in a specialized post anesthesia care unit (PACU) and follow specific discharge guidelines [27].

Taking into account that general anesthetic is employed in more challenging patients and procedures, the recovery is best arranged via PACU. By doing so the standard of anesthesia recovery is maintained, and last minute confusion of patient disposition is avoided, but this does prolong the turnover time, as the recovery unit is often designed to be in close proximity to the operating rooms and not the electrophysiology suite. Nonetheless, avoidance of patient complications offsets turnover prolongation both financially and ethically.

Conclusion

Anesthesia for Electrophysiology ablation procedures can be challenging and rewarding task. These anesthetics will require maximal planning between the anesthesiologist and the cardiologist to ensure expedient and safe delivery of patient care. Addressing key tasks during the pre-procedure time-out, such as need for invasive monitoring lines, prolonged or unstable arrhythmia potential, need for avoidance of muscle relaxation, performing intraoperative TEE or esophageal temperature monitoring, and anticoagulation goals eliminates unnecessary confusion and may prevent complications.

An induction of general anesthesia can be performed with drugs that anesthesiologist deems appropriate for the patient, such as Propofol, Etomidate, Ketamine, or combination thereof. If no long-term muscle relaxation is desired for the procedure, either Succinylcholine or a small dose of intermediate-acting non-depolarizing muscle relaxant (NDMR) can be used for intubation. Alternatively, patient can be intubated with a judicious administration of induction and narcotic drugs, which can be augmented with addition of intratracheal lidocaine.

Endotracheal tube has advantage over LMA as it simplifies access for esophageal temperature monitoring and TEE insertion.

Intraoperative vasopressor use should be dictated by the depth of anesthetic needed for immobility if NDMR is not administered, patient's comorbidities, and cardiac function throughout the procedure. Depending on a specific patient needs, Phenylephrine, Norepinephrine, Vasopressin, and Epinephrine – all have a place as a vasoactive drug of choice.

The process of extubation must be controlled and well-planned to ensure that the patient is not agitated and reflexively flexing his or her legs immediately after the vascular access sheaths have been removed. Deep extubation can be considered in patients with an otherwise easy airway and no additional aspiration risk. PACU staff need to be alerted if groin hematoma formation is a concern for a more vigilant monitoring. Finally, any other procedure-related concerns, residual anticoagulation and last ACT value, potential for arrhythmias post procedure, and any pre-existing neurological deficits that may mask discovery of a CVA need to be clearly communicated.

References

1. Continuum of depth of sedation: definition of general anesthesia and levels of sedation/analgesia. ASA Quality Management and Department Administration; 2009. p. 1–2.
2. Bubien RS, Fisher JD, Gentzel JA, Murphy EK, Irwin ME, Shea JB, et al. NASPE expert consensus document: use of IV (conscious) sedation/analgesia by nonanesthesia personnel in

patients undergoing arrhythmia specific diagnostic, therapeutic, and surgical procedures. Pacing Clin Electrophysiol. 1998;21(2):375–85.

3. Kezerashvili A, Fisher JD, DeLaney J, Mushiyev S, Monahan E, Taylor V, et al. Intravenous sedation for cardiac procedures can be administered safely and cost-effectively by non-anesthesia personnel. J Interv Card Electrophysiol. 1998;21(1):43–51.

4. Conway A, Page K, Rolley JX, Worrall-Carter L. Nurse-administered procedural sedation and analgesia in the cardiac catheter laboratory: an integrative review. Int J Nurs Stud. 2011;48:1012–23.

5. Kottkamp H, Hindricks G, Eitel C, Muller C, Siedziako A, Koch J, et al. Deep sedation for catheter ablation of atrial fibrillation: a prospective study in 650 consecutive patients. J Cardiovasc Electrophysiol. 2011;22:1339–43.

6. Di Biase L, Conti S, Mohanty P, Bai R, Sanchez J, Walton D, et al. General anesthesia reduces the prevalence of pulmonary vein reconnection during repeat ablation when compared with conscious sedation: results from a randomized study. Heart Rhythm. 2011;8(3):368–72.

7. Di Biase L, Saenz LC, Burkhardt DJ, Vacca M, Elayi CS, Barrett CD, Natale A. Esophageal capsule endoscopy after radiofrequency catheter ablation for atrial fibrillation documented higher risk of luminal esophageal damage with general anesthesia as compared with conscious sedation. Circ Arrhythm Electrophysiol. 2009;2(2):108–12.

8. Standards for basic anesthetic monitoring. ASA Standards and Practice Parameters. 2010;1–3.

9. Anesthesia gas monitoring: evolution of a de facto standard of care. ProMed Strategies. 2009:1–10.

10. Liu E, Shehata M, Liu T, Amorn A, Cingolani E, Kannarkat V, et al. Prevention of esophageal thermal injury during radiofrequency ablate on for atrial fibrillation. J Interv Card Electrphysiol. 2012;35:35–44.

11. Deneke T, Bunz K, Bastian A, Pasler M, Anders H, Lehmann R, et al. Utility of esophageal temperature monitoring during pulmonary vein isolation for atrial fibrillation using duty-cycled phased radiofrequency ablation. J Cardiovasc Electrophysiol. 2011;22(3):255–61.

12. Di Minno MN, Ambrosino P, Dello Russo A, Casella M, Tremoli E, Tondo C. Prevalence of left atrial thrombus in patients with non-valvular atrial fibrillation. A systematic review and meta-analysis of the literature. Thromb Haemost. 2016;115(3):663–77.

13. Calkins H, Kuck KH, Cappato R, Brugada J, Camm AJ, Chen SA, et al. 2012 HRS/EHRA/ECAS expert consensus statement on catheter and surgical ablation of atrial fibrillation: recommendations for patient selection, procedural techniques, patient management and follow-up, definitions, endpoints, and research trial design. Europace. 2012;14:528–606.

14. Hahn RT, Abraham T, Adams MS, Bruce CJ, Glas KE, Lang RM, Reeves ST, Shanewise JS, Siu SC, Stewart W, Picard MH. Guidelines for performing a comprehensive transesophageal echocardiographic examination: recommendations from the American Society of Echocardiography and the Society of Cardiovascular Anesthesiologists. J Am Soc Echocardiogr. 2013;26(9):921–64.

15. Kim MY, Ng FS, Ariff B, Hanna GB, Whinnett Z, Kanagaratnam P, Tanner M, Lim PB. Extensive intramural esophageal hematoma after transesophageal echocardiography during atrial fibrillation ablation. Circulation. 2015;132(19):1847–9.

16. Fleisher LA, Fleischmann KE, Auerbach AD, Barnason SA, Beckman JA, Bozkurt B, Davila-Roman VG, Gerhard-Herman MD, Holly TA, Kane GC, Marine JE, Nelson MT, Spencer CC, Thompson A, Ting HH, Uretsky BF, Wijeysundera DN. 2014 ACC/AHA guideline on perioperative cardiovascular evaluation and management of patients undergoing noncardiac surgery. J Am Coll Cardiol. 2014;64(22):e77–137.

17. Wutzler A, Huemer M, Boldt LH, Parwani AS, Attanasio P, Tscholl V, Haverkamp W. Effects of deep sedation on cardiac electrophysiology in patients undergoing radiofrequency ablation of supraventricular tachycardia: impact of propofol and ketamine. Europace. 2013;15(7):1019–24.

18. Sharpe MD, Dobkowski WB, Murkin JM, Klein G, Guiraudon G, Yee R. Alfentanil-midazolam anaesthesia has no electrophysiological effects upon the normal conduction system or accessory pathways in patients with Wolff-Parkinson-White syndrome. Can J Anesth. 1992;39(8):816–21.
19. Sharpe MD, Dobkowski WB, Murkin JM, Klein G, Guiraudon G, Yee R. The electrophysiologic effects of volatile anesthetics and sufentanil on the normal atrioventricular conduction system and accessory pathways in Wolff-Parkinson-White syndrome. Anesthesiology. 1994;80(1):63–70.
20. Sharpe MD, Dobkowski WB, Murkin JM, Klein G, Yee R. Propofol has no direct effect on sinoatrial node function or on normal atrioventricular and accessory pathway conduction in Wolff-Parkinson-White syndrome during alfentanil/midazolam anesthesia. Anesthesiology. 1995;82(4):888–95.
21. Sharpe MD, Cuillerier DJ, Lee JK, Basta M, Krahn AD, Klein GJ, Yee R. Sevoflurane has no effect on sinoatrial node function or on normal atrioventricular and accessory pathway conduction in Wolff-Parkinson-White syndrome during alfentanil/midazolam anesthesia. Anesthesiology. 1999;90(1):60–5.
22. Erb TO, Kanter RJ, Hall JM, Gan TJ, Kern FH, Schulman SR. Comparison of electrophysiologic effects of propofol and isoflurane-based anesthetics in children undergoing radiofrequency catheter ablation for supraventricular tachycardia. J Am Soc Anesth. 2002;96(6): 1386–94.
23. Andrade JG, Khairy P, Guerra PG, Deyell MW, Rivard L, Macle L, Thibault B, Talajic M, Roy D, Dubuc M. Efficacy and safety of cryoballoon ablation for atrial fibrillation: a systematic review of published studies. Heart Rhythm. 2011;9:1444–51.
24. Abuissa H, Roshan J, Lim B, Asirvatham SJ. Use of the Impella™ microaxial blood pump for ablation of hemodynamically unstable ventricular tachycardia. J Cardiovasc Electrophysiol. 2010;21(4):458–61.
25. Miller MA, Dukkipati SR, Chinitz JS, Koruth JS, Mittnacht AJ, Napolitano C, Reddy VY. Percutaneous hemodynamic support with Impella 2.5 during scar-related ventricular tachycardia ablation (PERMIT 1). Circ: Arrhythm Electrophysiol. 2012:CIRCEP-112.
26. Abiomed.com [Internet]. Danvers, massachusetts. [Cited 2015 Dec 6]. Available from: http://www.abiomed.com/products/impella-5-0/.
27. Apfelbaum JL, Silverstein JH, Chung FF, Connis RT, Fillmore RB, Hunt SE. Practice guidelines for postanesthetic care: an updated report by the American Society of Anesthesiologists Task Force on Postanesthetic Care. Anesthesiology. 2013;118(2):1–17.

Further Reading

Bhatt HV, Syros G, Greco M, Miller M, Fischer GW. Ablation therapy for atrial fibrillation: implications for the anesthesiologist. J Cardiothorac Vasc Anesth. 2015;29(5):1341–56.
Calkins H, Brugada J, Packer DL, Cappato R, Chen S, Crijns HJG. HRS/EHRA/ECAS expert consensus statement on catheter and surgical ablation of atrial fibrillation: recommendations for personnel, policy, procedures and follow-up. Heart Rhythm. 2007;4(6):816–59.
Geršak B, Zembala MO, Müller D, Folliguet T, Jan M, Kowalski O, Erler S, Bars C, Robic B, Filipiak K, Wimmer-Greinecker G. European experience of the convergent atrial fibrillation procedure: multicenter outcomes in consecutive patients. J Thorac Cardiovasc Surg. 2014;147(4):1411–6.
Mountantonakis SE, Elkassabany N, Kondapalli L, Marchlinski FE, Mandel JE, Hutchinson MD. Provocation of atrial fibrillation triggers during ablation: does the use of general anesthesia affect inducibility? J Cardiovasc Electrophysiol. 2015;26(1):16–20.

Chapter 15
Ventilation Strategies Including High Frequency Jet Ventilation

Alexander Bailey and Michael Duggan

Abstract The number of diagnostic and therapeutic interventions performed out-side of the operating room requiring anesthesia services has expanded several fold over the last several decades. With advances in medical research, new technology, and the increasing survival of complicated and elderly patients the role of the anesthesiologist in providing non-operating room anesthesia will continue to expand. Recent studies and advances in non-traditional ventilation techniques including lung-protective ventilation, jet ventilation and non-invasive ventilation have a promising outlook for current and future utilization in non-operating room anesthesia. It will continue to be the responsibility of the anesthesiologist to provide the same standard of care that a patient would receive in the operating room, including the use of capnography and assessment of adequate ventilation, to ensure safe outcomes in a higher risk patient population in the non-operating room environment.

Keywords High-Frequency Jet Ventilation • Low-Frequency Jet Ventilation • Non-Operating Room Anesthesia • Lung-Protective Ventilation • Ventilator-Induced Lung Injury • Atrial Fibrillation • Pulmonary Vein Isolation • Radiofrequency Catheter Ablation • Capnography • Monitored Anesthesia Care • Non-Invasive Ventilation

Introduction

The number of diagnostic and therapeutic interventions performed outside of the operating room requiring anesthesia services has expanded several fold over the last several decades. With advances in medical research, new technology, and the

A. Bailey, MD
Department of Anesthesiology, Emory University Hospital, Atlanta, GA, USA

M. Duggan, MD (✉)
Division of Cardiothoracic Anesthesiology, Department of Anesthesiology,
Emory University Hospital, 1364 Clifton Rd NE, Atlanta, GA 30322, USA
e-mail: mjdugga@emory.edu

© Springer International Publishing Switzerland 2017
B.G. Goudra, P.M. Singh (eds.), *Out of Operating Room Anesthesia*,
DOI 10.1007/978-3-319-39150-2_15

increasing survival of complicated and elderly patients the role of the anesthesiologist in providing non-operating room anesthesia (NORA) will continue to expand. The areas of activity that anesthesia providers may be involved in currently and in the future include diagnostic imaging, cardiac interventions, intervention radiology and gastrointestinal and urology suites. With this expanded role it requires attention to the same requirements for safe anesthetic care for patients that are followed in the operating room. An area often overlooked by anesthesia providers is the method of ventilation and its effects in NORA. Recent study and advances in non-traditional ventilation techniques including jet ventilation have a promising outlook for current and future utilization in NORA [1, 2].

Offsite Environment Challenges

Procedures requiring NORA are often complex, can take a significant time to complete and usually involve high acuity patients. These factors require that anesthesia providers play an integral role in patient care and patient safety initiatives [1]. A major challenge to patient care includes the problems that arise from the physical environment in which NORA is often delivered, including: space limitations, availability of gas supplies, suction, and electrical supply. Something as simple as ambient lighting may be overlooked [3]. Equipment may be mobile, unfamiliar or found in different locations when compared to standard operating rooms and requires an adaptable and vigilant anesthesiologist.

- In the NORA environment, pipeline gas supplies may not be available and the sole supply of gas may be the cylinder mounted on the anesthesia machine. An anesthesia provider must know how long the cylinder gas supply will last as this gas supply is finite and based on size of the cylinder and total fresh gas flow used [3].
- There is typically no anesthesia workroom nearby if items are needed in an emergency so any out of the operating room (OOR) site should be stocked with additional equipment and medications that anesthesia providers would routinely need to manage a hemodynamically unstable patient, unplanned event or difficult airway [1].
- Access may be limited to the patient once the procedure has started, especially in the cardiac catheterization lab or interventional radiology suite due to imaging equipment. Movement of the procedural table and fluoroscopy may be unpredictable and this may require the use of long intravenous lines and breathing circuits [1].
- It is important to establish communication prior to the initiation of anesthesia because unlike the operating room environment, proceduralists may not be used to anticipating the actions and needs of an anesthesia providers. In the OOR setting much of the procedure can only be ascertained from the fluoroscopy screen and communication should be collaborative to optimize patient care and safety [1].

Standard Ventilation for NORA

When traditional intermittent positive pressure ventilation (IPPV) is employed under general anesthesia, most anesthesia machines used in both the operating room and OOR settings are capable of volume control or pressure control ventilation modes. Newer variations provide additional modes as well such as volume guaranteed-pressure control ventilation and various types of pressure support.

- Depending on patient's characteristics, tidal volumes are adjusted to provide between 6 and 8 mL/kg, based on predicted body weight (PBW) rather than actual body weight (ABW)
- PBW for males: 50 kg + 2.3 kg (height[in] – 60) and females: 45.4 kg + 2.3 kg (height[in] -60) [4]
- Care must be exercised to not over-ventilate obese, short or female patients
- Delivering a tidal volume of 600–800 mL for an average person is associated with movement of the chest wall, lungs, heart, and abdomen [5].

Recently, lung protective ventilation (LPV) strategies have been studied and developed to minimize the risks of ventilator-induced lung injury (VILI) that may be associated with mechanical ventilation in critically ill patients. These strategies have encouraged anesthesiologists to consider LPV in susceptible non-injured lungs as well, especially in the complex patient population that may require diagnostic and therapeutic interventions outside of the operating room. VILI involves a complex interaction of over-distention (volutrauma), increased transpulmonary pressure (barotrauma), cyclic opening and closing of alveoli (alelectotrauma) and inflammatory mediators (biotrauma) [6].

- LPV typically consists of tidal volumes of 6–8 mL/kg based on patient's PBW and other characteristics, PEEP of ≥ 5 cmH$_2$O and recruitment maneuvers and may play a role in OOR ventilation strategies [4].
- LPV can improve lung mechanics, gas exchange and decrease the incidence of postoperative pulmonary complications, including ALI/ARDS, pulmonary infection and atelectasis in previously non-injured lungs [7].
- LPV involves the mindfulness of the anesthesia provider of targeted intraoperative tidal volume selection based on patient lung risk factors, gender and height [4].

Jet Ventilation for NORA

High-frequency jet ventilation (HFJV) is a technique that is most frequently used in the intensive care unit and in the OR during airway and laryngeal surgeries but has seen recent clinical penetration in areas outside of the intensive care unit (ICU) and operating rooms.

- In the operating room HFJV is often used for tracheal resection and complex reconstruction
- In the ICU it has been used for adult patients with acute respiratory distress syndrome [8].
- In the pediatric population it has shown benefit in children with persistent pulmonary hypertension of the newborn [9].

The use of HFJV in NORA is gaining application for providing mechanical ventilation where conscious sedation may not provide the necessary depth of patient comfort, safety and most favorable working conditions for the procedure. The ability to provide mechanical ventilation under general anesthesia with minimal movement of the thorax and abdomen is appealing to procedures where even slight motion artifact from spontaneous or intermittent positive pressure ventilation may significantly affect the duration and success of the procedure. A small tidal volume repeated at a high frequency allows the chest and abdomen to remain relatively motionless while supplying adequate oxygenation and ventilation [5]. Each patient must be evaluated for HFJV but any patient that is hemodynamically stable enough to tolerate induction and general anesthesia with IPPV is likely an appropriate candidate for HFJV [2].

Types of Jet Ventilation

Jet ventilation may be high- or low-frequency with similar general principles between the two methods. Both utilize jet-streams originating from high-pressure sources controlled by flow interruption devices, either hand-held or electronically controlled. Expiration is dependent on passive lung and chest-wall recoil. While much of the gas exchange in low-frequency jet ventilation (LFJV) is achieved by means of convective ventilation or bulk flow, successful gas exchange in HFJV is achieved by a relatively greater contribution of other mechanisms of gas exchange due to the smaller tidal volumes utilized in HFJV. Unlike conventional ventilation, tidal volumes during HFJV are often smaller than anatomical and equipment dead space and therefore alternative mechanisms of ventilation occur. These include laminar flow, Taylor-type dispersion, Pendelluft or collateral ventilation, molecular diffusion and cardiogenic mixing [10].

- LFJV is usually applied by a hand-triggered device and is often limited to short diagnostic procedures such as laryngoscopy or bronchoscopy or as an important management strategy of a "can't intubate, can't ventilate" situation during a difficult airway [10].
- During LFJV, a jet frequency of 8–10 breaths per minute allows sufficient time for exhalation via passive recoil of the lung and chest wall while preventing air-trapping and buildup of pressure in small airways [10].
- HFJV is achieved by commercially available jet ventilators that deliver a continuous flow of pressurized gas that is chopped into adjustable jets by a high-frequency flow interrupter valve [10].

- All ventilators are equipped with an airway pressure alarm and automatic shut-down that will stop gas flow in the presence of unintentional high airway pressures [10].

High Frequency Jet Ventilation

Several different ventilators are commercially available in the United States and internationally to provide HFJV, including the Monsoon jet ventilator (Acutronic Medical Systems, Fabrik im Shiffli, Switzerland) and the Life Pulse high frequency jet ventilator (Bunnell Incorporated, Salt Lake City, UT). The variables that can be manipulated are respiratory rate, inspiratory time and driving pressure [2]. Oxygen delivery depends on the set FiO_2 as well as the degree of room air entrainment. The tidal volume is not set but is rather a function of driving pressure, cannula/airway resistance, inspiratory time, entrainment volume, and the impedance of the respiratory system [10].

Respiratory Rate/Frequency

- The respiratory rate may be adjusted from 12 to 150 breaths per minute
- Often initiated at 120 breaths per minute based on clinical observation that it provides adequate CO_2 elimination
- Unlike traditional ventilation, the efficiency of CO_2 elimination will typically decrease as the respiratory rate increases [2]

Inspiratory Time

- Initially set at 30–40 % (I/E = 30–40 %) [11]
- As inspiratory time increases, lung volumes typically increase [2]

Driving Pressure

- The pressure the ventilator produces during inspiration is the driving pressure [2].
- It can be varied from 0 to 45 pounds per square inch (PSI) [2].
- The driving pressure is the most influential for CO_2 elimination, increases in driving pressure often lead to increased tidal volumes and airway pressure [10].
- It can be increased as needed to maintain normocarbia with an empiric starting setting of 15–20 psi [11].

Airway Considerations

- The high frequency jet ventilator may be connected to either an endotracheal tube (ETT) or laryngeal mask airway (LMA) with an elbow adapter in a circle system with the APL valve open allowing transition from IPPV to HFJV [2].
- The ventilator can also be connected to a catheter placed inside the ETT to help increase CO_2 elimination
- If the endotracheal cuff is deflated, an open system is created which may reduce the risk of barotrauma. However, an open system also entrains room air and often decreases lung volumes.

- The Monsoon jet ventilator continuously monitors a pause pressure (PP) before each breath is delivered. The pressure limit is adjustable and set by the user to help reduce the risk of barotrauma. A typical PP limit is 24 cmH$_2$O.
- Humidification can also be added to the system, especially for longer procedures, to help prevent airway desiccation and the risk of necrotizing tracheitis
- Ventilation can be assessed from arterial CO$_2$ (if invasive arterial blood pressure monitoring is being utilized) or by converting from HFJV to IPPV to measure end-tidal CO$_2$ (EtCO$_2$) as needed [2].
- While rare, hypercarbia or hypoxemia refractory to adjustments in the driving pressure and inspiratory time may call for a permanent transition to traditional ventilation strategies [2].

Anesthetic Considerations

- Total IV anesthesia (TIVA) remains mainstay of anesthetic maintenance as there is no practical method of delivering volatile anesthetics during HFJV. Propofol and/or remifentanil infusions are often used in conjunction with HFJV [2].
- Muscle relaxants are often not needed except to facilitate intubation and long-acting muscle relaxants are generally avoided because they interfere with the use of high output pacing to locate the phrenic nerves before cardiac ablation and HFJV is known to suppress chemical drive [2, 12].
- Unless otherwise indicated, induction is often delayed in cardiac ablations until after cardiac mapping is complete in an effort to give the electrophysiologist the greatest chance of detecting possible atrial trigger sites as it is not completely known how anesthetics could affect atrial triggers. This permits neurological assessment after trans-septal puncture to rule out left-sided emboli as well [2, 13].
- An esophageal temperature probe may be used to guard against possible thermal injury to the esophagus, especially if radiofrequency ablation is applied to the posterior wall of the left atrium [13].

Procedures Where HFJV Provides Benefit

Cardiac Arrhythmia Ablations

- Advances in cardiac electrophysiology have shown that pulmonary vein isolation (PVI) and ablation is an effective procedure for the treatment of some types of atrial fibrillation (AF) and successful treatment requires the ability to precisely identify and ablate the atrial foci [5].
- PVI involves the creation of serial circumferential radiofrequency ablation (RFA) lesions around the pulmonary vein ostia to electrically isolate them from the rest of the left atrium [13].
- Pulmonary vein isolation (PVI) and ablation for atrial fibrillation (AF) requires sustained contact between the ablation catheter and the pulmonary veins for improved results [2].

- IPPV may reduce catheter stability both through chest movement and changes in the dimensions of the left atrium and pulmonary veins [2].
- General anesthesia avoids the issues of under-sedation with patient discomfort as well as over-sedation with an obstructed breathing pattern for a procedure that may take up 6 h [2].

Interventional Radiology Procedures (Computed Tomography(CT)-guided Tumor Ablation)

- Due to technological advances in imaging techniques and minimally invasive approaches there has been an increase in radiofrequency ablations for tumor treatment, often requiring immobility of the abdomen and chest during treatment [5].
- RFA procedures often take several minutes requiring relative immobility, much longer than ventilation may be safely held in a spontaneously breathing or mechanically ventilated patient, but which may be achieved utilizing HFJV [5].
- Patients may benefit from reduced diaphragmatic and abdominal motion when HFJV is used during percutaneous RFA of hepatic or renal tumors under CT guidance as a result of more accurate application and use of the ablation catheter with less damage to normal surrounding tissue [5].

Extracorporeal Shock Wave Lithotripsy (ESWL)

- ESWL relies on the precise application of shock waves to break up kidney stones while minimizing collateral damage to adjacent tissue [5].
- HFJV has been associated with a reduced number of shocks needed to treat the stone as well as less energy to fragment the stone when compared to traditional mechanical ventilation [5].

Evidence for Superiority of Jet Ventilation

- Goode et al. retrospectively and prospectively compared IPPV to HFJV in posterior left atrial catheter ablation for AF and found that fewer ablation lesions were required in the HFJV group because of fewer incidences of ablation electrode dislodgement. In the 72 patients studied, there was a significant reduction in the average time required to complete the ablation from 260 to 170 min. HFJV was also associated with less fluctuations in LA volume, pressure, pulmonary vein blood flow velocity, and posterior LA motility which further facilitates the ablation procedure [11].
- An additional observational study by Hutchinson and Garcia et al. demonstrated that integrating contemporary technologies, including the utilization of HFJV, to enhance anatomical detail and ablation catheter stability improved 1-year outcomes after AF ablation. The patients who received HFJV also had lower PV reconnection rates despite lower fluoroscopy times, fewer ablation lesions and a shorter time to PVI [12].

- HFJV in adults has a relatively low potential for serious complications, including barotrauma, pneumothorax, and pneumo-mediastinum. Several studies have shown the use of this technique and its relative safety while others suggest it is best suited to patients with normal airways and normal lung and chest wall compliance [13, 14].
- Support for the use of general anesthesia over conscious sedation comes from the 2011 randomized study by Di Biase et al. When compared to conscious sedation, they found that general anesthesia was associated with a higher AF cure rate (88 % vs 69 %) in patients undergoing PVI in addition to a shorter procedure time (2.4 h vs 3.6 h) [14].
- A small feasibility study of 19 patients having CT-guided radiofrequency ablation of hepatic or renal lesions showed that the nine HFJV patients had no complications and received lower dose of radiation than the ten patients receiving IPPV [15].
- Early studies have shown an association between HFJV and a decrease in the amount of shocks needed to treat nephrolithiasis. Mucksavage et al. demonstrated in a retrospective study of 112 patients undergoing ESWL for nephrolithiasis that, when compared to IPPV, HFJV was associated with less shocks and less energy required to fragment the stone [16, 17].

Monitored Anesthesia Care with Assisted Ventilation

Importance of Using $EtCO_2$

Although capnography has long been embraced and incorporated into the standards of monitoring in the operating room, its utilization during the sedation outside of the operating room, especially when performed by non-anesthesiologists, has been limited. As NORA continues to expand, it should be considered the responsibility of anesthesiologists to convince other physicians that capnography is a vital tool for patient safety. This is particularly true since the American Society of Anesthesiologists (ASA) has issued revised standards to monitor ventilation by capnography in patients undergoing sedation, irrespective of the location of the procedure. Likewise, in the United States, the Centers for Medicare and Medicaid Services have revised guidelines that require sedation and analgesia services be under the guidance of the anesthesia service [18, 19].

- Detailed analysis of the closed claim database of the ASA has confirmed that respiratory depression is the most prominent adverse effect of sedation and that significant respiratory compromise can occur despite normal oxygen saturation as measured by pulse oximetry [19].
- Several studies have shown the importance of capnography illustrating less hypoxia when capnography is utilized and the forewarning of impending respiratory depression due to hypoxia [19].

- Capnography triggers early intervention and decreases the incidence rates of severe hypoxemia under procedural sedation as well [18].
- Clinical information can be obtained from three sources in capnography: numerical value of $EtCO_2$, shape of the capnogram, and the difference between $EtCO_2$ and $PaCO_2$ [18].
- Each change from the baseline $EtCO_2$ value, the waveform shape, or respiratory rate should alert the sedation provider to closely monitor the patient for respiratory depression or airway obstruction [18].
- Use of capnography for monitoring the adequacy of ventilation and developing policies and procedures governing the application of sedation by anesthesia providers, including minimal qualifications and training for non-anesthesia providers, can enhance the safety of NORA [19].

Non-invasive Ventilation for Assisted Ventilation

Non-invasive ventilation (NIV) may be applicable in patients where general anesthesia (GA) and positive pressure ventilation is considered best avoided because of hemodynamic changes and risks associated with invasive mechanical ventilation. Several small retrospective and case studies from Europe have explored the use of NIV in OOR cardiac procedures requiring sedation and minimal support of ventilation. Although limited and requiring further study, safe results have been reported in select patients supported by NIV undergoing catheter ablations of atrial fibrillation with deep sedation and orthopneic patients undergoing percutaneous aortic valve implantation and aortic valvuloplasty with minimal sedation [20, 21].

- ASA preoperative fasting guidelines, at least 2 h for liquids and 6 h for solids, are recommended to minimize risk of pulmonary aspiration
- Sedation should be titrated to specific patient characteristics, documented sedation scales and procedural requirements to maintain spontaneous ventilation and a cooperative patient throughout the length of the procedure
- Inspiratory positive airway pressure (I-PAP), expiratory positive airway pressure (E-PAP) and inspiratory oxygen fraction (FiO_2) can be adjusted throughout the procedure to maintain an arterial oxygen saturation (SaO_2) >92 % and an arterial CO_2 tension ($PaCO_2$) <50 mmHg [21].
- I-PAP between 8 and 12 cmH_2O, E-PAP of 4–6 cmH_2O, and a FiO_2 between 0.35 and 0.50 have been described to maintain an appropriate SaO_2 and $PaCO_2$ [21].
- No problems due to mask-related difficulties, NIV discomfort or significant respiratory or hemodynamic complications were reported [21].

However, limitations exist for patients receiving NIV for procedures under sedation

- Airways are not protected so careful monitoring of the patient's level of sedation is mandatory and the risk of aspiration must be thoroughly examined [21].
- Cooperation of the patient is essential [21].

- Close monitoring of the patient's vital signs, including oxygen saturation and capnography, must be performed through the length of the procedure [21].
- It is difficult to predict each patient's response to a particular sedative, consequently, sedation should be performed by an anesthesia provider

In these select studies, NIV proved effective in preventing respiratory failure due to sedation while maintaining spontaneous ventilation and may be used in other settings where general anesthesia is either not needed or poorly tolerated due to patient risks [21].

Conclusion

As NORA and the area of activity outside of the operating room for anesthesiologists continues to grow larger new methods and procedures will continue to challenge the anesthesia provider to update their skill and technique. It remains the responsibility of the anesthesiologist to provide the same standard of care that a patient would receive in the operating room, including the use of capnography and assessment of adequate ventilation, to ensure safe outcomes in a potentially more multifaceted and riskier patient population in an unfamiliar environment. New ventilation strategies may play role in NORA as well, specifically jet ventilation, especially when conscious sedation may not provide the necessary depth of patient comfort, safety and most favorable working conditions for the procedure and proceduralist. NORA and ventilation will remain an active area of interest in the field of anesthesiology with significant overlap into other fields of medicine and surgery which will continue to benefit from additional research and study.

References

1. Shook DC, Gross W. Offsite anesthesiology in the cardiac catheterization lab. Curr Opin Anaesthesiol. 2007;20(4):352–8.
2. Raiten J, Elkassabany N, Gao W, Mandel JE. Medical intelligence article: novel uses of high frequency ventilation outside the operating room. Anesth Analg. 2011;112(5):1110–3.
3. Feldman JM, Kalli I. Equipment and environmental issues for nonoperating room anesthesia. Curr Opin Anaesthesiol. 2006;19(4):450–2.
4. Bender SP, Paganelli WC, Gerety LP, Tharp WG, Shanks AM, Housey M, et al. Intraoperative lung-protective ventilation trends and practice patterns: a report from the multicenter perioperative outcomes group. Anesth Analg. 2015;121(5):1231–9.
5. Raiten J, Elkassabany N, Mandel JE. The use of high-frequency jet ventilation for out of operating room anesthesia. Curr Opin Anaesthesiol. 2012;25(4):482–5.
6. Kilpatrick B, Slinger P. Lung protective strategies in anaesthesia. Br J Anaesth. 2010;105 Suppl 1: i108–16.
7. Sutherasan Y, Vargas M, Pelosi P. Protective mechanical ventilation in the non-injured lung: review and meta-analysis. Crit Care. 2014;18(2):211.

8. Chan KP, Stewart TE, Mehta S. High-frequency oscillatory ventilation for adult patients with ARDS. Chest. 2007;131(6):1907–16.
9. Konduri GG, Kim UO. Advances in the diagnosis and management of persistent pulmonary hypertension of the newborn. Pediatr Clin North Am. 2009;56(3):579–600, Table of Contents.
10. Evans E, Biro P, Bedforth N. Jet ventilation. Contin Educ Anaesth Crit Care Pain. 2007;7(1):2–5.
11. Goode Jr JS, Taylor RL, Buffington CW, Klain MM, Schwartzman D. High-frequency jet ventilation: utility in posterior left atrial catheter ablation. Heart Rhythm. 2006;3(1):13–9.
12. Hutchinson MD, Garcia FC, Mandel JE, Elkassabany N, Zado ES, Riley MP, et al. Efforts to enhance catheter stability improve atrial fibrillation ablation outcome. Heart Rhythm. 2013;10(3):347–53.
13. Elkassabany N, Garcia F, Tschabrunn C, Raiten J, Gao W, Chaichana K, et al. Anesthetic management of patients undergoing pulmonary vein isolation for treatment of atrial fibrillation using high-frequency jet ventilation. J Cardiothorac Vasc Anesth. 2012;26(3):433–8.
14. Di Biase L, Conti S, Mohanty P, Bai R, Sanchez J, Walton D, et al. General anesthesia reduces the prevalence of pulmonary vein reconnection during repeat ablation when compared with conscious sedation: results from a randomized study. Heart Rhythm. 2011;8(3):368–72.
15. Abderhalden S, Biro P, Hechelhammer L, Pfiffner R, Pfammatter T. CT-guided navigation of percutaneous hepatic and renal radiofrequency ablation under high-frequency jet ventilation: feasibility study. J Vasc Interv Radiol. 2011;22(9):1275–8.
16. Warner MA, Warner ME, Buck CF, Segura JW. Clinical efficacy of high frequency jet ventilation during extracorporeal shock wave lithotripsy of renal and ureteral calculi: a comparison with conventional mechanical ventilation. J Urol. 1988;139(3):486–7.
17. Mucksavage P, Mayer WA, Mandel JE, Van Arsdalen KN. High-frequency jet ventilation is beneficial during shock wave lithotripsy utilizing a newer unit with a narrower focal zone. Can Urol Assoc J. 2010;4(5):333–5.
18. Kodali BS. Capnography outside the operating rooms. Anesthesiology. 2013;118(1):192–201.
19. Metzner J, Domino KB. Risks of anesthesia or sedation outside the operating room: the role of the anesthesia care provider. Curr Opin Anaesthesiol. 2010;23(4):523–31.
20. Sbrana F, Ripoli A, Formichi B. Safety and utility of noninvasive ventilation during deep sedation for catheter ablation of atrial fibrillation. J Cardiothorac Vasc Anesth. 2014;28(1):e6–8.
21. Guarracino F, Cabrini L, Baldassarri R, Cariello C, Covello RD, Landoni G, et al. Non-invasive ventilation-aided transoesophageal echocardiography in high-risk patients: a pilot study. Eur J Echocardiogr. 2010;11(6):554–6.

Part V
Anesthesia for Neuroradiology

Chapter 16
Anesthesia in the MRI Suite and for CT Scan

Gregory E.R. Weller

Abstract Complex imaging technology offers exceptional diagnostic and thera-peutic procedural capabilities. Both magnetic resonance imaging (MRI) and com-puted tomography (CT) are non-operating room locations that can represent significant challenges for the delivery of safe patient care. Over the past decade, requests for anesthesiology services in these remote imaging environments have dramatically increased. This chapter examines many of the complexities and haz-ards that are relatively unique to MRI and CT, such as the ferromagnetic missile effect, thermal injury, difficulties with patient monitoring in a strong electromag-netic environment, ionizing radiation, and magnetic and radio-opaque contrast agents. Options and rationales for sedation and anesthesia care in these remote loca-tions are presented, along with methods to address the particular hazards and chal-lenges found in each of these imaging suites. Patient safety and occupational safety are thoroughly addressed. Anesthesiologists should become familiar with these concepts, as the clinical demand for our safe and efficient services in these unique environments continues to grow.

Keywords MRI/Magnetic resonance imaging • MRI Zones • MRI Safety • Magnetic fields • CT/Computed tomography • Imaging • Contrast • Gadolinium • Quench • Radiation • Ferromagnetic objects • Cardiovascular implantable elec-tronic device (CIED)

Introduction

Modern advances in complex imaging technology offer exceptional diagnostic capabilities. Magnetic resonance imaging (MRI) and computed tomography (CT) are non-operating room locations that represent significant challenges for the deliv-ery of safe patient care. Over the past decade, requests for anesthesiology services

G.E.R. Weller, MD, PhD
Department of Anesthesiology & Perioperative Medicine,
Penn State Hershey Medical Center, 500 University Drive,
PO Box 850, Hershey, PA 17033, USA
e-mail: gweller@hmc.psu.edu

© Springer International Publishing Switzerland 2017
B.G. Goudra, P.M. Singh (eds.), *Out of Operating Room Anesthesia*,
DOI 10.1007/978-3-319-39150-2_16

Table 16.1 Common indications for imaging

MRI	CT
Seizures	Head or body trauma
Hypotonia	Suspected intracranial hemorrhage
Failure to thrive	Seizures
Developmental delay	Mental status changes/encephalopathy
Hydrocephalus, suspected shunt	Focal neurological findings
malfunction	Vertigo, apraxia, headache, visual field defects
Sensorineural hearing loss	Increased ICP
Tumors & staging	Hydrocephalus, suspected shunt malfunction
Skeletal abnormalities	Tumors & staging, mass effect
Metabolic disease	Differentiation of solid, cystic, inflammatory,
Vascular anomalies (aneurysms, vascular	vascular, and fatty lesions
malformations, hemangiomas)	Bone lesions
ENT issues	Mediastinal mass
Nerve lesions	Thoracic and abdominal masses or fluid
Spinal cord compression	collections, abscesses, and cysts
Meningomyelocele	Spinal cord disease, e.g. meningomyelocele
Tethered cord	Foreign body localization
Back pain	
Osteonecrosis	
Cardiac or aortic disease	

in these remote imaging environments have dramatically increased. Clinical indications for MRI and CT scanning are numerous, as presented in Table 16.1.

In addition to the usual concerns for out-of-the-OR anesthesia, the MRI and CT environments present some unique complexities and hazards for anesthesiologists and their patients, including ionizing radiation, strong magnetic fields, cryogens, awkward patient access, the need for the anesthesiologist to remain disconcertingly far away from the patient, and cumbersome but necessary safety processes. All anesthesiologists should be educated regarding the unique safety aspects of the MRI and CT environments [1]. Table 16.2 lists websites that may be of interest.

Physics

CT

- X-Rays are high-frequency, high-energy electromagnetic radiation that carries sufficient energy to displace electrons from their atoms (ionization).
- **Ionizing radiation** can directly or indirectly damage DNA, causing radiation-induced cell damage or death, leading to a wide range of problems including cataracts, sterility, radiation burns, teratogenesis, and cancer.
- The radiation dose from a CT scan is much higher than for plain X-ray films (see Table 16.3). High radiation exposures are of particular concern in pediatric patients, since CT scans are known to increase the risk of leukemia and brain tumors [2].

Table 16.2 Websites of interest

Name	URL	Comments
ASA Statement on Nonoperating Room Anesthetizing Locations	http://www.asahq.org/quality-and-practice-management/standards-and-guidelines	Sets minimal guidelines for anesthesia care in out-of-the-OR sites
APSF Clinical Safety – MRI	http://www.apsf.org/resources_safety_suite.php	Information from the Anesthesia Patient Safety Foundation on MRI safety
Joint Commission Sentinel Event Alerts	http://www.jointcommission.org/sentinel_event.aspx	Alerts intended to draw attention to specific current safety & care concerns of national import (see SEA#38 & #47)
MRISafety.com	http://www.mrisafety.com	Has large database of equipment & devices tested for MR environments
Simply Physics	http://simplyphysics.com	Lots of MRI information, including an excellent collection of photographs of MR projectile incidents
ACR Guidance Document for Safe MRI Practices	http://www.acr.org/Quality-Safety/Radiology-Safety/MR-Safety	American College of Radiology's MR safety guidelines
OSHA Ionizing Radiation website	https://www.osha.gov/SLTC/radiationionizing/index.html	U.S. Dept of Labor Occupational Safety & Health Administration; Health effects and standards information

Table 16.3 Ionizing radiation doses

Source	Exposure
Cross-country airplane flight	3 mrem
Dental bitewing X-Ray	0.5–5 mrem
Chest X-Ray	5–15 mrem
Abdominal X-Ray	40–60 mrem
Mammogram	70 mrem
Head CT scan	200 mrem
Chest CT scan	800 mrem
Abdominal CT scan	1000 mrem
PTCA	500–5000 mrem
Annual dose from smoking (1 pack/day)	20 mrem/year
Annual dose from natural sources	300 mrem/year

mrem millirem, *PTCA* percutaneous transluminal coronary angioplasty

- Radiation exposure is inversely proportional to the square of the distance from the source (inverse-square law).
- CT scanners employ an X-ray tube that rotates axially around the patient gantry. Emitted radiation passing through the patient is sensed by a detector array.
- CT measures electron density, differentiating between high-density tissues (calcium, bone, iron, and contrast-enhanced areas) and lower-density tissues (air, muscle, fat, water).

MRI

- Nuclear magnetic resonance (MR) refers to the phenomenon whereby atomic nuclei exposed to magnetic fields absorb and emit electromagnetic radiation.
- Magnetic resonance scanners have three interacting electromagnetic fields (**static**, **gradient**, and **radiofrequency fields**) that perturb the orientation and magnetic dipole moment of hydrogen nuclei, causing them to release energy that is detectable by the MR scanner [3].
- The main static magnetic field is generated by large electric currents flowing through loops of wires immersed in superconducting cryogenic fluid.
- Current clinical MR scanners use static magnetic fields of either 1.5 or 3 Tesla (T). These magnets are approximately 50,000 times the strength of the Earth's natural magnetic field. In other words, these are enormously powerful magnetic fields! 3 T scanners have superior sensitivity and resolution.
- Clinical MRI scanners measure at least three different properties of tissue samples: T1 relaxation, T2 decay, and proton density.
- Due to the complex spatial encoding of MR signals, any patient movement significantly degrades image quality. Anesthesia facilitates patient immobility for the scan.
- Cryogens, most commonly liquid helium, are utilized inside the scanner to cool the wire bundles to superconducting temperatures.
- A "**quench**" is the rapid release of cryogen from the scanner in the form of a gas. Quenching rapidly eliminates the static magnetic field (1–3 min), and is used only for emergencies. Liquid helium expands at a 750:1 ratio as it boils into gas; thus it must be vented to the outside via special escape valves and ventilation system. If the expanding helium gas escapes into the scanner room, hypoxia and asphyxiation may result. Quenching is used only in emergencies to remove a patient or equipment from the magnet.
- MR angiography and venography (MRA/MRV) are MRI imaging techniques that study blood vessels and vascular flow, in particular to evaluate stenoses or aneurysms.
- Three decades of clinical MRI use has revealed no known significant physiological impacts from MRI, unlike X-Ray or CT.
- There is little evidence from either *in vitro* or *in vivo* studies that there is any detrimental biological impact from exposure to clinically-relevant static 1.5 T or 3 T magnetic fields [4, 5].

Physical Layout

CT

- CT scanner rooms are lined with lead to restrict ionizing radiation.
- Large lead-infused windows in the control room allow direct visualization of patients and monitors in the scanner.
- For anesthesia cases, the CT scanner room should have oxygen (preferably built-in wall gas lines), vacuum suction, and available electric outlets.

MRI

- The MRI suite is designed around the MR scanner and its extremely powerful magnetic fields. Of paramount concern is the ability to restrict access to the scanner room and its magnetic fields.
- Faraday cage – The walls of MRI scanner rooms are sheathed in metal (copper or aluminum) forming a complete box around the scanner, shielding it from external radiofrequency interference.
- Large windows in the control room wall facilitate direct visualization of patients in the scanner. They are lined with fine copper mesh to maintain Faraday cage continuity.
- The American College of Radiology (ACR) sets standards for MRI suite design and access as well as safe practices in MR environments [6]. A major concern is ensuring screening and controlling access to the powerful magnetic fields, as a component of large-scale efforts to minimize the risk of harm from ferromagnetic object projectiles, or adverse effects related to implanted medical devices.
- The ACR guidance documents define the conceptual division of all MR suites into four **Zones** [6] (See Table 16.4).
  - Access to Zones III & IV is strictly controlled, due to the hazards of ferromagnetic objects in strong magnetic fields.
  - Only trained, approved personnel and properly screened patients may enter Zones III & IV.
- The scanner room should have built-in wall gases (oxygen, air, and nitrous oxide) and vacuum (suction) lines available for patient care.
- Direct observation of the patient may be at least somewhat compromised during MRI scans. The anesthesiologist's workstation in the control room should be positioned to optimize visualization of the patient and anesthesia monitoring equipment.
- Anesthesia care can and does occur in all four Zones.
- It is preferable to set up an **"anesthesia induction suite" within Zone II**, for the induction and emergence of anesthetized patients, away from the magnetic field hazards of Zones III & IV.

Table 16.4 MRI zones

Zone	Locations	Comments
I	Areas outside of MRI suite	Freely accessible to public No restrictions
II	Reception area Nursing station Interview & Waiting area	Buffer between Zones I & III Patient interviews & Screening occur here Patients are supervised by nurses Ideal for anesthesia inductions
III	MRI Control room ± Adjoining spaces & Hallways	Access is strictly controlled **Only** screened patients & personnel may enter Only screened equipment may enter Access must be restricted by barriers or locks
IV	MRI scanner room	Hazardous environment! Access is strictly controlled **Only** screened patients & personnel may enter No ferromagnetic items may enter Constant direct supervision by MR personnel

Based on the ACR Guidance Document on MR Safe Practices [6]

Contrast Enhancement

CT

- Radiocontrast agents are often employed during CT scans to improve tissue differentiation and visualization of vascular structures.
- CT contrast agents are typically **iodine-based**.
- There is a high rate of adverse events (up to 5 %) from the administration of CT contrast agents [7, 8], including hypersensitivity/anaphylactoid reactions, anaphylaxis, thyroid dysfunction, and kidney injury.
- Adverse reactions are most common with older, high-osmolar contrast agents. Newer, low-osmolar and iso-osmolar agents are considerably safer.
- Adverse reaction management: Call for assistance as appropriate. Respond with monitoring, oxygen, fluid resuscitation, antihistamines, bronchodilators, steroids, epinephrine, advanced airway management, and ACLS/PALS as needed.
- Radiocontrast agents can be **nephrotoxic**, causing iatrogenic acute renal failure, aka contrast-induced nephropathy, especially in patients with pre-existing renal disease (GFR <30 mL/min/1.73 m^2). Renal function should be checked pre-operatively.
- Oral contrast enhancement can be achieved with diatrizoate agents such as Gastrografin.

MRI

- **Gadolinium**-based contrast agents are often employed for the enhancement of MRI images.
- Clearance is by the kidney. Expect clearance to be lower in neonates and infants.
- MRI contrast can be nephrotoxic. In patients with renal impairment, gadolinium agents can cause **nephrogenic systemic fibrosis** [9].

    - Consider sending patients with significant renal dysfunction for dialysis following contrast-enhanced MRI scans.

- Other possible reactions to gadolinium agents include: rashes, hives, nausea/vomiting, headache, and anaphylaxis.
- Oral contrast enhancement is used rarely, to enhance the gastrointestinal tract for abdominal imaging.

Safety

CT

In general, the CT scanner presents fewer safety challenges for the anesthesiologist than the MRI suite. The main safety issue is the risk from ionizing radiation to the patient and medical personnel. In 2011, the Joint Commission released a Sentinel Event Alert regarding the radiation risks of diagnostic imaging [10], stating that physicians should ensure the "right test" (consider non-ionizing radiation if possible, e.g. ultrasound or MRI) and "right dose" (minimize radiation dose).

MRI

In 2008, the Joint Commission published a Sentinel Event Alert regarding MRI safety [11], citing 398 adverse MRI-related events in the prior decade, of which nine were fatalities. The Joint Commission's declaration of MR safety as a national priority helped stimulate ongoing efforts to improve patient and occupational safety in the MRI environment. Additionally, the ACR Guidance Document on Safe MR Practices [6], most recently updated in 2013, sets guidelines for promoting safety in MRI suites, including defining the MRI Zones, patient screening recommendations, and equipment and medical device labeling issues.

Be aware that the **MAGNET IS ALWAYS ON**! Even between cases, the large static magnetic field remains active. In the presence of a strong magnetic field, any objects containing **ferromagnetic** material will be attracted to the field source, and may become hazardous **high-velocity projectiles** (**missile effect**). A famous tragedy occurred in 2001, when a 6 year-old boy getting an MRI scan died from cranial trauma when an oxygen cylinder that was accidentally brought into the scanner room turned into a high-velocity missile [12]. Examples of objects susceptible to the missile effect include medical gas cylinders, chairs, ventilators, stretchers, wheelchairs, IV poles, stethoscopes, laryngoscopes, monitors, hemostats, phones, pagers, buckets, scissors, ID badges, jewelry, and keys.

Current MRI safety terminology is based on the American Society for Testing and Materials (ASTM) F2503-13 Standard Practice for Marking Medical Devices and Other Items for Safety in the Magnetic Resonance Environment (2005, revised 2013) [13]. Table 16.5 summarizes the current safety terminology.

MRI safety protocols require that all devices used in MR environments be labeled, either permanently on the item itself, or in the accompanying documentation (instructions, package inserts, or user manual) using color-coded, easily identifiable **safety icons** [13].

- **MR Safe**: the letters "MR" inside of a green square
- **MR Conditional**: the letters "MR" inside of a yellow triangle
- **MR Unsafe**: the letters "MR" enclosed by a red circle with a diagonal red bar (typical "prohibited" sign)

Screening must be rigorously enforced, with careful, methodical, in-person checks for ferromagnetic metal objects and implanted medical devices [1]. Handheld and walk-through detectors are available to facilitate screening. **Implanted medical devices** are potentially hazardous in the MR environment. Threats to medical devices include heating and burning, movement or dislodgement, interference, malfunction, or permanent damage. Many common medical devices have been tested for MR safety, but not all devices have been tested under all scanning conditions [14]. Examples of devices that are problematic in MR include: intracranial aneurysm clips, programmable VP shunts, spinal cord stimulators, epidural catheters, metallic foreign bodies, cochlear implants, orthodontics, heart valves, and stents.

Cardiovascular implantable electronic devices (**CIEDs**) including pacemakers and automated implantable cardioverter-defibrillators (AICDs) may become heated, dislodged, inhibited, or malfunction [15]. In general, MRIs should not be performed on patients with CIEDs [1]. However, some newer devices have been classified as MR-conditional, and development is underway to produce MR-safe devices [16]. Any patient with a CIED who requires an MRI must be carefully

Table 16.5 MRI safety terminology for devices, implants, and labeling

MR Safe	Item poses no known hazards in any MRI environments
MR Conditional	Item poses no known hazards in **specified** MRI environments under **specified** conditions of use. Conditional parameters may include static magnetic field strength, gradient and RF field variables, and item configuration.
MR Unsafe	Item poses unacceptable hazard in all MRI environments.

Based on ASTM F2503-13 Standard Practice for Marking Medical Devices and Other Items for Safety in the Magnetic Resonance Environment [13].

screened, the device's MR safety status thoroughly investigated, and risks/benefits weighed with multidisciplinary input. Consult the CIED/pacer clinic to interrogate and re-program CIEDs pre- and post-scan.

MRI scanners are **very loud**. Noise increases with magnetic field strength, up to 100 decibels. There are reports of hearing loss by patients from MR scans. All patients must have hearing protection (earmuffs or earplugs).

Temperature is an issue for patients in MRI. The scanner rooms are slightly cool (68–70 °F) to maintain image quality, creating a risk for **hypothermia**, especially in neonates and infants. For anesthesia cases, it is prudent to turn off the scanner's patient cooling fan, and consider applying warm blankets. MRI-compatible fiberoptic temperature probes are available. Contrarily, MRI scanners can also increase a patient's temperature, or cause **burns**, which comprised 70 % of the events reported in the 2008 Sentinel Event Alert [11]. The radiofrequency and gradient fields can induce electric currents in any conductive material, especially when looped. Consequently, avoid allowing any monitoring cables or wires to kink, loop, fray, or touch the patient's body (place a towel between all wires/cables and the patient).

Medical **codes** must <u>not</u> be conducted in Zone IV (MR scanner room). Instead, the patient must be emergently transferred back to Zone II, because code equipment (carts, monitors, defibrillators) are not MR-safe, and may malfunction or cause harm in the presence of strong magnetic fields.

There appear to be no adverse reproductive outcomes for **pregnant** women from MRI exposure [6, 17]. However, pregnant women may wish to consider avoiding MRI out of an abundance of caution, especially during fetal organogenesis.

Anesthesia Equipment

CT

- Standard monitors, anesthesia machines, infusion pumps, and other equipment may be employed in the CT suite without risk of electromagnetic interference or injury.
- High-quality lead shielding, including wraparound lead skirt, jacket, thyroid shield, leaded eyeglasses, and a radiation badge (dosimeter) are highly recommended.

MRI

- Regular (MR-unsafe) anesthesia equipment may be used freely in Zone II, and with caution in Zone III. Only MR-conditional or MR-safe anesthesia equipment may be used in Zone IV.
- Monitoring:
  - MR-safe pulse oximeters are fiber-optic, and often wireless.
  - ECG monitoring systems for MRI are non-ferrous, often wireless, and designed to minimize radiofrequency interference. Electromagnetic fields may cause artifacts in ECG tracings, inhibiting the reliable monitoring of

ischemia and arrhythmias. Cardiac MRI may require ECG gating, in which the image sequencing is synchronized to the patient's cardiac cycle.
- Invasive BP monitoring is possible using conventional transducers, with long extension tubing.
- The Invivo (Gainesville, FL) Expression patient monitoring system is MR-conditional, employing wireless, battery-powered ECG and pulse-oximetry monitors.

- Infusion pumps:
  - Most common hospital infusion systems are <u>not</u> safe for MRI.
  - A few MR-conditional or MR-safe infusion pumps are available, such as the MRidium 3860+ pump (IRadimed, Winter Springs, FL), and the Harvard Apparatus (Holliston, MA) remote-operated MRI Syringe Pump.
  - MR-unsafe infusion pumps can be used, by keeping them in Zone III, and employing long intravenous tubing extended into Zone IV through a wave guide.

- Miscellaneous:
  - MR-safe plastic laryngoscopes are available.
  - MR-safe aluminum medical gas cylinders are available.
  - Endotracheal tubes and LMAs are safe for MRI use.
  - Bivona tracheostomy tubes contain metallic fibers, and should be switched to Shiley tubes for MRI scans

- Anesthesia machines:
  - MR-conditional anesthesia machines have significantly advanced the administration of anesthesia for MRI.
  - Dräger Fabius MRI (Dräger Medical, Telford, PA)
  - GE/Datex-Ohmeda Aestiva 5 MRI (GE Healthcare, Waukesha, WI)
  - All servicing of MR-conditional anesthesia machines should be performed <u>outside</u> of Zone IV, including vaporizer changes, gas cylinder changes, and repairs.
  - If an MR-conditional machine is not available, a standard MR-unsafe anesthesia machine may be used, restricted to Zone III, and utilizing an elongated circuit extended into Zone IV through a wave guide.

Indications for Anesthesia

Indications for anesthesia for MRI and CT scan are similar, although fewer patients overall should require anesthesia for CT, as the scan durations are much shorter.

- Claustrophobia (usually not a problem for brief CT scans)
- Pain (usually not a problem for brief CT scans)
- Significant anxiety
- Movement disorders
- Autism

- Developmental delay
- Poorly controlled GERD or vomiting
- Unstable airways (e.g. craniofacial abnormalities, mediastinal mass, peritonsillar abscess)
- Inability to lie flat without respiratory support
- Children too young to remain adequately motionless (<10 years of age for MRI, <3 years for CT)

Anesthesia Techniques

General Considerations

- The anesthesiologist likely will be physically separated from patient during the scan.
- A single MRI scan (imaging of one body part) takes 20–45 min of scanner time.
- A CT scan takes 1–10 min of scanner time.
- The **goals** of anesthesia for MRI at CT are: patient safety, control of movement, anxiolysis or amnesia, and possibly analgesia. Ideally, this is accomplished with quick inductions and rapid recovery.
- Full ASA monitors should be employed [18].
- During an MRI scan, minor anesthetic issues (such as needing to change the IV drip rate, adjust ventilator settings, or re-position a nasal cannula) that require entering the scanner room should precipitate a discussion with the MRI technologist. If the issue is non-urgent, determine the next conveniently available pause in the image sequencing, allowing for entry into the scanner room and movement of the patient gantry without sacrificing a partially-completed sequence. For more urgent needs, such as patient movement or loss of monitoring signals, communicate with the technologist that urgent entry is needed, and proceed to care for the patient.
- If the MR or CT scan requires **oral contrast**, then appropriate options include either:

  - Contrast administration prior to general anesthesia, then rapid sequence induction
  - Anesthesia induction followed by intubation and placement of an orogastric tube, allowing contrast administration after securing the airway

- For CT scan, the anesthesiologist should remain in the control room during radiation emission. If staying in the scanner room, the anesthesiologist should wear full lead protective gear, including leaded eyeglasses, and remain as far from scanner bore as feasible (inverse-square law).
- **Vacuum papoose systems**, e.g. Med-Vac Infant Immobilizer (CFI Medical, Fenton, MI), mimic traditional swaddling, offering a great alternative for scanning

without sedation or anesthesia [19]. This concept works best with babies younger than 3 months, and is most successful if used approximately 30–45 min after a feeding.
• Post-operatively, patients deserve the same level of care as they would receive in the main ORs [1]. A dedicated recovery area in the Radiology suites is ideal, but if this is not available, consider transport to the main PACU.

Sedation Verses General Anesthesia

• The question of sedation versus general anesthesia (GA) for any given procedure is a topic for great debate.
• The author prefers general anesthesia for most cases.
• Sedation, while often successful, can present significant risks of hypoxemia, respiratory depression, agitation, excessive motion, and procedural failure [20, 21].
• Strongly consider GA for patients with:

  – Failed prior attempt at sedation
  – Obstructive sleep apnea (OSA) or central apneas
  – Recent respiratory illness (pneumonia, asthma exacerbation, bronchitis, URI)
  – Known or suspected difficult airway, craniofacial defects, airway masses
  – Poorly controlled GERD, vomiting, or aspiration risk
  – Complex or unstable cardiac disease
  – Multiple co-morbidities
  – Young age

• There is scant convincing data demonstrating the superiority of any specific anesthesia techniques over others in MRI and CT, and there are no strict guidelines governing the choice of anesthetic.
• Many techniques have been used successfully [21–26], and strategies vary tremendously based on the institution and the anesthesiologist.

Sedation/Monitored Anesthesia Care

• Options for specific anesthetic agents are numerous (See Table 16.6)
• Maintain vigilance for respiratory depression and/or loss of airway protective reflexes.
• Oral and intramuscular methods generally offer less predictable onset and depth of anesthesia.
• Chloral hydrate was heavily used in the past, but is falling out of favor due to poorly predictable side effects and adverse events [26, 27].

Table 16.6 Properties of specific anesthetic agents

Medication	Usual Dose	Timing	Comments
Chloral hydrate	30–100 mg/kg PO (max 1–2 g)	Onset: 10–20 min Duration: 1–6 h	Can get prolonged sedation (2–8 h) Can cause airway obstruction High rate of sedation failure
Dexmedetomidine	Load 0.5–2 mcg/kg over 10 min IV, then Infusion 0.5–2 mcg/kg/h	Onset: 10 min with load	Preserves respiratory drive Can cause bradycardia
Etomidate	0.1–0.3 mg/kg IV	Onset: 30–60 s	Can cause adrenal suppression Hemodynamically stable
Fentanyl	1–3 mcg/kg IV	Onset: 1–3 min Duration: 15–60 min	Significant respiratory depression
Ketamine	1–2 mg/kg IV bolus 10–30 mcg/kg/min IV 3–7 mg/kg IM 6–10 mg/kg PO	Onset depends on route IV 30–60 s IM 3–5 min PO 20–30 min	Preserves respiratory drive Has some analgesic properties Can cause increased secretions Can cause hallucinations/nightmares Avoid with increased ICP
Midazolam	0.025–0.25 mg/kg IV 0.5 mg/kg PO	Onset depends on route IV 1–3 min PO 10–20 min	Risk of paradoxical reaction
Propofol	1–4 mg/kg bolus 100–300 mcg/kg/min infusion	Onset: 30–60 s	Can cause respiratory depression Context-sensitive half-time Antiemetic properties

General Anesthesia

- The author's preferred anesthetic for **children** for CT or MRI:
    - GA using propofol TIVA with nasal cannula oxygen.
    - This technique is reliable, efficient, easily titratable, and almost always allows for maintenance of spontaneous ventilation.
    - Backup plan is GA with a laryngeal mask airway (LMA) or endotracheal tube (ETT), using propofol or sevoflurane.
- The author's preferred anesthetic for **adults** for CT or MRI:
    - For healthy, non-obese patients: GA using propofol TIVA with nasal cannula oxygen.
    - For patients with co-morbid conditions: GA with an LMA or ETT.
    - In adults, have a low threshold for employing an LMA or ETT.

- Choice of technique should take into consideration the patient's co-morbidities (especially airway risk), scan duration (longer scans need more airway protection), and experience of the anesthesiologist.
- There is little convincing data demonstrating the superiority of any particular technique.
- The most common problem with TIVA plus nasal cannula is mild airway obstruction during the scan, usually easily resolved with re-positioning, or placement of an oral or nasal airway.
- An LMA or ETT is needed for scans requiring **breath holds** (some cardiac, thoracic, and abdominal scans).
- Patients at increased risk for airway compromise should receive an LMA or ETT.
- Options for specific intravenous anesthetic agents are presented in Table 16.6.
- Propofol is the mainstay intravenous agent, but dexmedetomidine [25, 28] and sevoflurane are good alternatives.
- Narcotics are generally not required, unless pre-existing pain is a significant issue.

References

1. Practice advisory on anesthetic care for magnetic resonance imaging: an updated report by the American Society of Anesthesiologists Task Force on Anesthetic Care for Magnetic Resonance Imaging. Anesthesiology. 2015;122:495–520.
2. Pearce MS, Salotti JA, Little MP, et al. Radiation exposure from CT scans in childhood and subsequent risk of leukaemia and brain tumours: a retrospective cohort study. Lancet. 2012;380:499–505.
3. Pooley RA. AAPM/RSNA physics tutorial for residents. Radiographics. 2005;25:1087–99.
4. International Commission on Non-Ionizing Radiation Protection; Vecchia P, Hietanen M, Ahlbom A, et al. Guidelines on limits of exposure to static magnetic fields. Health Phys. 2009;96:504–14.
5. Hartwig V, Giovannetti G, Vanello N, et al. Biological effects and safety in magnetic resonance imaging: a review. Int J Environ Res Public Health. 2009;6:1778–98.
6. Expert Panel on MR Safety; Kanal E, Barkovich AJ, Bell C, et al. ACR guidance document on MR safe practices: 2013. J Magn Reson Imaging. 2013;37:501–30.
7. Andreucci M, Solomon R, Tasanarong A. Side effects of radiographic contrast media: pathogenesis, risk factors, and prevention. Biomed Res Int. 2014;2014:741018.
8. Davenport MS, Cohan RH, Ellis JH. Contrast media controversies in 2015: imaging patients with renal impairment or risk of contrast reaction. AJR Am J Roentgenol. 2015;204:1174–81.
9. Marckmann P, Skov L. Nephrogenic systemic fibrosis: clinical picture and treatment. Radiol Clin N Am. 2009;47:833–40.
10. The Joint Commission. Radiation risks of diagnostic imaging. Sentinel Event Alert, Issue 47, 2011. http://www.jointcommission.org/assets/1/18/SEA_47.pdf. Accessed 17 Dec 2015.
11. The Joint Commission. Preventing accidents and injuries in the MRI suite. Sentinel Event Alert, Issue 38, 2008. http://www.jointcommission.org/assets/1/18/SEA_38.pdf. Accessed 18 Dec 2015.
12. Martinez J, Ferraro S, Siemaszko C. Freak MRI accident kills W'Chester boy. New York Daily News. 2001.

13. ASTM International. Standard practice for marking medical devices and other items for safety in the magnetic resonance environment. Designation: F2503-13. West Conshohocken. 2013.
14. Shellock FG. Reference manual for magnetic resonance safety, implants and devices: 2015 Edition. Los Angeles: Biomedical Research Publishing Group; 2015.
15. Levine GN, Gomes AS, Arai AE, et al. Safety of magnetic resonance imaging in patients with cardiovascular devices: an American Heart Association scientific statement from the Committee on Diagnostic and Interventional Cardiac Catheterization, Council on Clinical Cardiology, and the Council on Cardiovascular Radiology and Intervention. Circulation. 2007;116:2878–91.
16. Harden SP. MRI conditional pacemakers: the start of a new era. Br J Radiol. 2011;84:773–4.
17. Kanal E, Gillen J, Evans JA, et al. Survey of reproductive health among female MR workers. Radiology. 1993;187:395–9.
18. ASA Standards on basic anesthetic monitoring. Approved by the ASA House of Delegates on October 21, 1986, last amended on October 20, 2010, and last affirmed on October 28, 2015. Schaumburg: American Society of Anesthesiologists.
19. Golan A, Marco R, Raz H, et al. Imaging in the newborn: infant immobilizer obviates the need for anesthesia. Isr Med Assoc J. 2011;13:663–5.
20. Sanborn PA, Michna E, Zurakowski D, et al. Adverse cardiovascular and respiratory events during sedation of pediatric patients for imaging examinations. Radiology. 2005;237:288–94.
21. Malviya S, Voepel-Lewis T, Eldevik OP, et al. Sedation and general anaesthesia in children undergoing MRI and CT: adverse events and outcomes. Br J Anaesth. 2000;84:743–8.
22. Bryan YF, Hoke LK, Taghon TA, et al. A randomized trial comparing sevoflurane and propofol in children undergoing MRI scans. Pediatr Anesth. 2009;19:672–81.
23. De Sanctis Briggs V. Magnetic resonance imaging under sedation in newborns and infants: a study of 640 cases using sevoflurane. Pediatr Anesth. 2005;15:9–15.
24. Pershad J, Wan J, Anghelescu DL. Comparison of propofol with pentobarbital/midazolam/fentanyl sedation for magnetic resonance imaging of the brain in children. Pediatrics. 2007;120:e629–36.
25. Mason KP, Fontaine PJ, Robinson F, et al. Pediatric sedation in a community hospital-based outpatient MRI center. AJR Am J Roentgenol. 2012;198:448–52.
26. Merola C, Albarracin C, Lebowitz P, et al. An audit of adverse events in children sedated with chloral hydrate or propofol during imaging studies. Pediatr Anesth. 1995;5:375–8.
27. Coté CJ, Karl HW, Notterman DA, et al. Adverse sedation events in pediatrics: analysis of medications used for sedation. Pediatrics. 2000;106:633–44.
28. Mahmoud M, Mason KP. Dexmedetomidine: review, update, and future considerations of paediatric perioperative and periprocedural applications and limitations. Br J Anaesth. 2015;115:171–82.

Chapter 17
Anesthesia for Procedures in the Neurointerventional Suite

Arne O. Budde and Sprague W. Hazard III

Abstract Procedures in the neurointerventional suite can be divided into opening procedures and closing procedures, such as angioplasty for stroke, embolization for cerebral arterio-venous malformations or coiling for cerebral aneurysm. Different equipment and medications are available for each type of procedure with unique possible side effects and complications.

Anesthesia plans must entail patient and provider safety, including radiation safety. Hemodynamic goals for individual procedures and patients may be very different and should be set and modified as necessary. Neuro-physiological monitoring requires the use and combination of medications that have the least effect on transmitted signals. Neuroprotective measures should be considered. Anticoagulation is often necessary. Various approaches to anticoagulation and reversal are available.

Keywords Neurointerventional • Stroke • Cerebral vascular malformations • Neuroprotection • Neuromonitoring • Anticoagulation • Hemodynamic monitoring • Radiation safety

Environment

Radiation Technology [36]

- Neuroradiology diagnostic and therapeutic procedures are done under high resolution fluoroscopy plus/minus digital subtraction angiography (DSA).

A.O. Budde, MD, DEAA (✉)
Anesthesiology and Perioperative Medicine, Penn State Milton S Hershey Medical Center, Center for Perioperative Services, 500 University Drive, Hershey, PA 17033, USA
e-mail: abudde@hmc.psu.edu

S.W. Hazard III, MD
Anesthesiology and Perioperative Medicine, Penn State Milton S Hershey Medical Center, 500 University Drive, Hershey, PA 17033, USA
e-mail: shazard@hmc.psu.edu

© Springer International Publishing Switzerland 2017
B.G. Goudra, P.M. Singh (eds.), *Out of Operating Room Anesthesia*,
DOI 10.1007/978-3-319-39150-2_17

- For DSA, a preliminary film is taken and all the bony structures are subtracted by a computer.
- The resultant images only display vessels containing injected contrast material, called a road map.
- Road mapping facilitates the placement of microcatheters into the distal circulation.
- For accuracy of this technique, the patient must not move and akinesia is a prerequisite.

Radiation Safety

- Ionizing radiation can cause cell death leading to tissue injury, in particular lens opacities, skin injury and infertility. Radiation exposure may also induce cancer neoplasms. Different recommendations exist for dose limits for tissue injury and cancer induction [27].
- Organs most affected are the eyes,-where radiation exposure can lead to cataract formation. Another organ of concern is the pregnant uterus where ionized radiation to the fetus can cause malformations and even fetal demise [9].
- Leaded protection gear should be used, including aprons, shields and glasses.
- Leaded glasses should be worn to protect the eyes from developing cataract. Lead glasses provide a higher degree of protection than transparent shields provide, in particular if the anesthesiologist is in close proximity to the patient [1].
- Prescription glasses with glass lenses provide some protection, while plastic lenses provide very little protection.

Material and Equipment

Material Used for Occlusive Procedures, Such as Aneurysm Coiling or AVM Embolization

- For procedures that aim at occluding a lesion or structure, such as a cerebral aneurysm or an arterio-venous malformation, different embolic material is available [36].
- Solid embolic material includes coils (usually titanium), Polyvinyl Alcohol (PVA) particles, detachable balloons and gelatin containing sponges (Gelfoam).
- Liquid embolic material [24] includes highly adhesive N-Butyl-Cyano-Acrylate (NBCA) and non-adhesive Ethylene-Vinyl-Alcohol Co-Polymer EVOH (Onyx).

Agents Used for Opening Procedures, Such as Vasospasm Treatment After Sub Arachnoid Hemorrhage (SAH)

Endovascular treatment for SAH induced cerebral vasospasm includes the following procedures and medications [8]:

- Percutaneous Transluminal Baloon Angioplasty: PTA is usually limited to proximal vessels with a diameter of more than 2–3 mm.
- Possible complications of PTA are reperfusion injury, embolism, thrombosis, displacement of surgical clips and vessel rupture.

Intra-arterial (IA) Pharmacological Therapy Final effects of IA drug therapy are vascular relaxation and vasodilation. Hypotension and increase in ICP may result from such treatment.

- Combinations of the drugs listed below may be used.
  - **Papaverine**

    Papaverine is a potent nonselective vasodilator.
    Intraarterial application reverses cerebral vasospasm.
    Papaverine improves CBF, cerebral circulation time and cerebral oxygenation.
    Increases in ICP during intra-arterial administration of Papaverine are common, i.e. ICP monitoring during the procedure is recommended.
    Other complications include cardiac side effects, thrombocytopenia, hypotension, neurological deficits, loss of visual acuity, mydriasis, and paradoxical worsening of vasospasm.

- **Phosphodiesterase III inhibitors** (Amrinone, Milrinone)

  Increase intracellular cAMP levels has positive inotropic and vasodilatory effects.
  Systemic effects are rare and have been reported only in case reports. These include increases in heart rate and one case of hypotension requiring dopamine administration.
  Increase in CBF has been demonstrated for both amrinone and milrinone.

- **Calcium channel antagonists** (Verapamil, Nimodipine, Nicardipine)

  Ca + channel antagonists inhibit Ca + influx into smooth muscle cells and have a vasodilatory effect.
  IA administration of Ca + channel antagonists can result in decreases in blood pressure and increases in ICP, particularly at higher doses.
  Blood pressure usually returns to normal shortly after stopping an IA infusion.
  Vasopressors may be needed to maintain hemodynamic stability during procedures.

- **Fasudil HCl**

  Fasudil is a potent vasodilator with relative specificity for cerebral arteries.
  Systemic hypotension may occur in addition to small increases in ICP.

- **Colforsine Daropate HCl**

   Colforsine increases intracellular cAMP via activation of Adenyl Cyclase.
   It has positive chronotropic, inotropic and vasodilatory effects.
   Colforsine has been successfully used to treat vasospasm.
   Transient changes in heart rate and blood pressure were seen.

Flow Augmentation Strategies

- NeuroFlo catheter, Intra-aortic balloon pump (IAPB) counterpulsation.

   Intra-aortic balloon catheters can be used to augment cerebral blood flow.
   Successful application of the NeuroFlo catheter as well as IABP in patients with
   cerebral vasospasm has been demonstrated in multiple recent trials

Recanalization of Ischemic Stroke [33]

- The only currently FDA approved therapy for recanalization following ischemic
  stroke is intravenous tissue plasminogen activator (tPA), given within 4.5 h of
  onset of symptoms.
- Other approaches to address a longer time window up to 8 h include intra-arterial
  thrombolysis, mechanical thrombectomy and a combination of those
  techniques.
- Agents used for intra-arterial thrombolysis are prourokinase and tPA. These
  should be used within 6 h of onset of acute ischemic stroke in a large proximal
  vessel or up to 24 h after onset of acute basilar artery occlusion.
- The use of endovascular ultrasound – called sonothrbmolectomy – has been shown
  to increase the recanalization rate, particularly when used in addition to tPA.

Mechanical Devices

- Mechanical devices can be used when intravenous or intra-arterial therapy failed
  or when thrombolysis is contraindicated. Contraindications include bleeding diathesis, warfarin use, elevated international normalized ratio (INR), major surgery
  within 14 days, thrombocytopenia, genitourinary or gastrointestinal bleeding
  and trauma associated with the onset of stroke symptoms.
- Mechanical Strategies for thrombectomy include:

   - Distal clot retrieval: The retrieving device is advanced over a microcatheter
     through the clot and then withdrawn.

- Proximal clot aspiration: The devices remove the clot from its proximal end by using aspiration methods or ultrasound.
- Stentrievers: The clot is temporarily stented against the vessel wall to achieve faster reperfusion. The stent and clot can then be removed together. The stent can also be permanently deployed.

Anesthesia Plan

- Patient positioning in relation to anesthesia machine monitors and radiology equipment requires flexibility and thinking outside the box compared to the operating room.
- The anesthesia work space is often to the left of the patients head, opposed to the traditional setup with the anesthesia machine to the patient's right.
- This makes anesthesia induction an unusual procedure with the circuit coming from the left of the anesthesia provider.
- The c-arm may be close to the patients head with limited access around the patient.
- Frequent "runs" of the fluoroscopic x-ray equipment around the patient including the patients head with airway, breathing circuit and intravenous as well as arterial lines may pose the integrity of the anesthesia delivery and monitoring system at risk.
- Line extensions for intravenous and arterial lines should be used and positioned cautiously. Attenstion should be paid to prevent pulling out of these lines unintentionally and/or unrecognized during the procedure.
- The same applies to the breathing circuit, which should be extended and carefully secured.
- A protective shield between the patient and the anesthesia provider protects against radiation exposure but may also be an obstacle to overcome when direct access to the patient is required. Lines and the anesthesia circuit have to be maneuvered around the shield and getting to the patient quickly may be difficult.
- Vital sign monitors and equipment are often shared with the proceduralist.
- Arterial blood pressure measurement may be transduced form a side port of the femoral arterial introducer sheath. However, a separate arterial line should be considered for close blood pressure monitoring during induction of general anesthesia.
- Pulse oximetry is often measured from two extremities simultaneously. An additional pulse oximeter probe on the extremity with the introducer sheath may help detect perfusion defects from thrombus formation or vascular dissection.
- Emergency equipment including airway management tools should be readily available. Relying on backup equipment from the main operating room may not be suitable.
- Patient recovery should be in or close to the procedure area. Transporting freshly extubated patients for long distances through the vaults of a hospital may be a setup for possible disaster.

Hemodynamic/Anesthetic Goals

Ischemic Stroke

- Maintain oxygen saturation >94 % [17]
- Maintain normothermia: treat hyperthermia (temperature >38 °C) with anti-pyretic medications and/or cooling devices [17]
- Patients eligible for acute reperfusion therapy must have BP controlled to <185/110 mmHg prior to, during and after reperfusion
- Strategies to lower BP include the following:
  - Labetalol 10–20 mg IV over 1–2 min repeat x times one
  - Nicardipine 5 mg/h IV, titrate up by 2.5 mg/h every 5–15 min -maximum 15 mg/h
  - If BP not controlled or diastolic BP >140 mmHg, IV sodium nitroprusside can be used
- The use of high-dose albumin is not well established.
- The usefulness of drug-induced hypertension in patients with acute ischemic stroke is not well established
- Hemodilution by volume expansion is not recommended
- Studies favor conscious sedation over general anesthesia during endovascular therapy for acute stroke however, randomized trials do not exist [31]
- Anesthetic technique during endovascular therapy should be individualized: considerations include patient comorbidities, ability to lay flat, tolerance to the procedure etc.

Intracerebral Hemorrhage (ICH)

- INTERACT2 – largest randomized clinical trial to date: intensive BP lowering in 2839 patients with SBP between 150 and 220 mmHg within 6 h of ICH [2]
- Early treatment targeted to an SBP level <140 mmHg improves chances of patients with ICH achieving better functional recovery [15]

Subarachnoid Hemorrhage (SAH)

- Minimize the degree and duration of hypotension during aneurysm repair [6]
- Induced hypothermia during aneurysm repair is not routinely recommended
- Avoid intraoperative hyperglycemia
- Do not administer large volumes of hypotonic fluids
- Avoid intravascular volume contraction
- Maintain normothermia (with standard or advanced temperature modulating systems) during acute phase of aneurysmal SAH

- Optimal hemoglobin goal in patients with aSAH who are at risk of cerebral ischemia is undetermined
- Hypothermia during aneurysm repair is not routinely recommended [6]

Neuromonitoring

- EEG: electrical activity of cortical cells received by a grid of scalp electrodes
- Amplitude and frequency of groups of cells can be affected by perturbations in metabolism (both global and regional) [23]
- Strong correlation between EEG flattening and reductions in CBF [35]
- SSEP: evoked potentials are more specific whereas EEG is passive and more generalized
- Peripheral nerve stimulated (e.g. median nerve) – evoked potential peaks travel from median nerve to brachial plexus, spinal cord, and terminates in the cerebral cortex [23]
- Correlation between regional CBF and SSEP's – changes begin at approximately 20 ml/min/100 g and are lost at 15–18 ml/min/100 g [4]
- SSEP's in intravascular procedures can determins the following: (1) adequacy of collateral flow (2) temporary occlusion testing (3) adequacy of MAP/CPP

  - SSEP from upper extremity supplied by the middle cerebral artery (aneurysm coiling of the ICA/MCA)
  - SSEP from lower extremity supplied by the anterior cerebral artery

- MEP: Measures the transcranial stimulation of the motor cortex and evaluates the descending response via cortospinal tract to innervated muscle group [26]
- Motor and sensory strips have distinct vascular innervations and therefore can be used independently or in combination depending on the area of interest
- MEP's – more rapid detection of ischemia – grey matter (higher metabolic requirements) more sensitive to ischemia [18]

Renal Protection

- The incidence of contrast induced nephropathy is approximately 2 % in the general population
- High-risk patients (diabetic patients, congestive heart failure, chronic renal impairment, and older age) incidence increases to 20–30 % [13]
- The precise mechanisms of Contrast induced nephropathy (CIN) is unknown

  - Adenosine, endothelin, and free radical-induced vasoconstriction increase following CIN
  - Nitric oxide and prostaglandin-induced vasodilatation decrease

- Contrast agents have direct toxic effects on kidney tubular cells (vacuolization, mitochondrial dysfunction, and apoptosis) [30]
- N-acetylcysteine (NAC) increases production of nitric oxide (potent vasodilator) and the concentration of glutathione (free radical scavenger) [13]
- Oral NAC, together with intravenous isotonic crystalloids, is recommended in patients at increased risk of CIN [19]
- Saline is more effective than half normal saline for the prevention of CIN [28]
- Saline is also more effective than aggressive oral water intake alone [5]
- Saline increases tubular fluid volume (reducing the concentration of contrast media) and causes a slight increases in tubular pH and reduction in reactive oxygen species (ROS) [30]
- For benefit, saline infusion must be maintained for the duration that contrast media is being excreted by the kidney
- Low pH is known to accelerate cellular apoptosis when free radical species are present [5]
- Na bicarbonate infusions increase in tubular bicarbonate anion concentration and can be protective.

Neuro Protection

- There are more than 1000 published reports of neuroprotective treatments for acute stroke and over 100 clinical trials [29]
- To date there are no pharmacological agents with neuroprotective actions that have proven to be efficacious in improving outcomes after ischemic stroke [17]
- Routine use of hypothermia for the treatment of patients with ischemic stroke is not recommended [17]

Anticoagulation/Reversal

- Patients with non-valvular atrial fibrillation (AF) with prior stroke, transient ischemic attack (TIA), or a CHA2DS2-VASc score of 2 or greater, oral anticoagulants are recommended
- Options include warfarin (INR 2.0–3.0) or new oral anticoagulants (NOACs) which include dabigatran, rivaroxaban or apixaban [16]
- More than 2.5 million Americans are chronically anticoagulated: indications including venous thromboembolism (VTE), mechanical heart valve(s), (AF) [37]
- NOAC use has increased dramatically ~1/3 of patients with atrial fibrillation (AF) using them for stroke prophylaxis [20]
- The annual incidence of stroke in patients with AF varies widely: between 1.9 and 18.2 % based on the CHADS2 risk score [11]
- Maintaining INR between 2 and 3 reduces the risk of stroke to an annual incidence of 1.6–2.2 % [7]

- All NOACs are at least non-inferior to warfarin in terms of efficacy, reducing the annual incidence of stroke to 1.2–1.7%/year [7, 12, 14]
- Major bleeding (intracranial and other) NOACs are also as least as safe as warfarin [7, 12, 14]
- Coagulation Cascade – injury to vessel wall, tissue factor is exposed
- Tissue factor reacts with factor VII → activates coagulation cascade
- Thrombin produced by series of proenzymes
- Thrombin converts fibrinogen to fibrin; activates factors V, VIII, and XI (which generates more thrombin stimulates platelets) factor XIII – cross-links fibrin stabilizing clot [10]
- Factor Xa acts upstream of thrombin in the clotting cascade → convergence point of the intrinsic and extrinsic pathways
- Inhibition of factor Xa prevents amplified thrombin generation
- One molecule of factor Xa can cleave over 1000 molecules of prothrombin to thrombin [21]
- Dabigatran etexilate (PRADAXA) – converted to active form by serum esterases; approved in October 2010 by FDA
- Mechanism of action: Binds to the active site of thrombin
- Rivaroxaban (Xarelto) first oral direct coagulation factor Xa inhibitor approved in the United States
- Mechanism of action: selectively inhibits free and clot-bound FXa as well as FXa – prothrombinase complex prevents thrombin formation
- Does not require a cofactor (such as antithrombin III) for activity
- APIXABAN (Eliquis) oral direct coagulation factor Xa inhibitor

Laboratory Tests

- Prothrombin time and International normalized ratio is not helpful in determining whether an anticoagulant effect from dabigatran is present [17]
- Rivaroxaban prolonged PT in a concentration-dependent manner however therapeutic concentrations weak effect on PT
- Significant variation in the PT depending on the thromboplastin reagent
- Apixaban prolonged PT concentration-dependent therapeutic concentrations weak effect on PT
- Rivaroxaban Apixaban prolongs Activated partial thromboplastin time (aPTT) (to varying degrees) dose-dependent manner
- Conclusion: PT and aPTT are insensitive to determine activity of oral Xa inhibitors [17]
- Specific assays for anti-factor Xa activity are available
- Ecarin Clotting Time (ECT) (derived from the Saw-scaled viper: *Echis carinatus*) Ecarin activates prothrombin (proteolytic cleavage)

Produces meizothrombin – an unstable precursor of thrombin

- Direct thrombin inhibitors inhibit the thrombin-like activity of meizothrombin
- Ecarin Clotting Time (ECT) test provides a direct measure (linear over the full range of concentrations) of the activity of DTIs
- Thrombin clotting time (TT) – provides a direct measure of the activity of Pradaxa → linear dose–response over therapeutic concentrations

Reversal

- INR is in therapeutic range about 70 % of the time [3]
- Intracerebral hemorrhage is the most common (70 %) anticoagulant -related intracranial hemorrhage (subdural second most common)
- The incidence of anticoagulant-related ICH 0.25–1.1 %/year: approaches 2 % when INR >2.0
- Anticoagulant-related ICH have a mortality rate 60 % (40 % not anticoagulated) [3]
- Acute subdural haemorrhage (SDH) – coagulopathy (INR >1.2 independently predicted in-hospital mortality [3]

Antidotes for Warfarin

- Vitamin K
- Recombinant factor VIIa (Novoseven) ®
- Fresh frozen plasma (FFP)
- Prothrombin complex conjugates (PCC)

FFP Limitations

- Large volume (15–20 ml/kg)
- Longer infusion
- Transfusion-related acute lung injury (TRALI)
- Time to thaw (15–45 min)
- ABO typing
- Infectious transmission

Vitamin K Limitations

- Delayed onset
- IV = faster than PO
- Baseline INR 6–10 → therapeutic range INR at 6 h (11/24 vs. 0/23) and at 12 h (16/24 vs. 8/23) [25]

- Anaphylactic reactions with IV form
- Anaphylaxis is not phytonadione but the *solubilizing vehicle* (polyethoxylated castor oil: PEO-CO)
- 6572 doses of IV phytonadione – 2938 patients incidence of anaphylaxis → 3 per 10,000 doses
- "The incidence of anaphylaxis after IV phytonadione is overall comparable or slightly less than other drugs known to cause anaphylaxis"
- Dosing = 10 mg IV infusion over 30 min [34].

Factor VIIa Imitations

- rFVIIa does not replace all clotting factors – INR may be lowered, clotting may not be restored in vivo
- rFVIIa is not recommended for vitamin k antagonist (VKA) reversal in ICH [17]

Prothrombin Complex Concentrate (PCC)

4 factor-concentrates – adequate amounts of vitamin K dependent factors II, VII, IX and X (Beriplex®, Octaplex®, Proplex T®, Kcentra ®)
3 factor-concentrates – significantly lower amounts of factor VII (less than one third of factor IX) (Prothrombinex-HT®, Profilnine® and Bebulin®)
Activated PCCs (Factor 8 inhibitor activity bypassing agent [FEIBA])

- PCCs that contain at least one activated factor
- FEIBA is the only aPCC available in the United States
- FEIBA – factor VII is activated
- Factor IX complex, human derived protein
- Contains factors II, VII, IX, X
- Non-therapeutic levels of factor VII (3 factor concentrates)
- Dosing is based on factor IX component
- Vitamin K should always be given with PCC due to transient effects [15]
- Not necessary to give FFP [15]
- PCCs may have fewer complications and correct the INR more rapidly than FFP [17]

Dosing for Prothrombin Complex Concentrate

- Dose of PCC for initial INR of 2.0–3.9, 4.0–6.0, and >6.0 was 25, 35, and 60 IU/kg, respectively [32]
- Reversal of NOAC's – aPCC (FEIBA), at a dose of 50–80 units/kg. If an aPCC

- If aPCC unavailable – unactivated 4-factor or 3-factor PCC reasonable alternative at 50 units/kg [22]
- Activated charcoal might be used if the most recent dose of dabigatran, apixaban, or rivaroxaban was taken <2 h
- Hemodialysis can be considered for reversal of dabigatran [15]
- Idarucizumab (Praxbind)® is the humanized monoclonal antibody fragment that binds to dabigatran (Pradaxa)®: FDA approved on October 16, 2015 and can be used for its reversal.
- Indications: patients requiring emergency surgery or urgent procedures patients with life-threatening or uncontrolled bleeding

References

1. Anastasian ZH, Strozyk D, et al. Radiation exposure of the anesthesiologist in the neurointerventional suite. Anesthesiology. 2011;114(3):512–20.
2. Anderson CS, Heeley E, et al. Rapid blood-pressure lowering in patients with acute intracerebral hemorrhage. N Engl J Med. 2013;368(25):2355–65.
3. Bershad EM, Suarez JI. Prothrombin complex concentrates for oral anticoagulant therapy-related intracranial hemorrhage: a review of the literature. Neurocrit Care. 2010;12(3):403–13.
4. Branston NM, Symon L, et al. Recovery of the cortical evoked response following temporary middle cerebral artery occlusion in baboons: relation to local blood flow and PO_2. Stroke. 1976;7(2):151–7.
5. Burgess WP, Walker PJ. Mechanisms of contrast-induced nephropathy reduction for saline (NaCl) and sodium bicarbonate ($NaHCO_3$). Biomed Res Int. 2014;2014:510385.
6. Connolly Jr ES, Rabinstein AA, et al. Guidelines for the management of aneurysmal subarachnoid hemorrhage: a guideline for healthcare professionals from the American Heart Association/american Stroke Association. Stroke. 2012;43(6):1711–37.
7. Connolly SJ, Ezekowitz MD, et al. Dabigatran versus warfarin in patients with atrial fibrillation. N Engl J Med. 2009;361(12):1139–51.
8. Dabus G, Nogueira RG. Current options for the management of aneurysmal subarachnoid hemorrhage-induced cerebral vasospasm: a comprehensive review of the literature. Interv Neurol. 2013;2(1):30–51.
9. Dagal A. Radiation safety for anesthesiologists. Curr Opin Anaesthesiol. 2011;24(4):445–50.
10. Di Nisio M, Middeldorp S, et al. Direct thrombin inhibitors. N Engl J Med. 2005;353(10):1028–40.
11. Gage BF, Waterman AD, et al. Validation of clinical classification schemes for predicting stroke: results from the National Registry of Atrial Fibrillation. JAMA. 2001;285(22):2864–70.
12. Giugliano RP, Ruff CT, et al. Edoxaban versus warfarin in patients with atrial fibrillation. N Engl J Med. 2013;369(22):2093–104.
13. Golshahi J, Nasri H, et al. Contrast-induced nephropathy: a literature review. J Nephropathol. 2014;3(2):51–6.
14. Granger CB, Alexander JH, et al. Apixaban versus warfarin in patients with atrial fibrillation. N Engl J Med. 2011;365(11):981–92.
15. Hemphill 3rd JC, Greenberg SM, et al. Guidelines for the management of spontaneous intracerebral hemorrhage: a guideline for healthcare professionals from the American Heart Association/American Stroke Association. Stroke. 2015;46(7):2032–60.
16. January CT, Wann LS, et al. 2014 AHA/ACC/HRS guideline for the management of patients with atrial fibrillation: a report of the American College of Cardiology/American Heart Association Task Force on Practice Guidelines and the Heart Rhythm Society. J Am Coll Cardiol. 2014;64(21):e1–76.

17. Jauch EC, Saver JL, et al. Guidelines for the early management of patients with acute ischemic stroke: a guideline for healthcare professionals from the American Heart Association/American Stroke Association. Stroke. 2013;44(3):870–947.
18. Krieg SM, Shiban E, et al. Predictive value and safety of intraoperative neurophysiological monitoring with motor evoked potentials in glioma surgery. Neurosurgery. 2012;70(5):1060–70; discussion 1070–71.
19. Lameire N, Kellum JA, et al. Contrast-induced acute kidney injury and renal support for acute kidney injury: a KDIGO summary (Part 2). Crit Care. 2013;17(1):205.
20. Lauffenburger JC, Farley JF, et al. Factors driving anticoagulant selection in patients with atrial fibrillation in the United States. Am J Cardiol. 2015;115(8):1095–101.
21. Laux V, Perzborn E, et al. Direct inhibitors of coagulation proteins – the end of the heparin and low-molecular-weight heparin era for anticoagulant therapy? Thromb Haemost. 2009; 102(5):892–9.
22. Liotta EM, Levasseur-Franklin KE, et al. Reversal of the novel oral anticoagulants dabigatran, rivoraxaban, and apixaban. Curr Opin Crit Care. 2015;21(2):127–33.
23. Loftus CM, Biller J, et al. Intraoperative neuromonitoring. New York: McGraw-Hill Education; 2014.
24. Loh Y, Duckwiler GR. A prospective, multicenter, randomized trial of the Onyx liquid embolic system and N-butyl cyanoacrylate embolization of cerebral arteriovenous malformations. Clinical article. J Neurosurg. 2010;113(4):733–41.
25. Lubetsky A, Yonath H, et al. Comparison of oral vs intravenous phytonadione (vitamin K1) in patients with excessive anticoagulation: a prospective randomized controlled study. Arch Intern Med. 2003;163(20):2469–73.
26. Macdonald DB. Intraoperative motor evoked potential monitoring: overview and update. J Clin Monit Comput. 2006;20(5):347–77.
27. Miller DL, Schueler BA, et al. New recommendations for occupational radiation protection. J Am Coll Radiol. 2012;9(5):366–8.
28. Murphy SW, Barrett BJ, et al. Contrast nephropathy. J Am Soc Nephrol. 2000;11(1):177–82.
29. O'Collins VE, Macleod MR, et al. 1,026 experimental treatments in acute stroke. Ann Neurol. 2006;59(3):467–77.
30. Persson PB, Hansell P, et al. Pathophysiology of contrast medium-induced nephropathy. Kidney Int. 2005;68(1):14–22.
31. Powers WJ, Derdeyn CP, et al. 2015 American Heart Association/American Stroke Association Focused Update of the 2013 Guidelines for the Early Management of Patients With Acute Ischemic Stroke Regarding Endovascular Treatment: A Guideline for Healthcare Professionals From the American Heart Association/American Stroke Association. Stroke. 2015;46(10):3020–35.
32. Preston FE, Laidlaw ST, et al. Rapid reversal of oral anticoagulation with warfarin by a pro-thrombin complex concentrate (Beriplex): efficacy and safety in 42 patients. Br J Haematol. 2002;116(3):619–24.
33. Raphaeli G, Mazighi M, et al. State-of-the-art endovascular treatment of acute ischemic stroke. Adv Tech Stand Neurosurg. 2015;42:33–68.
34. Riegert-Johnson DL, Volcheck GW. The incidence of anaphylaxis following intravenous phytonadione (vitamin K1): a 5-year retrospective review. Ann Allergy Asthma Immunol. 2002;89(4):400–6.
35. Sundt Jr TM, Sharbrough FW, et al. Correlation of cerebral blood flow and electroencephalographic changes during carotid endarterectomy: with results of surgery and hemodynamics of cerebral ischemia. Mayo Clin Proc. 1981;56(9):533–43.
36. Varma MK, Price K, et al. Anaesthetic considerations for interventional neuroradiology. Br J Anaesth. 2007;99(1):75–85.
37. Wysokinski WE, McBane 2nd RD. Periprocedural bridging management of anticoagulation. Circulation. 2012;126(4):486–90.

Part VI
Anesthesia for Other Out of Operating Room Procedures

Chapter 18
Anesthesia for Outpatient Dental Procedures

Carolyn Barbieri and Meghan Whitley

Abstract While a significant amount of dental procedures can be done in a dentist's office with local anesthetic, there are circumstances when the patient's medical comorbidities require additional monitoring and deeper levels of sedation than can be provided in an outpatient office. These may range in spectrum from mild anxiolysis performed by a dentist, to general anesthesia performed by an anesthesiologist. The content below offers an overview of human dental anatomy, dental notation, levels of sedation, common anxiolytics and anesthetic practices, adverse events, and guidelines for the management of dental anesthesia.

Keywords Dental Anesthesia • Human Dentition • Dental Identification • American Society of Anesthesiologists (ASA) guidelines for sedation and analgesia by non-anesthesiologists • Spontaneous Bacterial Endocarditis guidelines • Local Anesthetics • Nitrous Oxide • Ketamine • Chloral Hydrate • Arrhythmias with Dental Procedures

Introduction

With all of the advances in modern day medicine, dental disease remains the most common chronic disease of children and adults, according to the Centers for Disease Control and Prevention.

- Dental carries and the formation of cavities in teeth by bacteria are four times more common than asthma in children. Dental carries also affect adults; 90 % of people over the age of 20 have some degree of tooth or root decay (Dye et al. Vital Health Stat Ser (248):1–92, 2007) [3].

C. Barbieri, MD (✉)
Department of Anesthesiology and Perioperative Medicine, Penn State Milton S Hershey Medical Center, 500 University Drive, H187, Hershey, PA 17036, USA
e-mail: cbarbieri@hmc.psu.edu

M. Whitley, BS, DO
Anesthesiology and Perioperative Medicine, Penn State Milton S. Hershey Medical Center, 500 University Drive, Hershey, PA 17033, USA
e-mail: mwhitley@hmc.psu.edu

© Springer International Publishing Switzerland 2017
B.G. Goudra, P.M. Singh (eds.), *Out of Operating Room Anesthesia*,
DOI 10.1007/978-3-319-39150-2_18

237

- Periodontal disease, inflammation and infections of the gums or bone, affect 47.2 % of adults aged 30 years or older and 70.1 % of adults 65 years or older (Eke et al. J Dent Res 91(10):1–7, 2012) [4].

Human Dentition

Dental Anatomy

Human teeth are subdivided into two major parts, the crown and the root. The crown is the part of the tooth that is visible in the mouth and is responsible for slicing, ripping and grinding food (incisors, canines, and molars respectively). The root structure yields strength and stability to the tooth and surrounding structures. The anterior teeth, incisors, and canines, are single rooted teeth and have a conical shape. The posterior teeth, premolars and molars, are multi rooted teeth and provide stability by number of roots and direction of root implantation.

Every human tooth is composed of four different tissues that serve different functions. The outmost layer is enamel which makes up the protective surface of the crown of the tooth. The next later is the dentin which makes up the majority of the inner surface of the tooth. The dentin can only be seen on x-rays. The pulp is the central area of the tooth that contains the nerves and blood vessels. The pulp extends into both the crown and the root of the tooth. Lastly, the cementum makes up the outer surface of the root of the tooth, this is much softer than the enamel [23].

The periodontium is the structure surrounding the root of the tooth. The periodontium is composed of three structures, the gingival and alveolar mucosa, the periodontal ligament, and the alveolar bone. The gingival and alveolar mucosa comprises the soft tissue covering all of the periodontal structures. The periodontal ligament attaches the external surface of the root to the alveolar bone, acting as an anchor and shock absorber during mastication. The alveolar bone is the thickened ridge of bone that contains the tooth sockets. The alveolar bone can easily remodel, thus allowing orthodontic tooth movement. The alveolar bone abuts the deep supporting basal or skeletal bone of the mandible and maxilla. When teeth are lost or removed, the alveolar bone degenerates and the basal bone is evident in edentulous patients; forming the skeletal support for full or partial dentures.

Dental Identification

There are two universal dental identification systems, the Universal Numbering System and the Palmer Notation System. In both systems the primary teeth are designated by letters and the permanent teeth are designated by numbers.

Table 18.1 Universal numbering system – Primary dentition

Upper right									Upper left
A	B	C	D	E	F	G	H	I	J
T	S	R	Q	P	O	N	M	L	K
Lower right									Lower left

Table 18.2 Universal numbering system – Permanent dentition

Upper right														Upper left	
1	2	3	4	5	6	7	8	9	10	11	12	13	14	15	16
32	31	30	29	28	27	26	25	24	23	22	21	20	19	18	
Lower right														Lower left	

Universal Numbering System

The most widely uses system in the United States dental schools is the Universal Numbering system. The Universal Numbering system starts identification at the farthest back upper right tooth passes across the maxilla to the farthest back upper left tooth, then moving to the lower left of the mandible and moving across to the last lower right tooth [17].

- As can be seen in Table 18.1, the primary dentition is assigned letters from A to T starting at the upper right second molar and ending at the lower right second molar.
- As can be seen in Table 18.2, the permanent dentition is assigned numbers 1–32 starting in the upper right third molar and continuing to the lower right third molar.

Palmer Notation System

The Palmer Notation system is widely used in the United Kingdom and is the primary means of identification by orthodontists. The Palmer Notation system splits the dental arch into four quadrants, starting with the central incisor following distally and posteriorly, with all four quadrants designated by a symbol (⌐ ⌐ ⌐ ⌐) [5].

- The primary dentition is assigned letters to the teeth from A to E in all four quadrants starting with the central incisor and moving distally, as shown in Table 18.3.
- The permanent dentition is assigned numbers from 1 to 8 in all four quadrants starting with the central incisor and moving distally, as shown in Table 18.4.

Table 18.3 Palmer notation system – Primary dentition

				Upper right	Upper left				
E⅃	D⅃	C⅃	B⅃	A⅃	⌐A	⌐B	⌐C	⌐D	⌐E
E⌐	D⌐	C⌐	B⌐	A⌐	⌐A	⌐B	⌐C	⌐D	⌐E
				Lower right	Lower left				

Table 18.4 Palmer notation system – Permanent dentition

								Upper right	Upper left						
8⅃	7⅃	6⅃	5⅃	4⅃	3⅃	2⅃	1⅃	⌐1	⌐2	⌐3	⌐4	⌐5	⌐6	⌐7	⌐8
8⌐	7⌐	6⌐	5⌐	4⌐	3⌐	2⌐	1⌐	⌐1	⌐2	⌐3	⌐4	⌐5	⌐6	⌐7	⌐8
								Lower right	Lower left						

Dental Procedures

The majority of dental procedures are performed in the dental office. For most dental procedures, local anesthesia with or without sedation is sufficient. However, there are many patient medical conditions and procedural needs that may require additional monitoring and deeper levels of sedation than can be completed in the outpatient office.

Medical Conditions [2, 19, 21]

- Ischemic heart disease
- Congenital heart disease
- Pulmonary impairment with oxygen requirements
- Bleeding disorders
- Craniofacial abnormalities
- Orofacial trauma
- Mental retardation or severe behavioral disturbances
- Malignant Hyperthermia or at increased risk

Levels of Sedation

There are varying degrees of sedation that patients can receive for dental procedures. Sedation and analgesia comprise a continuum of states ranging from minimal sedation (anxiolysis) through general anesthesia.

Minimal Sedation (Anxiolysis)

- Drug induced state which patients respond normally to verbal commands
- Cognitive function and coordination may be impaired

- Pulmonary and cardiovascular function is unaffected
- No vital sign monitoring is necessary, only visual observation
- Sedation must be provided by second qualified provider (BLS certified)

Moderate Sedation (Conscious Sedation)

- Drug induced depression of consciousness during which patients respond purposefully to verbal commands
- Cognitive function is impaired, but should remain conscious throughout
- Spontaneous ventilation is maintained
- Cardiovascular function is maintained
- Vital signs are monitored (heart rate, oxygen saturation, blood pressure and respiratory rate)
- Sedation must be provided by second qualified provider (BLS & ACLS certified)

Deep Sedation (Analgesia)

- Drug induced depression of consciousness during which patients cannot be easily aroused, but arousable after repeated verbal or painful stimuli
- Cognitive function is depressed
- Ventilation may be impaired and may require assistance; there may be partial or complete loss of reflexes
- Cardiovascular function is maintained
- Vital signs are monitored (heart rate, oxygen saturation, blood pressure and respiratory rate)
- Sedation must be provided by second qualified provider (BLS & ACLS certified)

General Anesthesia

- Drug induced loss of consciousness during which patients are not arousable
- No cognitive function is present
- Ventilation may be impaired and may require assistance; there may be partial or complete loss of reflexes
- Cardiovascular function is impaired
- Standard ASA monitors are required
- General anesthesia must be provided by an anesthesiologist, anesthesia resident or anesthetist

Pharmacology of Dental Anesthesia

A number of medications are utilized by clinicians to assist with anxiolysis and maintenance of sedation and analgesia for dental procedures. These various medications are available through different routes of administration which can be tailored based on the cooperation of the patient, desired effect, and duration of action required. We will highlight some of the common agents which will be encountered in office-based dental suites.

Midazolam

- Can be administered PO, sublingual, IV, intranasal, IM, or PR
- Onset is 15–30 min with duration of 60–90 min with PO administration
- Intranasal route can be irritating
- Risk of airway obstruction and respiratory depression when combined with opioids (recommend reduction in midazolam dose by at least 25 %) or when used alone [1, 11]
- Retrograde amnesia with initial use may improve compliance with further dental procedures.
- Flumazenil may be administered for benzodiazepine reversal, but may require re-dosing due to its short half-life.

Chloral Hydrate

- Sedative used for less stimulating procedures, in neonates through children less than three [11]
- Can be administered PO or PR, but there is a risk of incomplete absorption
- Onset is 30–60 min with duration of 60–120 min
- Dose 50–100 mg/kg with maximum dose of 2 g
- May cause airway obstruction and respiratory depression at higher doses (75–100 mg/kg).
- There are significant differences in half life based on age. This ranges from 10 h in toddlers to as long as 40 h in preterm infants and therefore, may require prolonged recovery time [1, 11].

Meperidine (Demerol)

- Can be administered PO, IV, Subcutaneous or IM
- Onset is 30–60 min with duration of 2–4 h with PO administration
- Dose 1–2 mg/kg with maximum dose of 50 mg
- Risk of respiratory depression and seizures due to its active metabolite, normeperidine [11]

Ketamine

- Can be administered IV or IM; however, PO has also been described [11].
- Dose is 3–10 mg/kg when used alone, but should be decreased to 3–6 mg/kg when combined with midazolam [10].

Hydroxyzine

- Administered PO or IM
- First-generation H1 antagonist utilized for its sedation side effect.
- Dose 1–2 mg/kg, maximum dose 100 mg
- Onset within 15–30 min with duration of 2–4 h
- Increased risk of QT prolongation noted [18].

Nitrous Oxide

- Can be considered minimal sedation when administered in a 50:50 ratio with oxygen
- Is considered moderate sedation when administered in a greater than 50:50 ratio with or without the administration of sedatives or analgesics
- Onset is less than 5 min with rapid return to baseline
- Risk of hypoxia increases significantly with supplemental PO or IV agents. Hypoxemia can occur with as minimal as 30 % nitrous when chloral hydrate is also administered [10].
- Requires specialized equipment for delivery, including a nasal mask, monitoring including FiO_2 sensing, and a scavenging system [11].
- Studies have shown an increased risk of spontaneous abortion and decreased conception rates in personnel routinely exposed to nitrous without scavenging equipment; however, this risk was not shown when the equipment was used [12].

Local Anesthetics

- Local anesthetic selection is based on the patient's medical history, mental status, expected procedure duration, and planned administration of other adjuncts.
- Local anesthetics typically available for dental procedures are contained below in Table 18.5 with maximum doses and anticipated duration of action [8, 14].

Table 18.5 Local Anestetics for Dental Anesthesia

Local anesthetic	Maximum dose (mg/kg) with epinephrine	Maximum dose (mg/kg) without epinephrine	Duration (min)
Atricaine	–	7	60–230
Bupivicaine	2	3	240–480
Lidocaine	5	7	60–240
Mepivicaine	5	7	60–240
Prilocaine	7	10	60–120

Complications

Subacute Bacterial Endocarditis (SBE)

- Transient bacteremia (not present within 15 min) is noted in up to 65 % of dental extractions and 16 % of dental restorations and nasotracheal intubations. The two most common organisms responsible are Streptococcus viridans and Staphylococcus aureus [16].
- While there is a risk with general dental maintenance such as flossing, the risk is greater with mucosal/gingival tissue perforation, or procedures involving the periapical region of the tooth [7].
- The American Heart Association (AHA) 2007 guidelines limited SBE prophylaxis to only those at greatest risk of adverse complications from endocarditis [6].

Patients Requiring SBE Prophylaxis [22]

- History of prior infective endocarditis
- Prosthetic cardiac valves or prosthetic material used in valve repair
- Cyanotic congenital heart disease (CHD) with shunts or conduits
- Acyanotic (repaired) CHD within the first 6 months of repair with prosthetic material due to inadequate time for endothelialization
- Acyanotic (repaired) CHD with residual defects present near prosthetic material which presumably impedes endothelialization
- History of heart transplant with valvulopathy

SBE Prophylaxis Dosing and Administration

- Ideally, antibiotics should be given 30–60 min prior to surgery; however, they can be given up to 2 h after the procedure if needed [6, 7].
- The standard antibiotic used for SBE prophylaxis is PO amoxicillin (50 mg/kg up to 2 g). However, the AHA offers alternatives for patients unable to tolerate PO or with penicillin allergies with appropriate dosages [23].
- In the event a patient requiring SBE prophylaxis is already on another antibiotic, the American Dental Association recommends a different class of antibiotics be administered for SBE prophylaxis [7].

- There is no increased risk of prosthetic joint infections with dental procedures. SBE prophylaxis should not be administered to these patients [20].

Arrhythmias Associated with Dental Procedures

- A number of case reports have described arrhythmias associated with dental procedures.
- Some of the implicating factors described include iatrogenic epinephrine administration, as well as pain and anxiety since catecholamine levels can increase 40 fold with stress [15].
- Other confounding factors include arrhythmias associated with hypoxia, hypercapnia and volatile anesthetic administration.
- The impetus for arrhythmias has also been attributed to trigeminal nerve stimulation which can be alleviated or decreased by local infiltration to cranial nerve V or removing the surgical stimulus [16].

General Anesthesia for Dental Procedures

General anesthesia can be induced for dental procedures or can unintentionally occur on the continuum of sedation. In patients who lack the ability to cooperate, have anticipated difficult airways, or need for significant dental work requiring a long surgical procedure time, general anesthesia may be necessary.

General Anesthesia Techniques

- General Anesthesia may be maintained using volatile anesthetics or total intravenous anesthesia (TIVA).
- Propofol has been used with opioids or ketamine for analgesic supplementation with the benefit of less post-operative nausea and vomiting and no need for a scavenger system [9].
- Konig et al. described no difference in emergence delirium or post-operative pain with propofol versus sevoflurane for anesthetic maintenance [10, 13].

Intubation Techniques

- Nasal intubation is generally preferred over oral intubation due to the concern for displacement with tube repositioning, potential obstruction due to dental equipment, and tube migration resulting in endobronchial intubation
- A thorough history must be elicited regarding a history of epistaxis, or recent nasal or head trauma which all would preclude nasal tracheal intubation.

- The patient should also be consented regarding the potential of epistaxis or mucosal damage, infection or creating a false passage with nasal intubation.
- In order to decrease the risk of epistaxis and mucosal damage, vasoconstrictors such as oxymetazoline (Afrin) can be administered. The recommended dose in children ages 2–5 is 2–3 drops of 0.025 % solution [10].
- Serial nare dilation can be utilized prior to attempted intubation to accommodate a nasotracheal tube.
- Bleeding can also be limited by decreasing tube size by 0.5–1, as well as warming the endotracheal (ETT) and covering the ETT tip on initial entry into the nare [10].
- Endotracheal intubation can be accomplished with Magill forceps or fiberoptic visualization.
- Special care should also be taken to secure the nasal ETT in order to prevent Alar damage for lengthy procedures.

References

1. Anderson B, Lerman J, Coté C. Pharmacokinetics and pharmacology of drugs used in children. In: Coté C, Lerman J, Anderson B, editors. Coté and Lermans' practice of anesthesia for infants and children. 1st ed. Philadelphia: Elsevier; 2013.
2. Dougherty N, Romer M, Lee RS. Trends in special care training in pediatric dental residencies. ASDC J Dent Child. 2001;68(5–6):384–7, 303.
3. Dye BA, Tan S, Smith V, Lewis BG, Barker LK, Thornton-Evans G, et al. Trends in oral health status: United States, 1988–1994 and 1999–2004. Vital Health Stat Ser, series 11. 2007;(248):1–92.
4. Eke PI, Dye B, Wei L, Thornton-Evans G, Genco R. Prevalence of periodontitis in adults in the United States: 2009 and 2010. J Dent Res. 2012;91(10):1–7.
5. Ferguson J. The Palmer notation system and its used with personal computer applications. Br Dent J. 2005;198:551–3.
6. Gertler R, Miller-Hance W. Essentials of cardiology. In: Coté C, Lerman J, Anderson B, editors. Coté and Lermans' practice of anesthesia for infants and children. 1st ed. Philadelphia: Elsevier; 2013.
7. Guideline on antibiotic prophylaxis for dental patients at risk of infection [document on the Intenet]. American Academy of Pediatric Dentisty: Clinical Guidelines; 1990 [updated 2014; cited 2015 Dec 20]. Available from: http://www.aapd.org/media/policies_guidelines/g_antibioticprophylaxis.pdf.
8. Guideline on use of local anesthesia for pediatric dental patients [document on the Internet]. American Academy of Pediatric Dentisty: Clinical Guidelines; 2005 [updated 2015; cited 2015 Dec 20]. Available from: http://www.aapd.org/media/policies_guidelines/g_localanesthesia.pdf.
9. Hausman L, Rosenblatt M. Office-based anesthesia. In: Barash P, Cullen B, Stoelting R, Cahalan M, Stock M, Ortega R, editors. Clinical anesthesia. 7th ed. Philadelphia: Lippincott Williams & Wilkins; 2013.
10. Herlich A, Martin B, Vecchione L, Cladis F. Anesthesia for pediatric dentistry. In: Davis P, Cladis F, Motoyama E, editors. Smith's anesthesia for infants and children. 8th ed. Philadelphia: Elsevier; 2011.
11. Kaplan R, Cravero J, Yaster M, Coté C. Sedation for diagnostic and therapeutic procedures outside the operating room. In: Coté C, Lerman J, Anderson B, editors. Coté and Lermans' practice of anesthesia for infants and children. 1st ed. Philadelphia: Elsevier; 2013.

12. Katz J, Holzman R. Occulational health. In: Barash P, Cullen B, Stoelting R, Cahalan M, Stock M, Ortega R, editors. Clinical anesthesia. 7th ed. Philadelphia: Lippincott Williams & Wilkins; 2013.
13. Konig M, Varughese A, Brennen K, Barclay S, Shackleford T, Samuels P, et al. Quality of recovery from teo types of general anesthesia for ambulatory dental surgery in children: a double-blind, randomized trial. Paediatr Anaesth. 2009;19(8):748–55.
14. Lin Y, Liu S. Local anesthetics. In: Barash P, Cullen B, Stoelting R, Cahalan M, Stock M, Ortega R, editors. Clinical anesthesia. 7th ed. Philadelphia: Lippincott Williams & Wilkins; 2013.
15. Manani G, Facco E, Casiglia E, Cancian M, Zanette G. Isolated atrial fibrillation (IAF) after local anaesthesia with epinephrine in an anxious dental patient. Br Dent J. 2008; 205(10):539–41.
16. Olutoye O, Watcha M. Eyes, ears, nose and throat surgery. In: Gregory G, Andropoulos D, editors. Gregory's pediatric anesthesia. 1st ed. Oxford: Wiley-Blackwell; 2012. p. 777–809.
17. Oral Health Topics A-Z "Tooth Numbering Systems" [document on the internet]. American Dental Association; 2014 [cited 2015 Dec 20]. Available from: https://web.archive.org/web/20061102074427/http://www.ada.org/public/topics/tooth_number.asp.
18. Sakaguchi T, Itoh H, Ding W, Tsiju K, Nagaoka I, Oka Y, et al. Hydroxyzine, a first generation H(1)-receptor antagonist, inhibits human ether-a-go-go-related gene (HERG) current and causes syncope in a patient with the HERG mutation. J Pharmacol Sci. 2008;108(4):462–71.
19. Shenkin JD, Davis MJ, Corbin SB. The oral health of special needs children: dentistry's challenge to provide care. ASDC J Dent Child. 2001;68(3):2001–5.
20. Sollecito T, Abt E, Lockhart P, Truelove E, Paumier T, Tracy S, et al. The use of prophylactic antibiotics prior to dental procedures in patients with prosthetic joints. J Am Dent Assoc. 2015;146(1):11–6.
21. Waldman HB, Perlman SP. Children with both mental retardation and mental illness live in our communities and need dental care. ASDC J Dent Child. 2001;68(5–6):360–5.
22. Wilson W, Taubert K, Gewitz M, Lockhart P, Baddour L, Levinson M, et al. Prevention of infective endocarditis: guidelines from the American Heart Association. J Am Dent Assoc. 2008;139 Suppl 1:S3–9, S11–24.
23. Wright JT. Normal formation and development of defects of the human dentition. Pediatr Clin North Am. 2000;47(5):975–1000.

Chapter 19
Anesthesia for Electroconvulsive Therapy

Nicole Jackman and Jonathan Z. Pan

Abstract Electroconvulsive therapy (ECT) is commonly used to treat major depression and other psychiatric disorders. Although the mechanism of action is not clear, ECT is safe and effective, if managed appropriately. A sufficient long seizure induced by lowest possible amplitude of current is most likely to produce optimal effect, yet with fewer side effects. ECT elicits significant physiological responses, including cardiovascular (*e.g.* hypertension and tachycardia) and central nervous system (*e.g.* increase of intracranial pressure and cerebral blood flow). Thus anesthesia preoperative evaluation should identify patients with higher risks, who should be consulted beforehand with proper plan of care. General anesthesia is usually planned for ECT procedure. Although different anesthetic regimens can be used, the goal is to minimize the anesthetic factors on the efficacy of ECT treatment, while maintaining adequate depth of anesthesia and ensuring patient's safety. In many hospitals, ECT is often performed at remote sites; anesthesiologist should be aware and well prepared for escalation of care if emergency occurs.

Keywords ECT • Depression • Psychiatric disorder • Seizure • General anesthesia • NORA (non-operating room anesthesia) • Adverse response • Anesthetic • Preoperative evaluation • Patient safety

Electroconvulsive Therapy (ECT)

Electroconvulsive therapy (ECT) is used to treat psychiatric disorders after failure of pharmacologic medical management or as an emergent procedure in gravely debilitated patient populations [1]. While a widely accepted definition of failed pharmacologic therapy or treatment resistance does not exist, a lack of clinical response, intolerance of side effects, and acute deterioration in the psychiatric condition are all reasons to consider the initiation of ECT. Indications for ECT include primarily

N. Jackman, MD, PhD • J.Z. Pan, MD, PhD (✉)
Department of Anesthesia and Perioperative Care, University of California, San Francisco,
521 Parnassus Ave, San Francisco, CA 94143, USA
e-mail: jonathan.pan@ucsf.edu

© Springer International Publishing Switzerland 2017
B.G. Goudra, P.M. Singh (eds.), *Out of Operating Room Anesthesia*,
DOI 10.1007/978-3-319-39150-2_19

unipolar and bipolar depression, mania, but also schizophrenia, schizoaffective disorders, mixed affective disorders, and catatonia [2, 3]. Further applications include depression secondary to neurological disorders such as multiple sclerosis and obsessive-compulsive disorder, although the efficacy in these contexts remains to be determined. Notably, clinical improvement can occur within several treatments and as such is important in gravely affected populations including acutely suicidal patients and the severely catatonic. Importantly, the American Psychiatric Association (APA) states "[ECT] should not be reserved for use only as a 'last resort.' Such practice may deprive patients of an effective treatment, delay response and prolong suffering" [1].

History

Cerletti and Bini first reported the use of ECT in humans in Rome in 1938 after numerous studies on electrical induction of seizures in dogs [4, 5]. The first patient was a male with schizophrenia and delusions. In this report, a bitemporal shock was applied to the patient, a seizure was induced, respirations ceased, he became cyanotic and tachycardic then 48 s later he emitted a deep sigh, his cyanosis diminished and heart rate began to normalize. The patient had a series of 11 treatments and was discharged in good condition and well-oriented. For approximately 30 years ECT was practiced in the US and abroad without general anesthesia and neuromuscular blockade, which are now incorporated into routine practice [6, 7]. The initial use of neuromuscular blockade occurred in 1951, and the utilization of the hypnotic barbiturate methohexital occurred in the early 1960s. Now, ECT is considered a low-risk procedure routinely performed under general anesthesia with a mortality rate that is similar to that of brief general anesthesia and is estimated to be between 0.01 and 0.1 % with a complication rate of 0.3 % [1].

Proposed Mechanisms of Action

The mechanism of action of ECT is currently unknown, however, hypotheses for the improvement in psychiatric disorders are via the following mechanisms: the release of neurotransmitters (specifically dopamine, serotonin, and GABA) during the induced seizure or reestablishment of neurotransmitter levels after seizure activity (i.e., recalibrating the thermostat); altered cerebral glucose metabolism and blood flow; modulation of the hypothalamic-pituitary-adrenal axis, changes in synaptic transmission and plasticity; and cell proliferation [8].

Seizure Characteristics

A shock is applied to one or both cerebral hemispheres to induce a seizure. Importantly, the seizure must be of sufficient duration (20–60 s) for optimal effects, with therapeutic benefit often apparent after a total of 400–700 s of seizure activity. This can occur after 2–3 weeks of treatment with 2–3 sessions of ECT per week [9]. Short seizure duration, then, is a predictor of poor outcome. The psychiatrist determines the pattern, amplitude, and duration of the electrical impulse, yet the anesthetic plan may be the difference between a clinically significant seizure and a sub-optimal seizure. Changing from unilateral to bilateral electrode placement, increasing the stimulus intensity, or potentiating the seizure pharmacologically may facilitate the induction of seizures of an adequate length [10, 11]. A sufficiently long seizure, generated with the lowest possible amplitude of current has the best chance of fewer untoward side effects. Seizure duration is monitored by both electroencephalography and motor activity. A seizure longer than 120 s is classified as "prolonged" and the anesthesiologist should administer pharmacological agents to terminate the seizure.

Cardiovascular Effects

Seizures are characterized by an initial tonic phase noted by bradycardia (and rarely asystole), premature atrial and ventricular contractions, hypotension, and salivation that occur secondary to activation of the parasympathetic autonomic system. This phase may last only 10–15 s, followed by a myoclonic phase lasting 30–60 s marked by sympathetic activation and associated tachycardia (HR >130 bpm), hypertension (SBP increases of 30–70 mmHg and diastolic BP increases of 10–50 mmHg), premature ventricular contractions, and rarely, ventricular tachycardia and changes in the electrocardiogram, including ST-segment depression and T-wave inversion. Transient atrial and ventricular tachyarrhythmias occur in 10 % of patients with known or suspected cardiovascular disease. ECT induced cardiovascular mortality has been reported as 0.03 %. Notably, tachycardia peaks 1–2 min after the electrical stimulus is applied, hypertension peaks 1–3 min later and may continue into emergence and the post-procedural period [7, 12].

Cerebral Effects

Electrical stimulation produces large increases in cerebral blood flow and thus intracranial pressure (ICP) [13]. It has been reported that after electrically induced seizures CBF increases ~300 % and cerebral metabolism increases ~200 %. Additionally, there is evidence of a temporary increase in the vascular permeability of the blood brain barrier. These effects should be considered in all patients presenting for ECT with cerebral aneurysms, arteriovenous malformations (AVMs), intracranial lesions/tumors, and those with increased intracranial pressure of unknown etiology. As such, there has been concern that those with increased ICP are at risk for herniation and even death. However, not all intracranial lesions are created equal. Small slow growing lesions without edema pose less risk when compared to a large, highly-vascularized, aggressive tumor with radiological or clinical evidence of edema and mass effect.

Other effects Intraocular pressure increases as a result of ECT and also secondary to the administration of succinylcholine [14]. Care should be taken in those with increased intraocular pressures and patients at high-risk for retinal detachment. Glucose homeostasis is also affected and elevated blood glucose has been noted in patients after ECT, most likely as a function of the stress response. The clinical significance of this finding remains to be elucidated. Patients should hold oral hypoglycemics and short acting insulin on the day of the procedure and decrease their home long acting insulin in preparation for the procedure [15].

Patient Considerations

As with all anesthetics, pre-operative evaluation requires a focused history and physical to determine whether the patient is in an optimal state to proceed with brief general anesthesia, with attention to the cardiovascular, neurologic/cerebrovascular, and airway/pulmonary co-morbidities. Pre-operative evaluation may require consultation with cardiologists, neurologists, and other specialists to medically optimize a patient prior to this elective procedure and ascertain whether the potential benefits of treatment outweigh the risks. A 12-lead ECG should be done on all patients above the age of 60 [7].

According to the APA Task Force Report, there currently are no absolute contraindications to ECT. Strong relative contraindications include a known pheochromocytoma, recent myocardial infarction (<3 months) or stroke (<1 month), and increased intracerebral pressure of any cause. Other relative contraindications include angina, poorly controlled heart failure, severe valvular disease; aortic and cerebral aneurysms or other vascular malformations subject to rupture with increased blood pressure; bone fractures, severe osteoporosis; high risk pregnancy (for which an Obstetrics consult and fetal monitoring would be recommended); intraocular processes including glaucoma, and retinal detachment; and significant pulmonary disease including asthma/COPD. Thorough pre-procedural evaluation should be performed for all ASA IV patients, and ECT may be safer in the operating suite where the anesthesiologist would have access to more emergency equipment, medications, and resources in the event of life-threatening physiology [1].

Special Patient Populations

Patients with pacemakers/Automatic Implantable Cardioverter-Defibrillator (AICD) Patients with pacemakers/AICDs can have ECT as the device is far from the field of electrical stimulation, thus only small amounts of electricity reach the device. One retrospective study noted that anesthesia proceeded uneventfully in patients with pacemakers receiving ECT and no pacemaker malfunctions were noted in 146 treatments. One should have a magnet accessible to disable AICD functionality and/or use the magnet to set a pacemaker to a fixed rate if necessary.

Patients with severe heart disease should be medically optimized, if possible, prior to initiation of ECT. Electrolyte abnormalities should be corrected and hypertension well-controlled [16].

Pregnant patients In 2001, the APA stated its support of ECT as an appropriate treatment modality in the pregnant patient as neglected psychiatric illness can have a negative impact on the fetus by affecting development, gestational age at the time of delivery, and birth weight [17]. ECT is safe and effective for pregnant patients and some would argue that it is safer than pharmacologic agents [18]. Most anesthetic agents and all induction agents are US FDA category B or C; methohexital, thiopental, etomidate, propofol, ketamine and sevoflurane can all be utilized in the pregnant woman. Only benzodiazepines have been categorized as category D (with positive evidence of risk to fetus, however potential benefits may outweigh potential risk), and cocaine is the only category X (contraindicated) anesthetic agent. Ideally, ECT should occur during the second and third trimesters as rapid organogenesis is occurring in the fetus during the first trimester. An obstetrical exam should occur prior to the initiation of ECT with documentation of fetal heart rate. Adequate preoxygenation is essential as the pregnant woman will desaturate faster than her non-pregnant peers as her functional residual capacity (FRC) starts to decrease secondary to the upward displacement of the gravid uterus. The pregnant woman is always regarded as having a full stomach and at increased risk of aspiration as early as the 12th week. Therefore the administration of a non-particulate antacid (Bicitra/sodium citrate 30 ml) and/or histamine-2 receptor blockers (ranitidine 50 mg IV 30–60 min prior to the procedure) should be considered. After 20 weeks gestation a wedge should be placed under the right hip for left uterine displacement of the uterus from the aorta and inferior vena cava (IVC). After 24 weeks gestational age, the patient should be intubated for airway protection with a rapid-sequence induction with cricoid pressure and maintenance via sevoflurane which can reduce the risk of uterine contractions. Non-invasive fetal heart monitoring is advised after ECT performed in the second and third trimester. Complications include premature labor due to increased levels of oxytocin produced after ECT and spontaneous abortion, and thus prophylactic tocolytic therapy may be useful in women with a history of premature labor who need ECT. Other complications include uterine contractions, vaginal bleeding, fetal arrhythmias specifically fetal bradycardia, and abruption of the placenta. The most prudent way to optimize the chance of a safe anesthetic in obstetric patients is vigilance and close monitoring of both the mother and fetus before, during, and after ECT. Finally, it would be wise (depending on gestational age) to perform ECT on the pregnant patient in sites with immediate access to obstetrical care in the event that an emergency caesarian section is required. Certainly ECT is not without risk, and should be reserved for those with grave disability and psychiatric disorders recalcitrant to pharmacotherapy.

Anticoagulated patients One small retrospective study found no adverse effects attributed to ECT performed in patients on long-term warfarin therapy [19]. However, there is a single case report of hematuria in an anticoagulated patient status post ECT [20]. The presumed mechanism was that a vascular malformation and induced hypertension.

Children & adolescents ECT is not used in children and adolescence except in rare cases such as adolescent depression or catatonic schizophrenia unresponsive to antidepressants or antipsychotic medications. A recent literature review states that other forms of noninvasive brain stimulation in children and adolescents is safe with mainly mild transient side effects and relatively few serious adverse events, however these studies excluded ECT [21]. Human research protections likely will not permit study of ECT in the pediatric population, given the ethics and other potential problems associated with this intervention during brain maturation.

Cerebral aneurysms and intracranial masses The sympathetic surge after an induced seizure can augment the wall stress placed on an aneurysm increasing the probability of enlargement or rupture. Nitroprusside and beta-blockers may blunt this increase in blood pressure. Increased intracranial pressure has long been considered an absolute contraindication to ECT, notably due to case reports of clinical deterioration of patients after ECT. Notably, early reports featured adverse events with the subsequent discovery of an intracranial process. Nevertheless, proceeding with ECT in patients with increased intracranial pressure without mass effect can be concerning given the changes in cerebral blood flow. Patients could be optimized with pre-ECT steroids like dexamethasone to decrease peritumoral edema, diuretics such as furosemide, and hyperventilation if necessary [22].

Procedure Considerations

Typically, ECT is administered as follows: treatment is given after a period of fasting per anesthesia society guidelines. Patients should be instructed to take their regular medications the morning of the procedure if the medications are not thought to interfere with seizure generation or duration (i.e. benzodiazepines, theophylline should be held or discontinued if possible) [23]. Important drug interactions should not be ignored. Indirectly acting sympathomimetics such as ephedrine can cause a hypertensive crisis in patients receiving Monoamine oxidase inhibitors (MAOIs). Lithium prolongs the action of succinylcholine. Patients should be encouraged to empty their bladder before the procedure as incontinence is common. Sedatives such as midazolam may interfere with seizure generation, delay emergence and cognitive clearing after the procedure and should thus be avoided. Glycopyrolate or another anticholinergic agent can be given prior to ECT to decrease salivation and blunt the initial period of parasympathetic activation. Standard monitors (EKG, blood pressure (BP) cuff, pulse oximetry) must be routinely utilized. Stimulus electrodes are placed either bifrontotemporally (bilateral) or with one electrode placed frontotemporally and the second electrode placed on the ipsilateral side (unilateral). In unilateral ECT, the BP cuff should be on the same side as the electrodes to ensure that a bilateral seizure occurs [7].

An IV induction agent is administered, typically methohexital, followed by succinylcholine for muscle relaxation (Note: full relaxation is not necessary) [6]. Importantly, a BP cuff placed on an arm or leg is inflated above systolic blood pressure prior to administration of succinylcholine. Ventilatory assistance is provided with bag mask ventilation on 100% FiO$_2$ with the goal of hyperventilation (hypocapnia, EtCO$_2$ ~ 30–35 mmHg) which lengthens seizure duration [24]. After induction of anesthesia, a bite block is placed to minimize oral trauma and the electrical stimulus is applied. Seizure threshold varies greatly among patients and the lowest amount of electrical energy to induce an adequate seizure should be used. Seizure monitoring is necessary and may be accomplished by an EEG and by the "BP cuff" technique, which allows motor activity to be visualized in the limb with the cuff acting as a tourniquet to prevent entry of neuromuscular blocking agent to points distal to the cuff. Bag mask ventilation can be resumed after the stimulus applied, and the patient's airway managed and ventilation supported to prevent obstruction until the patient wakes [1, 7].

Pharmacologic Considerations

Induction Agent

An adequate seizure in ECT is defined as one lasting greater than 30 s, thus it is important to be cognizant of the pharmacologic agents, which can alter seizure threshold and duration [6, 25]. Thus thoughtful preparation is warranted for a successful treatment (one with a minimal amplitude stimulus applied, minimal number of shocks needed to achieve a clinically acceptable seizure, and minimization of untoward side effects). According to Miller, Methohexital (0.5–1.5 mg/kg) is believed to be the gold standard agent to use for induction prior to ECT, as it blunts the hemodynamic response to ECT without a change in seizure duration. Methohexital has minimal anticonvulsive properties on its own and has been compared to thiopental, propofol and etomidate and is viewed to be a superior agent [26, 27]. Propofol (0.75–2.5 mg/kg) and thiopental (1–2.5 mg/kg) both similarly blunt the hemodynamic response, but also minimally decrease seizure duration [28]. Of note, shortened seizure durations were observed with propofol doses of greater than 1.0 mg/kg. Nevertheless, they can still be utilized with good effect. Etomidate (0.15–0.3 mg/kg) results in seizures of a longer duration compared to propofol and thiopental. However, its use is associated with myoclonus, PONV, and a longer time to wake than methohexital, and etomidate does not effectively blunt the hypertension and tachycardia associated with the sympathetic discharge with ECT. Interestingly, both ketamine (0.7–3 mg/kg) and volatile anesthetics (sevoflurane 6–8% for induction, followed by 1–2 MAC) can increase seizure duration, presumably because less induction agent is needed [29]. Likely, sevoflurane is most advantageous in the pregnant patient and most frequently intravenous agents are utilized. Initially, all dosing should be calculated using patient weight but modified based on previous response to ECT. All agents can be utilized and the variability in emergence and recovery should not be the sole factor in selection of induction agents.

Neuromuscular Blockade

Prior to the participation of anesthesiologists in ECT in the 1950s the most common associated injuries included vertebral body compression fractures, broken limbs secondary to tonic-clonic seizures, and broken teeth as a result of to direct electrical stimulation of the masseter muscles. Paralysis need not be complete (as intubation is rarely required) – and often 0.5 mg/kg of the depolarizing agent succinycholine provides sufficient neuromuscular blockade for this short procedure [6]. Rarely larger doses are needed (up to 1.5 mg/kg; for severe osteoporosis or pre-existing skeletal injury). If there is a contraindication to succinylcholine, one can then consider mivacurium (0.15–0.2 mg/kg) or atracurium (0.3–0.5 mg/kg) as short-acting non-depolarizing agents. Of course, additional resources and equipment for airway management will be needed for supportive measures given prolonged paralysis. Mivacurium can result in clinically significant hypotension due to histamine release and is metabolized by pseudocholinesterase, thus patients with pseudocholinesterase deficiency are at risk for prolonged paralysis. If atracurium is utilized, reversal of neuromuscular blockade with atropine and edrophonium is required. Rocuronium and vecuronium should not routinely be utilized as a non-fasiculating dose/precurarization before succinycholine, but could be used as a single agent in settings where sugammadex is available.

Hemodynamic Modulation

Beta blockers can be administrated to blunt the sympathetic effects of ECT [30]. Atenolol is often administered pre-procedurally, whereas labetalol (0.05–0.4 mg/kg) and esmolol (1–2 mg/kg) are utilized during ECT. There is evidence to suggest that labetalol and esmolol may reduce seizure duration. Alternatively, calcium channel blockers such as nifedipine (0.1 mg/kg IV, 10 mg SL) and nicardipine (2.5–5 mg; ~40 µg/kg) have been used without effects on seizure generation or duration, although nicardipine is the agent of choice due to it's shorter duration of action [31, 32]. Diltiazem may reduce seizure duration. Nitroglycerin, nitroprusside, and clonidine (0.05–0.3 mg 60–90 min prior to induction) can blunt the hemodynamic response associated with ECT and may be warranted in the patient with high risk of myocardial ischemia or cerebrovascular injury. Of note, the alpha$_2$ adrenergic receptor agonist dexmedetomidine administered pre-ECT increases sedation but does not blunt hemodynamic changes associated with the sympathetic surge [33]. When using sodium nitroprusside or nitroglycerin continuous blood pressure monitoring via an arterial line is recommended.

Adjuvants

Anticholinergics can play a role in blunting the initial parasympathetic response [34]. Glycopyrrolate or atropine can be administered to reduce the incidence of bradycardia and decrease oral secretions. Glycopyrrolate is thought to be superior given its anti-sialogue effects, that it is not centrally acting, and use results in less post-ECT tachycardia compared to atropine. Routine administration of atropine is not recommended.

Analgesics (Opioids and NSAIDs)

Opioids are useful as they allow a lower dose of the induction agent to be used, thus allowing for a faster wakeup and if using propofol or thiopental, a dose related decrease in the induction agent. In this context, opioids such as remifentanil (1 µg/kg over 30–60 s), alfentanil (10–25 µg/kg), and fentanyl (1.5 µg/kg) with agents other than etomidate can lead produce longer seizures using this dose-sparing effect [35]. NSAIDs, specifically PO ibuprofen or IV ketorolac can also be utilized to reduce the frequency and severity of post-ECT headaches [36].

Medications and Techniques to Decrease the Seizure Threshold

Hyperventilation (hypocarbia) will lengthen seizure duration and thus the effectiveness of ECT [24]. Intravenous caffeine, theophylline, and aminophyllines (xanthines) have been demonstrated to be an effective method of increasing seizure length, but the clinical efficacy has not been elucidated [37]. Certainly use of caffeine may produce some adverse reactions in at-risk cardiac patients, but all methods of seizure enhancement run the risk of producing unacceptably long seizures and/or status epilepticus. A well-trained anesthesiologist should attempt to break a prolonged seizure using benzodiazepines or propofol.

Complications/Adverse Events

There is no relationship between ECT and permanent brain injury, although transient cognitive changes and memory impairment do occur and are the most commonly reported side effects [38]. Because ECT induces a seizure, all patients will experience some post-ictal confusion lasting from minutes to hours. Reassurance, support, and reorientation is all that is needed during this phase, however emergence agitation can be treated with a short-acting benzodiazepine such as midazolam. Memory impairment is frequently reported and patients may note retrograde amnesia (difficulty in recalling information known/learned prior to ECT), anterograde amnesia (difficulty in retaining new information), or both. Typically, both retrograde and anterograde amnesia disappear after a period of days to weeks, although some patients have reported that memory did not return to their previous baseline after ECT. General somatic complaints (headaches, nausea, muscle soreness) are also common. Other adverse events include reactions to anesthetic and neuromuscular blocking agents, and dental and/or oral trauma despite the use of a bite block. Dexmedetomidine has been utilized for management of post-ictal/emergence delirium [39, 40].

Conclusion

ECT remains a "low-risk" procedure performed in NORA locations. All providers should thoroughly review and optimize (if possible) patient's chronic medical conditions, practice safe anesthetic technique as if one were in an operating room, and have the back-up personnel and resources to escalate care if a complication were to occur.

References

1. Rasmussen K. The practice of electroconvulsive therapy: recommendations for treatment, training, and privileging (second edition). J ECT. 2002;18(1):58–9.
2. Lisanby SH. Electroconvulsive therapy for depression. N Engl J Med. 2007;357(19):1939–45.
3. Agarkar S, et al. ECT use in unipolar and bipolar depression. J ECT. 2012;28(3):e39–40.
4. Endler NS. The origins of Electroconvulsive Therapy (ECT). Convuls Ther. 1988;4(1):5–23.
5. Khan A, et al. Electroconvulsive therapy. Psychiatr Clin North Am. 1993;16(3):497–513.
6. Wagner KJ, et al. Guide to anaesthetic selection for electroconvulsive therapy. CNS Drugs. 2005;19(9):745–58.
7. Ding Z, White PF. Anesthesia for electroconvulsive therapy. Anesth Analg. 2002;94(5):1351–64.
8. Rosenquist PB, Miller B, Pillai A. The antipsychotic effects of ECT: a review of possible mechanisms. J ECT. 2014;30(2):125–31.
9. Segman RH, et al. Onset and time course of antidepressant action: psychopharmacological implications of a controlled trial of electroconvulsive therapy. Psychopharmacology (Berl). 1995;119(4):440–8.
10. Loo C, Simpson B, MacPherson R. Augmentation strategies in electroconvulsive therapy. J ECT. 2010;26(3):202–7.
11. Sackeim HA, et al. Effects of electrode placement on the efficacy of titrated, low-dose ECT. Am J Psychiatry. 1987;144(11):1449–55.
12. Swartz CM. Physiological response to ECT stimulus dose. Psychiatry Res. 2000;97(2–3):229–35.
13. Saito S, et al. Regional cerebral oxygen saturation during electroconvulsive therapy: monitoring by near-infrared spectrophotometry. Anesth Analg. 1996;83(4):726–30.
14. Edwards RM, et al. Intraocular pressure changes in nonglaucomatous patients undergoing electroconvulsive therapy. Convuls Ther. 1990;6(3):209–13.
15. Ghanizadeh A, et al. The effect of electroconvulsive therapy on blood glucose, creatinine levels, and lipid profile and its association with the type of psychiatric disorders. Neurochem Int. 2012;61(7):1007–10.
16. MacPherson RD, Loo CK, Barrett N. Electroconvulsive therapy in patients with cardiac pacemakers. Anaesth Intensive Care. 2006;34(4):470–4.

17. Mander AJ, Norton B, Hoare P. The effect of maternal psychotic illness on a child. Br J Psychiatry. 1987;151:848–50.
18. Spodniakova B, Halmo M, Nosalova P. Electroconvulsive therapy in pregnancy – a review. J Obstet Gynaecol. 2015;35(7):659–62.
19. Mehta V, et al. Safety of electroconvulsive therapy in patients receiving long-term warfarin therapy. Mayo Clin Proc. 2004;79(11):1396–401.
20. Blevins S, Greene G. Hematuria with electroconvulsive therapy: a case report. J ECT. 2009;25(4):287.
21. Krishnan C, et al. Safety of noninvasive brain stimulation in children and adolescents. Brain Stimul. 2015;8(1):76–87.
22. Patkar AA, et al. ECT in the presence of brain tumor and increased intracranial pressure: evaluation and reduction of risk. J ECT. 2000;16(2):189–97.
23. Rasmussen KG, Zorumski CF. Electroconvulsive therapy in patients taking theophylline. J Clin Psychiatry. 1993;54(11):427–31.
24. Sawayama E, et al. Moderate hyperventilation prolongs electroencephalogram seizure duration of the first electroconvulsive therapy. J ECT. 2008;24(3):195–8.
25. Lihua P, et al, Different regimens of intravenous sedatives or hypnotics for electroconvulsive therapy (ECT) in adult patients with depression. Cochrane Database Syst Rev. 2014;(4): CD009763.
26. Avramov MN, Husain MM, White PF. The comparative effects of methohexital, propofol, and etomidate for electroconvulsive therapy. Anesth Analg. 1995;81(3):596–602.
27. Singh PM, et al. Evaluation of etomidate for seizure duration in electroconvulsive therapy: a systematic review and meta-analysis. J ECT. 2015;31(4):213–25.
28. Rasmussen KG. Propofol for ECT anesthesia a review of the literature. J ECT. 2014;30(3):210–5.
29. Rasmussen KG, Jarvis MR, Zorumski CF. Ketamine anesthesia in electroconvulsive therapy. Convuls Ther. 1996;12(4):217–23.
30. Castelli I, et al. Comparative effects of esmolol and labetalol to attenuate hyperdynamic states after electroconvulsive therapy. Anesth Analg. 1995;80(3):557–61.
31. Avramov MN, et al. Effects of nicardipine and labetalol on the acute hemodynamic response to electroconvulsive therapy. J Clin Anesth. 1998;10(5):394–400.
32. Zhang Y, et al. The use of nicardipine for electroconvulsive therapy: a dose-ranging study. Anesth Analg. 2005;100(2):378–81.
33. Fu W, White PF. Dexmedetomidine failed to block the acute hyperdynamic response to electroconvulsive therapy. Anesthesiology. 1999;90(2):422–4.
34. Kramer BA. Anticholinergics and ECT. Convuls Ther. 1993;9(4):293–300.
35. Recart A, et al. The effect of remifentanil on seizure duration and acute hemodynamic responses to electroconvulsive therapy. Anesth Analg. 2003;96(4):1047–50, table of contents.
36. Leung M, Hollander Y, Brown GR. Pretreatment with ibuprofen to prevent electroconvulsive therapy-induced headache. J Clin Psychiatry. 2003;64(5):551–3.
37. Stern L, et al. Aminophylline increases seizure length during electroconvulsive therapy. J ECT. 1999;15(4):252–7.
38. Mander AJ, et al. Cerebral and brain stem changes after ECT revealed by nuclear magnetic resonance imaging. Br J Psychiatry. 1987;151:69–71.
39. Cohen MB, Stewart JT. Treatment of post-electroconvulsive therapy agitation with dexmedetomidine. J ECT. 2013;29(2):e23–4.
40. O'Brien EM, et al. Dexmedetomidine and the successful management of electroconvulsive therapy postictal agitation: a case report. J ECT. 2010;26(2):131–3.

Chapter 20
Anesthesia and Sedation for Interventional Pain Procedures

Jonathan Anson and Bunty Shah

Abstract Chronic pain patients requiring anesthetic care for interventional pain procedures provide unique challenges to the anesthesiologists. This patient population often presents with significant psychiatric comorbidities and complex polypharmacy. Concurrent anxiety, hyperalgesia, and claustrophobia can make anesthetic management of these patients difficult. Interventional pain procedures often require patient awareness and feedback for specific aspects of the procedure to avoid serious complications. Inappropriate or mis-timed sedation can increase the risk of procedural complications. Therefore, anesthesiologists must be intimately familiar with the critical portions and potential pitfalls of each planned procedure. This chapter focuses on preoperative evaluation and optimization, important intraoperative events, and potential complications for a wide range of interventional pain procedures.

Keywords Chronic pain • Radiofrequency ablation • Transforaminal injection • Spinal cord stimulator • Medial branch block • Intrathecal pump • Interventional pain procedures • Sympathetic blockade

Introduction

Chronic pain patients presenting for anesthesia and sedation for interventional pain procedures provide unique challenges to the anesthesiologists. They may potentially have significant comorbid psychiatric conditions, including anxiety and depression, requiring pharmacologic therapy with benzodiazepines and antidepressants. Additionally, these patients are frequently prescribed high doses of opioid analgesics and may experience hyperalgesia. The result can be a patient with a complicated pharmacologic regimen, low pain threshold, and an inherent tolerance to medications typically used for anesthesia and sedation. The anesthetic plan must

J. Anson, MD (✉) • B. Shah, MD
Anesthesiology and Perioperative Medicine, Penn State Milton S. Hershey Medical Center, 500 University Drive, P.O. Box 850, Hershey, PA 17033, USA
e-mail: Janson@hmc.psu.edu; bshah@hmc.psu.edu

© Springer International Publishing Switzerland 2017
B.G. Goudra, P.M. Singh (eds.), *Out of Operating Room Anesthesia*,
DOI 10.1007/978-3-319-39150-2_20

take into consideration the requirements for patient interaction during specific portions of the procedures. Communication between the patient and anesthesia provider is essential. Complications such as drug toxicity are significant risks and must be identified promptly to prevent significant morbidity.

Focused History and Physical

Prior to administering sedation for an interventional pain procedure, a focused history and physical must be performed. Past medical history, smoking history, and substance abuse history should be obtained. The patient's medical record should be reviewed and prior anesthetic records obtained. These patients often have multiple interventional procedures, and a review of prior anesthetic records can help guide management for subsequent procedures. Routine laboratory testing is not indicated for low risk patients. Selective laboratory tests (such as coagulation studies) are indicated if there is clinical suspicion for high bleeding risk. Medication lists should be reviewed with a particular emphasis on anticoagulants, anti-platelet therapy, benzodiazepines, opioids, and antidepressants. Physical examination should at a minimum include an airway assessment, a cardiopulmonary exam, and a focused neurologic exam (relevant to planned interventional procedure) to assess for any pre-existing neurologic deficits.

Is the Patient in an Optimum State to Proceed with Anesthesia?

As with any procedure, the patient's NPO status should be confirmed prior to administering sedation. Patients should be screened for narcotic induced gastroparesis. Often, these patients are prescribed high dose opioids or other medications that may impact their level of consciousness and awareness. Additionally, a subset of this patient population may abuse recreational drugs on top of their prescribed regimen. Careful attention should be paid on the day of surgery to ensure the patient is truly capable of participating in the informed consent process.

Procedures Commonly Requiring Sedation

- Lumbar interlaminar epidural steroid
- Lumbar diagnostic medial branch blocks.
- Medial branch radiofrequency ablation (RFA)
- Lumbar transforaminal epidural steroid injections
- Intrathecal infusion pump and catheter system implantation
- Spinal cord stimulator pulse generator and lead implantation

Procedures for Which Anesthesia or Deep Sedation Is Relatively Contraindicated

- Cervical and thoracic epidural steroid injections
  - Presence of spinal cord with attendant risk of damage and paralysis, especially when patients become disinhibited and move spontaneously
  - Under these circumstances it's safer to administer light sedation with the patient following commands or general anesthesia

Patient Positioning

Many interventional pain procedures are performed in the prone position, proving additional challenges to the anesthesia provider. There may be an elevated level of anxiety for the prone patient who cannot see what is occurring. Positioning the face in a pillow combined with surgical drapes over the head may lead to claustrophobia. Communication with the patient is the key to alleviating these anxieties. Pressure points must be padded, and comfortable positioning must be accomplished to avoid patient's movement during the procedure. The prone position does not allow direct access to the airway. Airway obstruction or apnea from over-sedation can be challenging to treat in the prone position.

Commonly Used Anesthesia Techniques

Monitored anesthesia care (MAC) with standard American Society of Anesthesiologists monitors is the most common anesthesia technique for interventional pain procedures. Short acting opioids and benzodiazepines are the medications of choice. Induction agents such as propofol and ketamine are generally avoided in these cases due to a need to maintain communication with the patient and to avoid over-sedation in the prone position. In addition to general MAC principles used for all types of surgeries, individual interventional pain procedures may have specific considerations that must be kept in mind (see Table 20.1 for summary of procedures):

Medial Branch Radiofrequency Ablation

With the patient in the prone position, the tip of the radiofrequency probe is guided to the junction of the transverse process and lateral neck of the superior articular process in an orientation parallel to the nerve branch. After needle positioning is confirmed visually, sensory and motor testing is carried out. Sensory testing involves

Table 20.1 A summary of key anesthetic considerations for specific interventional pain procedures

Procedure	Anesthesia type	Patient position	Required patient participation	Potential complications
Epidural Steroid Injection	MAC	Prone	Must move lower extremities after lidocaine test dose	Paraplegia secondary to arterial steroid injection
Medial Branch Block	MAC	Prone	Critical during sensory and motor testing	Intrathecal or epidural injection
Radiofrequency Ablation	MAC	Prone	Critical during sensory and motor testing	Thermal motor nerve injury
Intrathecal Pump	MAC, spinal, or GA	Lateral	Over-sedation or spinal anesthesia may mask new neurologic deficits	Neurologic injury, baclofen toxicity
Spinal Cord Stimulator	MAC	Lateral or prone	Communication of paresthesias/coverage	Post-dural puncture headache, arrhythmia

A summary of key anesthetic points including anesthesia type, positioning, and potential complications

Abbreviations: *MAC* monitored anesthesia care, *GA* general anesthesia

administering an electric current to reproduce the patient's baseline pain and confirm the diagnosis. Motor testing is conducted to ensure the needle tip is far enough away from the motor fibers to avoid inadvertent injury. It is critical that the patient is able to communicate with the proceduralist during sensory and motor testing. Over-sedation at this point of the procedure can have devastating consequences. Permanent motor deficits may result from thermal injury of motor nerves if patients can't effectively participate in sensory and motor testing. The patient should be counselled preoperatively regarding the importance of minimal sedation during sensory and motor testing. Careful communication and re-assurance during the procedure is critical. Lidocaine is typically administered through the cannula once proper position is confirmed, however, thermal ablation may be painful and more sedation may be required during this part of the procedure.

Prior to proceeding to radiofrequency ablation of the medial branch nerves in the thoracic, lumbar or cervical spines, it is standard practice to perform two sets of diagnostic medial branch nerve blocks. If both sets are positive, it is presumed with reasonable certainty that the facet joints are the pain generators and that thermal destruction of these nerves would provide the patient with considerable pain relief. Diagnostic medial branch nerve blocks are typically performed using local anesthetics of relatively short duration including lidocaine and bupivacaine. After the injection is performed, the patients are asked to engage themselves in activities, which, under normal circumstances, would provoke pain [1]. If excessive sedation is administered to these patients, they may not be alert enough to appreciate and record their pain levels during the duration of action of the administered local anesthetic. As a result of this, there exists the possibility that patients will perceive decreased pain scores that may be attributable to the sedatives administered rather than the local anesthetic itself. A physician relying on information from these diagnostic blocks may perform a radiofrequency ablation with less than expected subsequent pain relief.

Lumbar Transforaminal Epidural Steroid Injections

This procedure is performed when patients experience pain in a specific dermatome. A spinal needle is advanced under the pedicle, medial to the pars interacticularis using fluoroscopic guidance. At this point a mixture of local anesthetic and steroids is injected. The anterior thoracolumbar spinal cord is heavily dependent on the anterior spinal artery, which is in turn highly dependent on the contribution from the large and variably located radiculomedullary artery (artery of Adamkiewicz). Injection of a particulate steroid into this artery can result in paraplegia. Therefore, prior to injecting any particulate steroid, a test dose of 1 % lidocaine is administered. One minute after the test dose the patient is asked to move their lower extremities. Successful leg movement rules out intravascular needle position. It is absolutely critical that this test dose and movement test not be inhibited or impacted by oversedation. Prior to the test dose, the anesthesiologist and pain physician should communicate to ensure an appropriate level of sedation, and the patient should be counselled about the test dose preoperatively.

Spinal Cord Stimulation

A spinal cord stimulator (also known as a dorsal column stimulator) delivers low voltage electrical stimulation to the tracts in the spinal cord to inhibit the transmission of pain signals to the brain. This, in turn, elicits a paresthesia in the corresponding dermatomes. The goal is to produce paresthesias that overlap the painful areas, so patients feel a mild tingling sensation where they used to feel pain. A percutaneous trial is performed in the outpatient setting. An epidural lead is placed using fluoroscopic guidance and this is connected to an external device. If the 3–10 day trial is successful, the lead is removed and the patient is scheduled for a permanent spinal cord stimulator implantation.

This procedure requires a skin incision, therefore, preoperative antibiotics are indicated within one hour of incision. Initially, an epidural Touhy needle is inserted until it contacts the lamina, which can be painful. However, the anesthesiologist must not be overly aggressive with sedation. Deeply sedated patients may suddenly startle and move when the needle enters the epidural space. This can lead to accidental dural puncture with subsequent headache requiring an epidural blood patch. Dural puncture also increases the risk of infection in these patients, therefore the procedure is typically cancelled if this occurs. The best way to prevent this negative outcome is to avoid sedating the patient to the point of disinhibition. Careful communication and reassurance goes a long way.

The final stimulating lead position is usually in the T8–T9 region. Migration or misplacement to the level of T1–T4 can cause cardiac rate and rhythm disturbances secondary to stimulation of the cardiac accelerator fibers. Vigilant continuous ECG monitoring is required at this point of the procedure, and the lead should be withdrawn if tachyarrhythmias occur.

At the end of the procedure, the spinal cord stimulator is programmed using a radiofrequency signal. The signal used may reset or otherwise interfere with other implanted devices in the patient (such as pacemakers, defibrillators, or deep brain stimulators). Given this risk, all indwelling devices should be professionally interrogated post-procedure before the patient is discharged.

Intrathecal Pump Insertion

Intrathecal pumps infuse medications directly into the spinal space via a programmable rate. They are most commonly used in the management of severe pain or muscle spasticity. Anesthetic management depends primarily on individual patient factors, as the procedure can be performed under MAC, spinal anesthesia, or general anesthesia. The most painful portion of the procedure involves tunneling a trocar from the skin to the intrathecal pump pocket. The procedure is performed in the lateral position on a bean bag, and attention should be paid to properly pad bony prominences. These patients must be carefully monitored post-operatively for new neurologic defects or signs of intrathecal medication overdose. Local anesthetic administration through the pump should be avoided during pump insertion, as this may delay the diagnosis of neurologic complications. A similar risk is present if performed under spinal anesthesia. Intrathecal baclofen overdose can present with a multitude of symptoms including: seizure, somnolence, respiratory depression, loss of consciousness, and rostrally progressing hypotonia. Intrathecal baclofen overdose requires airway support. Although there is no specific baclofen antagonist, physostigmine may reverse some of its central effects. In severe cases, lumbar puncture with 30–40 ml cerebrospinal fluid withdrawal may be indicated to reduce the intrathecal baclofen concentration.

Anticipated Adverse Events

Vasovagal Episodes

Vasovagal episodes occur in up to 8.7 % of interventional spine procedures [2]. Risk factors for vasovagal episodes include: male gender, high preoperative pain score, and age less than 65 years old. Moderate sedation (defined as 1–4 mg midazolam and 25–100 mcg fentanyl) may actually have a preventative effect in patients with a history of prior vasovagal episodes [2]. A large retrospective review examined a series of patients with a prior history of vasovagal episodes during an interventional pain procedure. The study demonstrated 21 out of 90 patients receiving *no* sedation had repeat vagal response, while 0 out of 44 patients receiving moderate sedation had repeat vagal incidents during the subsequent procedure [2].

IVP Dye/Contrast Allergy

Contrast is frequently used in X-ray guided procedures to confirm proper needle placement. Severe allergies can result in anaphylactic reactions marked by broncho-spasm and cardiovascular collapse. For these reasons, it is important to properly identify those patients who are at risk for the development of an allergy to iodinated contrast agents. Furthermore, the nature and severity of the patient's allergy to iodinated contrast agents should be elucidated prior to proceeding with any proce-dure in which iodinated contrast agents may be used.

In cases of mild reactions (including cutaneous rashes or hives) pre-medication with steroids in combination with diphenhydramine may be sufficient to prevent uncomfortable but non-life threatening reactions. On the other hand, patients with documented severe allergies to iodinated contrast agents, such as bronchospasm and hemodynamic collapse, should be identified beforehand and all members of the patient care team alerted so that inadvertent administration of iodinated contrast agent does not occur. In cases in which contrast is required (such as interlaminar and transforaminal epidural steroid injections) the pain physician may opt to use a non-iodinated contrast agent, such as a gadolinium based contrast agent.

There is a widely held misconception that seafood allergies predispose patients to adverse reactions to contrast media. Shellfish allergy, however, does not confer an increased risk of allergic reaction related to intravenous contrast administration compared to the presence of other allergies [3]. Gadolinium based contrast is not as easily visualized on fluoroscopy compared with iodinated contrast media. Thus, inappropriately withholding iodinated contrast media can potentially prevent the prompt identification of unfavorable needle tip positioning.

High Spinal/Epidural Anesthesia

In the event that an intrathecal administration of local anesthetic occurs during a cervical interlaminar or transforaminal epidural steroid injection, total spinal anes-thesia may result. This requires supportive airway and hemodynamic management and immediate abandonment of the procedure. If the patient is in a prone position during one of these procedures, they must immediately be repositioned supine so that ventilator and hemodynamic support may be instituted as the individual situa-tion dictates. To avoid this situation, interventional pain physicians often inject contrast after anteroposterior and lateral radiographic images are obtained to confirm proper needle placement. Furthermore, injection of contrast agent and the resultant pattern of contrast spread can indicate intrathecal or epidural spread, and intravascular uptake. Despite these precautions, contrast spread pattern identification is variable and operator dependent and may not reliably alert the interventional pain physician to inadvertent intrathecal administration of medication. A test dose of local anesthetic is utilized prior to steroid administration in transforaminal epidural steroid injections. In the case of a lumbar level injection, the absence of lower extremity motor blockade after the test dose is regarded as negative for accidental intrathecal injection.

Intra-arterial Injection

Intra-arterial injection of local anesthetics into a high-pressure vascular system may result in seizures or convulsions. Prior to local anesthetic injection, contrast media is given under live fluoroscopy to observe for a vascular uptake pattern. If necessary, the needle tip is re-positioned until the visualized contrast pattern is consistent with the desired epidural spread. Nevertheless, intra-vascular injection may still occur and the anesthesiologist must be prepared to initiate supportive care in the event of airway or hemodynamic compromise. This may include the use of endotracheal intubation and positive pressure ventilation, bag-mask ventilation, or the administration of vasopressors (epinephrine, norepinephrine). Communication between the surgical and anesthesia teams is crucial to maximize preparedness prior to local anesthetic injection.

Local Anesthetic Toxicity

Local anesthetic toxicity (LAST) leading to cardiovascular collapse can occur from intravascular injection of local anesthetics. During interventional pain procedures it can also occur with improper programming of an intrathecal infusion pump containing local anesthetic such as bupivacaine. Immediate or delayed airway compromise, convulsions, and cardiopulmonary arrest may result. It is important for the anesthesiologist to recognize that cardiac arrest secondary to LAST may be refractory to most conventional resuscitation efforts. The use of lipid emulsion therapy for treatment of bupivacaine related cardiotoxicity is the first line medical therapy [4]. Guidelines for the treatment of LAST using 20 % lipid emulsion therapy are published by the American Society of Regional Anesthesia (ASRA) [4]. Notable features of the ASRA LAST checklist include the avoidance of certain medications including propofol, local anesthetics, calcium channel blockers, vasopressors and beta blockers (medications which may be indicated in other cardiopulmonary arrest scenarios) [4]. Additionally, ASRA recommends that initial doses of epinephrine be reduced to less than 1 mcg/kg and that a facility capable of providing cardiopulmonary bypass be notified, as epinephrine can decrease the effectiveness of lipid therapy [4]. Bolus lipid emulsion therapy followed by infusion therapy may be indicated until arrhythmias cease.

Hypotension from Sympathetic Blockade

Sympathetic blockade is commonly performed for conditions related to abnormal activity of the sympathetic nervous system or sympathetically mediated pain. One common indication is complex regional pain syndrome. During this procedure, a needle is place at the anterolateral portion of one of the upper lumbar vertebral bodies to target the ipsilateral lumbar sympathetic chain. The needle resides in close proximity to the aorta. Contrast administration is used to minimize the incidence of intravascular injection. With a successful sympathetic block, sudden hypotension may ensue, especially if the patient has been fasting in preparation for the procedure. The anesthesiologist must take note of the patient's pre-injection blood pressure and prepare for volume resuscitation or vasopressor administration if necessary. It is preferred to have intravenous crystalloid infusing prior to the administration of the local anesthetic. Though many patients will tolerate the hypotension associated with the procedure with little to no consequence, patients with pre-existing coronary artery disease or stenotic cardiac valve lesions may decompensate with resultant ischemia if not identified and treated appropriately.

Conclusion

Pre-procedure planning, preparation, and communication are key components to ensuring sedation for patients undergoing interventional pain procedures is carried out safely, and treatment outcomes are optimized. This chapter is intended to familiarize anesthesiologists with specific considerations for pain procedures and the potential complications associated with these procedures. It is crucial to understand, however, that the above information is to be applied in context, and sedation plans should be altered to individual patient needs. It is also important to emphasize that the majority of interventional pain procedures are **elective** procedures and this fact should be considered when deciding on whether or not to proceed with procedures when preoperative concerns arise. As pain interventions and procedures continue to evolve, so to will the need for anesthesiologists to understand the demands and safety considerations for these procedures.

References

1. Bogduk N. International spine intervention society practice guidelines for spinal diagnostic and treatment procedures. 2nd ed. 2013. p 3.
2. Kennedy DJ, Schneider B, Smuck M, Plastaras CT. The use of moderate sedation for the secondary prevention of adverse vasovagal reactions. Pain Med. 2015;16:673–9.
3. Schabelman E, Witting M. The relationship of radiocontrast, iodine, and seafood allergies: a medical myth exposed. J Emerg Med. 2010;39(5):701–7.
4. Weinberg GL. Lipid emulsion infusion: resuscitation for local anesthetic and other drug overdose. Anesthesiology. 2012;117(1):180–7.

Part VII
Special Situations

Chapter 21
Pediatric Off Site Anesthesia

Kara M. Barnett, Mian Ahmad, Todd Justin Liu, and Rayhan Ahmed Tariq

Abstract There is an increase in need for sedation for pediatric patients undergoing procedures and scans outside of the operating room. Overall, sedation is safe if the anesthesia provider is trained in rescuing the patient. Common complications include apnea and airway obstruction. Full monitoring should be provided, including capnometry. It is also crucial to have all emergency supplies and medications on hand. In many cases, propofol sedation is a safe anesthetic in patients who are sedation candidates. Other possible anesthetics include sedation with drugs like ketamine and versed or general anesthesia with an LMA or endotracheal tube.

Keywords Pediatric • Pediatric anesthesia • Pediatric sedation • Laryngospasm • MRI • CT scan • Nuclear medicine • Radiation • Gatrointestinal procedures • Ophthalmologic procedures • ER procedures • Propofol • Ketamine • Malignant hyperthermia • Oncology • Bone marrow • Lumbar puncture • Down's syndrome • Airway • Mental retardation

K.M. Barnett, MD (✉)
Department of Anesthesiology and Critical Care Medicine, Memorial Sloan Kettering Cancer Center, 1275 York Avenue, New York, NY 10065, USA
e-mail: barnettk@mskcc.org

M. Ahmad
Drexel University College of Medicine, Hahnemann University Hospital,
245 N. 15th St, Philadelphia, PA 19102, USA
e-mail: mian.ahmad@drexelmed.edu

T.J. Liu, BA, MD
Anesthesiology and Critical Care Medicine, Memorial Sloan Kettering,
1275 York Avenue, New York, NY 10065, USA
e-mail: liut@mskcc.org

R.A. Tariq, MD
Department of Anesthesiology and Perioperative Medicine, Drexel University College of Medicine, 245 N. 15th NCB. MS310, Philadelphia, PA 19102, USA
e-mail: rayhan.tariq@gmail.com

© Springer International Publishing Switzerland 2017
B.G. Goudra, P.M. Singh (eds.), *Out of Operating Room Anesthesia*,
DOI 10.1007/978-3-319-39150-2_21

Introduction

- There is an increase in need for sedation for pediatric patients [1].
- Sedation is used to control behavior but the provider must be able to rescue the patient if there is a complication [2].
- The goals of out of OR anesthesia for pediatric patients are:

    - Adequate anesthesia for the procedure/scan
    - Minimal or complete absence of movement (especially for radiologic and nuclear medicine scans)
    - Quick onset of action
    - Short half-life allowing for a quick wake-up and discharge
    - Minimal respiratory depression/obstruction
    - Minimal nausea/vomiting
    - Ability to titrate the medication to effect
    - Cost effective

- A majority of the sedation provided for pediatric patients outside the OR is for radiological procedures. Sedation is also used for many out of the operating room procedures such as hematologic/oncologic procedures, surgical and gastro-enterologic [3, 4].
- Overall, performing anesthesia out of the operating room for pediatric patients is safe [4].

Assessing the Child

- Is the child a candidate for a MAC anesthetic, a general anesthetic with an LMA or a general anesthetic with an endotracheal tube? Below are questions to consider while forming your anesthetic plan.

    - What does the scan or procedure require in terms of immobility and duration?
    - How old is the child chronologically and developmentally?
    - Has the child adequately fasted? Does the child have an aspiration risk such as actively vomiting, having a bowel obstruction or gastroparesis?
    - Is the child at risk for airway obstruction such as sleep apnea or a genetic syndrome like Hurler's, etc.? Does the patient have a potential or known difficult airway? What anesthetic equipment will you have readily available?
    - Does the child have reactive airway disease or currently have a recent upper respiratory infection? Are you worried about laryngospasm, bronchospasm or stridor?
    - Does the patient have any other concerning comorbidities like a congenital heart defect or neuromuscular disorder?

- Does the patient have a drug or food allergy that will change your anesthetic plan (such as an a allergy to propofol)?
- Does the patient currently have peripheral or central venous access? Will the patient need access?

Challenges in Pediatric Population

- **Children are not little adults**
  - **Drugs and metabolism**
    - The kidneys and liver in young children are immature. However, pediatric patients often require more anesthetic drug. Children have an increased minimum alveolar concentration and a larger volume of distribution for water-soluble drugs like succinylcholine.
  - **Respiratory**
    - Children have an elevated respiratory rate that decreases with age.
    - In younger children, the alveoli are immature and airways are smaller with a higher resistance.
      - Children have a decreased functional residual capacity and increased oxygen consumption. During apnea, there is a limited oxygen reserve and desaturation occurs more quickly than in adults.
    - Children are more prone to bronchospasm and laryngospasm.
    - Premature infants may have a decreased drive to breathe. A patient who is less than 60 weeks post conceptual age may need prolonged respiratory monitoring after anesthesia.
  - **Cardiac**
    - Children have a faster heart rate that decreases with age. They also have a lower blood pressure that increases with age.
    - Younger children have an active parasympathetic nervous system. Bradycardia can occur with hypoxia. It is essential to treat the hypoxia especially because cardiac output is dependent on heart rate.
  - **Temperature**
    - Children are more likely to get hypothermic. Use warm blankets or a warming blanket whenever possible.
- **Children can have more difficult airways**
  - Children have a larger head with a neck that naturally flexes.
  - Their tongue is larger and the tonsils and adenoids are more prominent. The epiglottis is also larger and floppier.

- The pediatric larynx is anterior and cephalad. It is at C4 in neonates versus C6 for adults.
- Children have a short neck with a short and narrow trachea. A right main stem intubation may easily occur with neck flexion.
- The pediatric cricoid cartilage is the narrowest part of the pediatric airway until age 5. In the adult, it is narrowest at the glottis. Consider having three different sized endotracheal tubes available when possible.
- The endotracheal tube can be more easily obstructed and kinked in a narrow airway.
- Consider a jaw thrust or placing a rolled towel or sheet under a child's shoulders to relieve airway obstruction when spontaneously ventilating.

Possible Complications

- As the amount of pediatric sedation cases outside of the operating room increases, the concern for the number of complications will naturally grow. Management for the treatment and prevention of these complications is critical for providers administering sedation.
- A recent paper discussed the rate of adverse events by studying 49,836 encounters. There were no deaths, but CPR was reported twice and aspiration four times. Unplanned intubation occurred at a rate of 11.4 per 10,000 [3].
- Pulmonary complications

  - Laryngospasm

    - Laryngospasm is one of the most significant complications to consider for pediatric patients undergoing procedures under sedation.
    - It occurred at a rate of 20.7 per 10,000 while oxygen desaturation (less than 90% for more than 30 s) occurred at a rate of 20.7 per 10,000 [3].
    - It is defined as the reflexive closure of the glottic opening, which can result in difficult ventilation.
    - It may present as a high-pitched upper airway sound, but severe laryngospasm may not make any sound at all since there is no air flow.
    - Presentation is worse in the setting of hyper-reactive airway/asthma, sickle cell, history of prematurity/bronchopulmonary dysplasia, hypocalcemia, less than 1 year of age and exposure to tobacco smoke.
    - There is an increased risk when a child has had an upper respiratory infection (URI). It is greatest in the first week but remains increased for up to 6–8 weeks. The anesthesia provider must consider the risks and benefits of proceeding with anesthesia in a child with a recent URI [5–7].
    - Airway manipulation with an endotracheal tube or supraglottic airway (e.g. LMA or oral airway) may increase the risk of laryngospasm when compared to mask anesthesia. However, a secure endotracheal tube prevents laryngospasm while in place, but the risk of laryngospasm is greater upon removal.

- Treatment of laryngospasm includes: providing 100 % FiO_2, and support-ive respiratory mechanics (consider a jaw thrust, chin lift, oral/nasal air-way). Minimize stimulation that may worsen the laryngospasm. Continuous gentle positive pressure may "break" the laryngospasm. Consider deepen-ing the sedation with a dose of propofol to blunt airway reflexes. Short acting muscle paralysis with succinylcholine may be needed if the other treatments do not work. Lightening the anesthetic plane may also reinstate normal respiratory mechanics and reflexes.
  - Negative pressure pulmonary edema is a possible complication after laryn-gospasm [8].

- Bronchospasm

  - Bronchospasm is defined as hyperreflexive pulmonary reflexes due to the contraction of bronchi resulting in an obstructive airway.
  - The associated risk factors and consideration are similar to those with laryngospasm.
  - Treatment includes beta-2 agonists, steroids or antihistamines, bronchodi-lating volatile anesthetics and epinephrine. Ketamine and propofol are also bronchodilators.
  - Wheezing significant enough to interrupt the procedure occurred at a rate of 9.5 per 10,000 [3].

- Aspiration

  - The most critical aspect to management is preventive care. Consider the ASA guidelines in terms of the patient's NPO (nil per os) status.
  - Aspiration of gastric contents or foreign bodies into the respiratory system can result in significant morbidity and mortality.
  - It can typically present as coughing emesis contents or secretions, result-ing in bronchospasm and hypoxemia. It may also present as tachypnea, tachycardia and decreased lung compliance.
  - Treatment includes suctioning and removal of the aspirate. Position the patient in order to limit further aspiration, such as trendelenburg and head tilted to the side. Administer 100 % FiO_2. Intubation may be necessary to secure the airway and prevent further aspiration, as well as support respira-tory status. Cricoid pressure may be useful. Consider fiberoptic lavage in order to remove material as needed. Place a gastric tube in order to empty the stomach. Consider administering bronchodilators. Prophylactic antibi-otics for pneumonia are usually not necessary.
  - Chest radiography is often not reflective of the clinical condition with aspi-ration. Clinical severity is often worse than it appears with radiography early on, and better than it appears with radiography in the later course [9].
  - Aspiration occurred at a rate of 0.9 per 10,000, while vomiting during sedation occurred at a rate of 10.6 per 10,000 [3].
  - A recent study from the Pediatric Sedation Research Consortium of 139,142 procedures showed that NPO status did not predict aspiration. Aspiration occurred at a rate of 0.97 events per 10,000 of NPO patients and 0.79 per 10,000 in those that were not NPO [4].

– Obstructive Sleep Apnea

- Obstructive sleep apnea (OSA) in pediatric patients is typically associated with adenotonsillar hypertrophy. Children with OSA have increased tissue edema and friability and an altered response to CO_2 and sedative agents [10].
- Children less than 3 years old are at a higher risk [11].
- If it is severe, treatment with surgical removal of tonsils and adenoids may be warranted.
- Airway obstruction occurred at a rate of 93.2 per 10,000 [3].

• Cardiac Complications: Bradycardia

– Pediatric patients have increased vagal tone and are more prone to bradycardic episodes than older patients.
– Pediatric hearts are less compliant and depend more on their heart rate than their stroke volume. Therefore, bradycardia may not be tolerated well in pediatric patients.
– Etiologies include hypoxia, hypercarbia, hypotension, hypovolemia, increased vagal tone and surgical stimulation [12].
– Diagnosis and treatment of the cause is critical for the management of bradycardia. Treat the underlying cause or stop the inciting event. Pharmacologic support of the heart may be needed with glycopyrrolate, atropine or epinephrine. Give supportive care with 100 % FiO_2.

• Malignant Hyperthermia

– Malignant Hyperthermia (MH) is a genetically inherited life threatening condition that results from a trigger drug, such as succinylcholine and volatile anesthetics.
– A trigger agent causes over activation of the ryanodine receptor causing uncontrolled skeletal muscle contraction. This leads to acidosis, hyperthermia and eventual hemodynamic collapse.
– The disease is related to central core disease and multi-minicore disease. Red flags for MH include a family history of "severe reaction to anesthesia" or neuromuscular disorder [13].
– Associated symptoms include masseter muscle spasm, rhabdomyalysis, hyperkalemia, hypercarbia and hyperthermia [14].
– In patients who are suspected to have MH or have a family of MH, it is best to avoid trigger agents. If a ventilator is being used for the procedure, the CO_2 absorber granules should be replaced and the ventilator needs to be flushed with oxygen for a prolonged period of time. Anesthetic vaporizers should be removed or disabled in order to avoid accidental delivery.
– Treatment of MH includes calling for help, discontinuing all trigger agents (including removing the circuit and anesthesia machine), hyperventilation and administering 100 % FiO_2. Dantrolene 2.5 mg/kg should be administered intravenously every 5 min with a maximum dose of 10 mg/kg. Consider bicarbonate, vasopressors, treatment of hyperkalemia and cooling the patient. Provide supportive care and avoid calcium channel blockers [13].

- Former Premature Infants

  - Pulmonary

    - Premature infants often have a history of bronchopulmonary dysplasia (BPD) or incomplete development of the pulmonary organ system, which increases the risk of pulmonary complications for procedures [15].
    - Prematurity increases the risk of postoperative apnea after sedation. The risk increases as the post conceptual age decreases.

      - Patients under 60 weeks post conceptual age may require at least 12 h observation after a procedure with sedation.
      - Even though a premature infant may appear to have returned to a fully intact respiratory drive mechanics immediately after sedation, the infant may still be at risk for apenic episodes and sudden infant death hours later [16].

    - Eyes

      - Retinopathy of prematurity can result in severe morbidity for premature infants.
      - Risk factors include low birth weight, prematurity, exposure to supplemental oxygen, mechanical ventilation, blood transfusion, and sepsis.
      - Anesthesia providers should limit supplemental oxygen therapy in patients at risk. Titrate oxygen levels to a pulse oximetry saturation of approximately 95 % [17].

- Allergic Reaction

  - Pediatric patients may not have had previous exposures to triggering agents; thus, they may be presenting for the first time with an allergic reaction.
  - Reactions may vary greatly from urticaria, erythema, bronchospasm and hyperreactivity, facial and/or laryngeal edema, and anaphylactic shock.
  - Treatments include diphenhydramine, steroids, epinephrine, H1 blockers, beta-2 agonists and supportive care.
  - Allergic reactions occurred at a rate of 3 per 10,000 [3].

- Intravenous Access

  - In addition to possibly having difficult veins to access, pediatric patients often resist intravenous (IV) cannula placement prior to sedation.
  - Some anesthesia providers advocate for inhalational sedation prior to or instead of IV sedation since it is a potentially less traumatic experience for children. Risks and benefits must be weighed when deciding between the two options.

    - Consider the patient and equipment availability when formulating an anesthetic plan.
    - Induction of anesthesia without IV access may prevent administration of certain medications if an emergency were to occur. The bioavailability of intramuscular administration is less predictable and has a slower onset of action.

- Less distress in the patient can prevent bronchospasm, laryngospasm, hemodynamic effects, and uncontrolled agitation that might result in a patient hurting him or herself or staff members.
- Propofol has a lower postoperative emesis rate and less airway obstruction than volatile anesthetics in the pediatric outpatient population [18].

Main Challenges and Setup in Pediatric Off-site Anesthesia

- Off-site anesthesia in pediatric patients is challenging because of the remoteness of the site while possibly caring for a challenging patient. For example, pediatric patients undergoing radiation therapy may have multiple co-morbidities while undergoing repeated procedures over a course of weeks or months.
- Sometimes the patient is not directly observable during a scan or radiation procedure.
- The anesthesia provider may work with personnel who have less or no familiarity with the anesthetic aspects of patients care in these settings.
- Off-site location means remoteness from available expert help.
- How rapidly can the case be shifted to an OR in case of an emergency?
- Needing to care for patients in a small procedure or treatment room that is not intended for anesthesia care.
- Working with unfamiliar or outdated anesthesia equipment.
- Ensure and check all emergency, airway, monitoring and suction equipment. See Table 21.1 for the setup of a pediatric cart offsite.
- See Table 21.2 for a pediatric offsite anesthesia checklist.
- Anesthesiologists are part of a multi-disciplinary team in pediatric off-site anesthesia, they must take a holistic approach towards patient care.
- NPO status

  - Challenging to have a young patient NPO for a procedure or scan especially if it is scheduled later in the day.
  - Consider the ASA guidelines [19] when instructing families when the patient should stop eating or drinking. See Table 21.3.
- Excessive fasting for patients who are not at an increased risk for aspiration may have excessive preoperative discomfort [20, 21].

Drugs

- Propofol

  - One of the mainstays for intravenous sedation by anesthesia providers.
  - It can provide significant amnesia and sedation for procedures but does not provide analgesia. It can be used safely by an anesthesia provider with an expertise in airway management.

Table 21.1 Pediatric off-site anesthesia cart setup

Table setup	Bair hugger	Shoulder roll
3 lead EKG	Pulse Ox	Appropriate sized BP cuff
Special cable for neonatal cuffs		Glucose (25 % or 50 %)
Monitor set to Neonate or Pediatric Mode	Flumazenil	Naloxone
Drugs	Glycopyrrolate, 0.2 mg/ml	Tetracaine, 0.45 %, 49 ml
Succinyl choline	Atropine	Epinephrine 10 mcg/cc
Ephedrine 10 cc of 5 mg/cc	Phenylephrine (1 syringe of 100ug/cc, 1 syringe of 10ug/cc)	Succinylcholine (4–6 mg/kg on IM needle)
Calcium Chloride (10 cc of 100 mg/cc, 10 cc of 10 mg/cc)	Sodium bicarbonate (8.4 % 1 mEq/cc for patients >1 year)	Ketamine – (0.5–5 mg/kg IV, 3–5 mg/kg IM)
Propofol – (2–3 mg/kg IV)	Rocuronium (0.6–1.2 mg/kg, dilute to 1 mg/cc for children <1 years)	Two syringes of saline flush
Lidocaine, 1 %, 50 ml	Lidocaine, 2 %, 50 ml	Xylocaine, 2 %, Jelly
Xylocaine, 5 %, ointment	Xylocaine prep 4 %, for topical spray	**Drawer One: Preps**
Alcohol prep	Oxymetazoline hydrochloride spray (Afrin)	Atomizer spray
Silicone lubricant	Catheter, 22-gauge angio × 1 in.	Stopcocks, three way
Gauze, 3 in. by 3 in.	Syringes, 3 cm [3]	Tongue depressors
Needle, 25-gauge × 3.5 in. spinal	Needles, 19-gauge, 1.5 in.	Albuterol Multi dose Inhaler
Cetacaine Spray	Eye-tape (Paper tape >1 year, Mepitec for <1 year or fragile skin)	Tega derm
Drawer Two: Laryngeal mask airways, suction catheters	No. 1 laryngeal mask (neonate/infants)	No. 2 laryngeal mask (babies/children)
No. 2.5 laryngeal mask (babies/children)	No. 3 laryngeal mask (children/small adults)	Laryngeal mask tube extensions
Yankauer suction tips	Catheter, suction, 8 F, pediatric	
Drawer Three: Blades, Handles		Combitube
Magill forceps (small)	Magill forceps (large)	Laryngoscope handle (regular)
Laryngoscope handle (short)	Macintosh blade no. 2 (child)	Miller blade no. 0 (Infants <3 months)
Miller blade no. 1 (children 3 months to 18 months)	Miller blade no. 1 (children 3–5 years)	Miller blade no. 2 (children >5 years)
	Drawer Four: Retrograde set and transtracheal jet ventilation (TTJV)	0.035 × 145 cm guidewire

(continued)

Table 21.1 (continued)

Needle, epidural with catheter	Catheter, 14-gauge intravenous (IV) (TTJV)	Nerve hooks
Catheter, red rubber, Robinson urethral	Clamps, Kelly	Sutures, silk
Needle, 18-gauge thin-wall	Surgical blade	**Drawer Five: Airways and tube exchangers**
Airway, Berman oral, 100 mm	Airway, Berman oral, 90 mm	Airway, Berman oral, 80 mm
Nasopharyngeal airway, 26 F	Nasopharyngeal airway, 28 F	Nasopharyngeal airway, 30 F
Nasopharyngeal airway, 32 F	Nasopharyngeal airway, 34 F	Catheter, 14-gauge × 2 in.
Catheter, 16-gauge × 2 in.	Catheter, 18-gauge × 2 in.	Needle, Benumof transtracheal (Cook)
Endotracheal Tube Exchanger	Syringes, 20 cc	Tube Exchanger Jet Ventilation Adapters
Drawer Six: Endotracheal tubes and lighted stylets	2.5–5.5 mm, uncuffed (Size based on the child's little finger or (age/4) + 4)	3.0–6.0 mm, cuffed (Subtract 0.5 size for cuffed tube)
Stylet, pediatric	Lighted stylet	Lighted stylet, Laerdal, disposable stylets
Lighted stylet, Laerdal, handle	**Drawer Seven: specialty blades, and miscellaneous**	Patil-Syracuse mask for FOB, appropriate pediatric size
Bronch swivel elbow	Bullard blade, adult	Bullard blade, small
CO_2 analyzer, Easy Cap, disposable	Scissors	Airway, Ovassapian
Tubing, O_2 supply	Airway, Williams, 10 cm	Airway, Williams, 9 cm
Tubing, suction connection	Augustine guide	WuScope, small
Belscope, small		

Table 21.2 Check list for pediatric off-site anesthesia

Are two sources of O_2 and a suction available?
Is the lighting sufficient?
Is Emergency Cart Available?
Are there enough electrical sockets available?
Is help readily available?
Standard machine check
Reset machine alarms for age appropriate vitals
Turn on machine suction

Table 21.3 ASA fasting guidelines [19]

Fasting required	Liquid/solid
2 h	Clears (e.g. water, clear juice without pulp, CT contrast)
4 h	Breast milk
6 h	Infant formula, nonhuman milk, light meal, juice pulp
Consider 8 h	Fatty meal

- It has a lower risk of postoperative nausea and vomiting.
- Bolus 1 mg/kg and repeat with 0.5 mg/kg as needed [22]. Also can consider an infusion of 100–200 mcg/kg/min for longer procedures [23].

- Ketamine

  - Unique sedative that is frequently used for pediatric sedation. Unlike most sedatives, ketamine causes an increase in sympathetic drive, which often results in an increase in heart rate and blood pressure. Furthermore, it preserves the respiratory drive better than many other agents.
  - Ketamine may cause hallucinations and dysphoric effects that may last beyond the immediate period of sedation. Consider administering midazolam to prevent emergence dysphoria [23].
  - Consider using an anticholinergic prior to the administration of ketamine due to an increase in oral secretions.
  - Cardiac depression can occur especially in the setting of an already activate sympathetic drive.
  - Postoperative nausea and vomiting is not uncommon.
  - Bolus 1–2 mg.kg IV or 3–4 mg/kg IM or 5–8 mg/kg can be used for general anesthesia induction [23].

- Dexmedetomidine

  - Dexmedetomidine is a newer sedative agent that has analgesic properties. It is an alpha-2 agonist similar to clonidine.
  - It does not carry the same level of respiratory depression found in many other agents.
  - Dexmedetomidine is associated with bradycardia, especially when administered as a bolus. It should be given slowly over 10 min. An anticholinergic may be necessary for treatment of the bradycardia.
  - Bolus 2 mcg/kg loading dose over 10 min and infuse at 0.2–1 mcg/kg/h.
  - There is evidence that a bolus of 0.5–1 mcg/kg of can decrease the incidence of emergence delirium [24].

- Midazolam

  - Midazolam is a versatile sedative agent with many routes of administration.
  - It is a short-acting amnestic agent. It is one of the most commonly used benzodiazepines in pediatrics.
  - A paradoxical reaction can occur especially in children.
  - Oral dose 0.5–0.75 mg/kg (maximum of 20 mg), rectal 0.25–0.5 mg/kg, intranasal 0.2–0.5 mg/kg, intravenous 0.025–0.05 mg/kg, intramuscular 0.1–0.15 mg/kg [23, 24]

- Fentanyl

  - Fentanyl is a synthetic opioid that is commonly used in both adult and pediatric populations for short acting pain relief.
  - Caution must be used because it will have a synergistic effect when used with other sedative agents, especially in regards to apnea.
  - Dose 1–2 mcg/kg IV with a titration to effect.

- Remifentanil

  - Remifentanil is an ultra short-acting opioid that has been become more popular recently for pediatric sedation.
  - Similar to all opioids, there is a significant risk of apnea.
  - It has very limited amnestic effects.
  - Dose 0.1 mcg/kg/min infusion with a titration to effect [23].

- Nitrous Oxide

  - Nitrous oxide is one of the oldest anesthetic agents yet its use is still prominent in today's practice.
  - As a non-pungent inhaled anesthetic, it is one of the best-tolerated agents for induction of anesthesia in pediatric patients.
  - Drawbacks include a reduction in inhaled oxygen concentration in order to administer it, an association with postoperative nausea and vomiting, and the potential to expand any airspaces (e.g. pneumothorax). There is also a controversy as to whether nitrous oxide's inactivation of plasma homocysteine via vitamin B12 inactivation with prolonged exposure could have hematologic complications for pediatric patients [25].

- Volatile Anesthetics

  - Inhaled volatile anesthetics have been used extensively in children.
  - Most anesthesia providers use sevoflurane for their pediatric patients because of its less odorous smell for inhaled induction and better bronchodilation to prevent reactive airway complications.
  - When considering the use of volatiles for pediatric patients outside of the operating room, the availability of proper anesthesia equipment and scavenging system may preclude their use.

- Succinylcholine

  - As the only clinically used depolarizing neuromuscular blocking agent, succinylcholine has a very important role in pediatrics. It has the shortest onset and ultra-short duration of action, which can both be very useful for airway management, especially when rapid sequence intubation is required.
  - There is an increased risk of succinylcholine use in pediatrics due to the possibility of undiagnosed muscular dystrophy that may cause a hyperkalemic response. Therefore, it is not recommended to use succinylcholine routinely.
  - Dose 1–3 mg/kg IV for intubation conditions, 4 mg/kg intramuscular

- Anticholingerics

  - Because children's hemodynamics are much more heart rate dependent than adults, anticholinergics are critical to have available as a rescue medication during pediatric sedation procedures.
  - Children can have high vagal tone and respond to noxious stimuli with profound bradycardia.

- Atropine and glycopyrrolate are useful due to their mechanism of action as a competitive inverse agonist of the muscarinic acetylcholine receptors.
  - Atropine dose 10–20 mcg/kg IV, 20–30 mcg/kg intramuscular
  - Glycopyrrolate dose 4 mcg/kg IV

- Ondansetron
  - Ondansetron is one of the most effect anti-emetic agents with a good safety profile within the pediatric population.
  - Dose of 0.1 mg/kg (up to 4 mg) has been found to significantly decrease post-operative nausea and vomiting as well as speed up home readiness in outpatient surgical settings [26].

- Local Anesthetics
  - Local anesthetics may be used for pain control once sedation has been begun.
  - Toxic doses of local anesthetics are calculated based on dose per body weight. Therefore, increased vigilance is warranted for young pediatric patients.
  - Local anesthetics bind sodium channels in the peripheral nervous system, but larger doses can lead to central nervous system and cardiovascular system toxicity. This can result in severe and or even life threatening arrhythmias and death.
  - Toxicity may also occur with direct intravascular injection.
  - Injection with epinephrine can decrease systemic absorption through vascular constriction and therefore increases the toxic dose of the local anesthetic.
  - Toxicity levels: Plain Lidocaine 5 mg/kg, Lidocaine with epinephrine 7 mg/kg; Plain Bupivacaine 2 mg/kg, Bupivacaine with epinephrine 3 mg/kg, Plain Mepivicaine 5 mg/kg, Mepivacaine with epinephrine 6 mg/kg; Ropivacaine with or without epinephrine 3.5 mg/kg

Pediatric Off-Site Anesthesia in a Non-pediatric Hospital

- Children may come to an adult hospital if particular services like advanced radiation treatment options are not available in the pediatric hospital or if a pediatric unit is too far [27].
- Biggest issue is unfamiliarity of the personnel with the requirements of a child and the uncomfortable feeling associated with it.
- Equipment and supplies may not be available readily or at all.
- Best solution is to have enough personnel in the department enlisted to handle these cases. These individuals should keep themselves up to date on pediatric anesthesia literature.
- A pediatric cart and its supplies need to be checked and updated on periodic basis.
- Areas that have these cases (radiology, ER etc.) should have periodic meetings with the dedicated anesthesia personnel and occasional debriefings after the procedures.

- Policies & Procedures of these departments may need to be modified to accommodate the needs of children, e.g. allowing the parents or care givers presence during the procedure.
- Nursing personnel may need to be trained and certified to take care of these children, especially recovery room nurses.

Radiological Scans and Nuclear Medicine Scans

- Radiological scans and nuclear medicine scans require immobility that young or developmentally delayed children may not be able to do without anesthesia. They all require a peripheral IV or central line access.
- Common off-site pediatric procedures requiring anesthesia and sedation are as follows:
    - Diagnostic radiology: CT, MRI, Bone Scan
    - Cardiovascular interventions: Angiography, Cardiac catheterizations
    - Radiation Oncology
    - Diagnostic & interventional procedures: Bronchoscopy, Eye examination, Endoscopy, Ultrasound, Transesophageal echo
    - Diagnostics exams: Lumbar puncture, Bone marrow aspiration, Biopsy, Evoked potentials

MRI

- MRI is the most common pediatric offsite procedure requiring sedation/anesthesia.
- A relatively longer scan in duration.
- No radiation is emitted but the anesthesia provider must monitor from outside the room in zone III or zone IV. Monitors and the patient should be easily viewed from a distance, either directly or via video camera [28].
- The anesthesia department should properly label equipment for the MRI as safe, unsafe or conditional. All equipment must be safe for use in the MRI suite [28].
- Fully monitor the patient vitals including capnography. There may be EKG or pulse oximetry artifact from the MRI magnetism.
- The patient and staff need to be screened for the presence of metal [28].
- If a patient does not have a peripheral IV or central line access prior to the procedure, the anesthesia provider can induce with sevoflurane by mask. An IV is required for contrast administration. Once access is established, the anesthesia provider can continue with a general anesthetic with either LMA or ETT or can convert to an infusion such as propofol.
- If a patient has a peripheral IV or central line, consider propofol sedation if the patient is an acceptable candidate. Bolus propofol until the patient is adequately

sedated and then begin an infusion. A dexmedetomidine infusion is also acceptable but requires a slow bolus and can cause bradycardia. Give supplemental oxygen via nasal cannula.
- Place ear plugs in the patient after the patient is sedated.

Nuclear Medicine Scan

- Nuclear medicine scans that a pediatric patient may need sedation for include Positron emission tomography (PET), CT scan, MIBG scan, and renal scan.
- Nuclear medicine scans vary in length. PET scans are relatively short while MIBG scans are relatively long. They require no movement.
- These children are injected before the scan so a peripheral IV or central access will be needed. The timing of the scan may need to be coordinated with the injection time.

    - PET/CT scans require PO contrast. The patient should be sedated after 2 h since the contrast is considered a clear liquid.
    - For both PET and PET/CT scans, the glucose analog tracer is injected intravenously approximately 45 min before scanning.
    - MIBG scans require an injection a day prior.

- Consider a propofol infusion with supplemental oxygen via nasal cannula if the patient is a candidate for MAC. Fully monitor the patient's vitals along with capnography.
- Except when a CT scan is being performed as part of the scan, the anesthesia provider is able to monitor in close proximity to the patient.
- The radioactive injection for MIBG scans is eliminated in the urine. Care must be taken if the patient urinates during the procedure.
- SPECT (single-photon emission computed tomography) is a technique in nuclear medicine to map blood flow. It can be used to identify a seizure source since that is where the maximum blood flow is during a seizure activity.
- A radioactive tracer is injected during the SPECT scan. The tracer usually contains radioactive technetium (Tc 99). The local tracer concentration peaks in the brain tissue about 2 min after injection, remains constant for about 2 h, and degrades with a half-life of 6 h.
- An Ictal SPECT scan is taken during the seizure and an interictal scan when no seizure is there. The ictal and inter-ictal images are then compared to each other and to MRI and analyzed.

CT Scan

- There is a 2 h wait after PO CT contrast ingestion per NPO guidelines [19].
- A peripheral IV or central access is required for IV contrast administration.

- These are relatively short scans that emit ionizing radiation, so that the anesthesia provider must be monitoring from a distance.
- Propofol is an ideal medication if the patient is a MAC candidate. Consider giving small boluses until the patient is adequately sedated. Can also consider sedation with midazolam. Give supplemental oxygen via nasal cannula. Fully monitor the patient along with end tidal CO_2.
- Consider general anesthesia if the scan is an emergency, if the patient is not NPO, has head trauma, cardiac or respiratory instability or if there is a need for breath holding during the scan [29].
- Because of the short duration, children over 3 or 4 years old may be able to do the scan without anesthesia with parental presence. Parents can stay with the patient wearing lead for protection.
- Give supplemental oxygen via nasal cannula with end tidal CO_2 monitoring.

Pediatric Off-Site Anesthesia for Radiation Oncology

- Working in the pediatric radiation therapy suite presents a unique range of challenges to the anesthesiologist. The anesthesia provider has to deliver anesthesia for a wide variety of complex conditions in a remote location where the patient is not directly observable during the procedure.
- Anesthesiologists are part of a multi-disciplinary team in radiation oncology, taking a holistic approach towards patient care.
- Radiation therapy uses x-rays, gamma rays or protons to either lessen or completely destroy the cancer cell burden. **Intensity-modulated radiotherapy** (IMRT) is the technique used in radiation-oncology involving photons [30].
- **Proton therapy** is the latest advancement in radiation therapy. It reduces the collateral radiation compared to the traditional photon based methods of radiation [31]. A typical session of proton therapy might run much longer as compared to the traditional techniques thus necessitating a change in anesthetic plan.
- The main goal in radiotherapy is to target a specific area so maximum dose can be delivered to the cancer tissue while the surrounding normal tissue is unaffected. As the side effects of radiation are directly proportional to the total dose, extraordinary effort is made to treat the tumor with minimum possible dose delivered to a localized area.
- Ideally to do so, the child should be as immobile as possible throughout the procedure. This is almost impossible for children under the age of four who are frightened in the unfamiliar environment.
- Children between ages of 4–8 can be managed without sedation if they are able to understand the explanation provided by the care giver. For such older kids, it might be helpful to use play therapy [32] prior to the procedure and allowing them to speak to their guardians via microphone during the procedure.
- Anesthesia is rarely required at age of 8 years and beyond [33].

- Child is evaluated by an anesthesiologist few days prior to start of the treatment to assess any comorbidities, primary effects of the tumor (Table 21.4), as well as the secondary effects of chemo or radiation therapy.
- There is currently insufficient data available to guide routine pre-anesthetic testing in children with cancer. The choice of diagnostic laboratory or diagnostic examination should be guided by the patient's specific history, physical examination and the nature of the procedure [36].
- During the subsequent visits a quick review of child's condition in last 24 h is carried out with questions like any vomiting, fever, cough or any untoward symptoms.
- A baseline set of vital signs is recorded and NPO history confirmed.
- Radiation therapy is a challenging and difficult time for both the children and their caregivers. The parents should be explained the entire anesthetic plan in as much detail as possible and with the permission of the parents, the children should be told about the radiation therapy session in age appropriate terms.
- The presence of the parents in the radiation oncology suite during the induction can ease the anxiety of the children.
- Planning for this kind of radiation therapy starts with a **simulation session** where the child is kept immobile while the tumor is mapped in a three dimensional manner. Since the child has to be moved to different locations during this process it is better to secure the airway for this relatively lengthy session.
- The mask made for the treatment of central nervous tumors or retinoblastoma during the simulation session should be designed in such a way that even during deep sedation airway stays open [37]. See Fig. 21.1 for a picture of a child with a mask.
- Subsequent actual treatment involves multiple sessions of short duration and can be managed under deep sedation.
- Multiple sessions of radiation therapy are often necessary to achieve desired result. The total radiation delivered is thus *fractionated* thereby decreasing side effects of radiation therapy.
- The sessions can range from a week to several months. In such cases it is advisable to have long-term central venous line.
- Radiation oncology suits are often located in the isolated parts of the hospital, so the anesthesiologist should ensure that full pediatric resuscitation facilities are available. There should be an effective way to communicate with rest of anesthesiology department and call for help and backup.
- Also pipeline gases and vacuum are not always available. Backup source of oxygen and suction should be arranged beforehand.
- The position of patient is supine for almost all the radiation therapy procedures due to advancements in radiotherapy techniques. In case of abdominal or peripheral radiotherapy a mold is not needed and the patients can be positioned appropriately via foam wedges.
- An airway is very rarely needed in a radiation oncology suite.
- There are no recommended guidelines nor any randomized studies guiding the use of anesthesia in radiation therapy. The ideal anesthetic plan should not only be safe but also allow rapid recovery and minimal disruption to the child.

Table 21.4 Primary diagnosis of 512 children undergoing radiation therapy (Duke University Medical Center) [33]

Diagnosis	Distribution of total Patients undergoing radiation therapy (%)	Primary effects/anesthetic considerations
Primary CNS tumor	28	CNS tumors accounted 29 % of all malignancies in children <15 years of age
		There is a potential for raised ICP. Factors that raise ICP should be considered such as hypoxia, hypercapnia and volatile anesthetic-induced increase in CBF
Retinoblastoma	27	Anesthetic management of retinoblastoma patients is unremarkable, but retinoblastoma caused by 13q deficiency might be associated with difficult intubation due to macroglossia [34]
Neuroblastoma	20	Neuroblastoma is the most common extracranial solid cancer in childhood
		It most frequently originates in one of the adrenal glands, but can also develop in nerve tissues elsewhere in the body
		Treatment therapies include surgery, radiation therapy, hematopoietic stem cell transplantation and biological-based therapy. Their effect of these treatment therapies should be considered
Acute leukemia	9	Patients with leukemia receive a course of chemotherapy which should be reviewed. Common anesthetic concerns of such patients include tumor lysis syndrome, coagulopathies, myelosuppression, Infection associated with neutropenia. The chemotherapeutic drugs used must be reviewed and their possible side-effects and interactions noted
Rhabdomyosarcoma	6	Embryonal rhabdomyosarcoma, the most common type, usually occurs in children under 6 years of age
		Alveolar rhabdomyosarcoma occurs in older children and is less common
		Chemotherapy is generally given to all rhabdomyosarcoma patients. These drugs can cause anemia and neutropenia
Wilms' tumor	4	In addition to the 'routine' issues, consequences of *para-neoplastic phenomena* should be considered, such as hypertension and coagulopathy, of proximal IVC or atrial extension of tumor thrombus, and of preoperative and previous treatment with chemotherapeutic drugs [35]

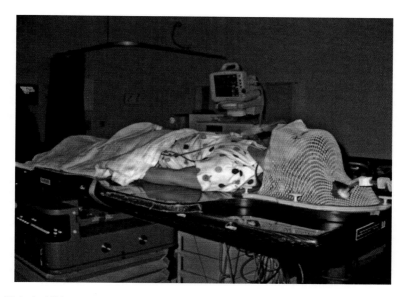

Fig. 21.1 A child undergoing radiation therapy. Note the thermoplastic mould and the Nasal cannula for monitoring $ETCO_2$ (With Permission *Clinical Oncology*, Thorp [30])

- The majority of institutes use total intra-venous anesthesia with propofol (T.I.V.A) [37]. Child is induced with intravenous propofol 3–5 mg/kg while still in parent's lap and is moved to the treatment table as soon as consciousness is lost.
- ASA recommended standard monitors are attached and breathing monitored by continuous capnography via nasal cannula.
- Radiation therapy is not painful and analgesia is not required.
- Since immobility is of paramount importance and anesthesia providers have to leave the room because of radiation hazard, the infusion dose of propofol is adjusted to assure deep level of sedation without any airway obstruction before leaving the procedure room.
- For procedure lasting more than an hour *temperature monitoring* should be done by skin temperature crystal strips and active warming via a forced air total body warming blanket should be considered.
- Two video cameras are used to monitor the child and observe the monitor from the control room located just outside the procedure room.
- Table position usually needs to be changed during these treatments and there is opportunity to adjust the dose of propofol.
- This anesthetic technique provides a quick and safe anesthetic with rapid recovery, so that the child is able to be managed on an outpatient basis.
- Other techniques where either ketamine and midazolam or propofol and fentanyl or midazolam and fentanyl have also been employed but with higher complication rate or slower recovery.
- Buchsbaum et al. (2013) discuss their experience with 138 children undergoing proton therapy. After inducing patients with about 2.5 mg/kg propofol given

intravenously, they inserted a laryngeal mask airway (L.M.A). Anesthesia was maintained via sevoflurane 3 % and oxygen delivered via LMA. The rate of complication was minimal (0.0074 %) [38].

- An alternative is to use ketamine to produce a state of dissociated amnesia. It used to be a popular choice back in the 1980s but is rarely resorted to currently in anesthesia for radiation therapy. Ketamine is often used in the pediatric ER but is seldom used in the radiation oncology room because it can cause an increase in intracranial pressure in the already susceptible population.
- In case of a shorter procedure, intravenous sedation alone with opioids and/or benzodiazepines can be considered.
- Anghelescu et al. retrospectively evaluated 3833 radiation oncology procedures (3611 radiotherapy sessions and 222 simulations) in 177 patients. The overall rate of anesthesia-related complications was low (1.3 %). The highest rate of complication was found for the group that was administered Propofol plus adjuncts (opioids, benzodiazepines, ketamine). The cohort of children that got intravenous sedation with opioids, benzodiazepines, and barbiturates had no recorded complications. Other factors that were found to increase the rate of complication were the duration of procedure and the total dose of propofol [39].
- An earlier study at Duke University reported a similar low incidence of complications (1.2 %) in 512 children who received radiation therapy between 1983 and 1996. The most common complications noted were laryngospasm (n = 13), central line sepsis (n = 11), airway obstruction (n = 5), and arrhythmia (n = 3) [33].

Pediatric Off-Site Anesthesia in Interventional Radiology

- Discussion with IR team for level of sedation needed for the procedure.
- Consider midazolam/fentanyl if the patient is older and requires light sedation. The patient may require a deeper sedation with a propofol infusion or general anesthetic for younger patients and longer procedures.
- **Radiation Safety**: Anesthesia providers are at a high risk for exposure to radiation while providing anesthetic care in radiology suits. The eye is the most sensitive organ for radiation-induced damage. It is imperative that anesthesiologists working in radiation oncology suite be properly monitored with radiation badges and follow universal radiation safety measures [40]. Current data does not suggest a significant risk to the fetus for pregnant women working in the interventional radiology suite.

Pediatric Off-Site Anesthesia in Oncology Procedure Room

- Children with cancer or hematological disorders may undergo several painful procedures that require sedation out of the operating room. These include **bone marrow aspirations and biopsies, lumbar punctures** with possible chemotherapy administration, and **central line placements and/or removals**.

- A procedure room with an anesthesia machine and equipment is ideal.
- Pain associated with the procedure will necessitate a deep sedation or general anesthetic. Have a goal to provide adequate anesthesia that will wear off quickly and allow for timely patient discharge [41].
- Ideally administer propofol sedation if the patient is a candidate. The patient will need a peripheral IV or central line access. Give supplemental oxygen via nasal cannula and use standard ASA monitors including end tidal CO_2.
- Propofol is an ideal medication because of its fast onset and offset. Midazolam and fentanyl may prolong recovery. Consider oral pain medications if needed after the procedure.
- General anesthesia may be needed if a patient is an aspiration risk or has airway obstruction that cannot be corrected with a chin lift or nasal or oral airway.
- If the patient does not have venous access, can induce with sevoflurane and continue with a mask anesthesia after placing an intravenous line or place an LMA or ETT. Or a propofol infusion may be started.
- Consider administering ondansetron if a patient undergoes general anesthesia, receives cytarabine intrathecally, or if there is a history of nausea or vomiting with these procedures.

Pediatric Off-Site Anesthesia in Emergency Room

- Factures of long bones and joint dislocations are two of the most common reasons for anesthesiology consultation in the pediatric Emergency Room (ER).
- Most of the time emergency medicine personnel are able to sedate their patients. Anesthesiologists are very occasionally called to provide anesthesia and analgesia in the pediatric ER [42, 43].
- There are various possible options to provide analgesia in these painful conditions. These include intravenous regional blocks (Bier blocks), nitrous oxide, deep sedation with ketamine/midazolam (K/M) administration, fentanyl/propofol administration or fentanyl/midazolam (F/M) administration [44, 45].
- Ketamine-midazolam seems to have a better safety profile than fentanyl-midazolam or propofol-fentanyl [46, 47].
- Most of the time emergency medicine physicians use midazolam, fentanyl and ketamine to provide a deep level of sedation, which still may not be enough to relax the muscles to reduce the two fragments of bone. The use of propofol for procedures in pediatric ED is increasing [48].
- Propofol is a good choice under the circumstances but since this is usually a post trauma situation theoretically, stomach is considered to be full. Safest course of action under the circumstances is general anesthesia with endotracheal tube.
- Since the procedure is usually very short there is no need to have the entire anesthesia set up like anesthesia machine and ventilator. Patient can be hand ventilated using a "*Mapleson D circuit*" or "*pediatric ambu bag*" connected to an oxygen source.

- In addition to the standard monitors that the child is already attached to, a portable *capnography monitor* can be used to monitor the inspired and expired oxygen and carbon dioxide.
- Propofol can be administered in bolus form or as an infusion.
- A recent, large scale, survey of propofol administered by emergency physicians showed it to be safe with a low prevalence of adverse effects. Significant predictors of serious adverse events were weight less than or equal to 5 kg, ASA classification greater than II, use of adjunctive medications (benzodiazepines, ketamine, opioids, or anticholinergics), non-painful procedures, and primary diagnoses of upper respiratory illness or prematurity [49].
- Anesthesiologists can also be called into emergency room to provide sedation/analgesia/anesthesia for children with special needs or possible difficult airway that emergency medicine providers feel uncomfortable to handle.
- Procedure can be short like suturing a laceration, passing a nasogastric tube or draining a small abscess. These patients need to be evaluated very carefully and dealt with on individual basis. Details of management of this kind of child is dealt with elsewhere in this chapter.

Ophthalmology Suite

- Shorter exams under anesthesia (EUA) often do not require airway manipulation or even intravenous access.
- Longer procedures, such as cryoablation, may require an inhalational induction with LMA placement.
- The anesthesia providers and procedure team should discuss if muscle paralysis or a secured airway is needed.
- Challenges of administering anesthesia include:

    - Often there is limited space in the ophthalmologic suite.
    - Most procedures are short but highly stimulating requiring general anesthesia. The anesthesia providers must be aware of the risks of proceeding without a secured airway or IV access if they choose to proceed with only a mask airway.
    - Avoiding coughing and bucking which can cause an increase in intraocular pressure especially at emergence. Deep extubation or removal of the LMA may be indicated if the child is not considered a "full stomach" or difficult airway.
    - Avoiding drugs that can increase intraocular pressure such as ketamine and succinylcholine [17].

        - A "defasciculating dose" of nondepolarizing agents prior to succinylcholine does not eliminate the increase in intraocular pressure.
        - Many agents decrease intraocular pressure such as propofol and volatile anesthetics.
        - Many agents have no effect on intraocular pressure such as opioids and non-depolarizing neuromuscular blockers [17].

- Ophthalmologists often wish to measure the intraocular pressures immediately after induction and prior to airway instrumentation in order to attempt to get an accurate measurement of intraocular pressure [17].
- Preventing postoperative nausea and vomiting which can also increase intraocular pressure. Consider antiemetic prophylaxis and minimizing opioids. Strabismus surgery is particularly associated with PONV.
- Oculocardiac reflex (OCR) is most commonly associated with ophthalmologic surgery [50].

  - It causes profound disturbances in cardiac rhythm, most commonly bradycardia, but also asystole, PVC's, bigeminy and ventricular tachycardia.
  - It typically occurs from stretching or pulling of the ocular muscles. It can also occur with conjuctival stimulation, hypoxia, hypertension, increased intracerebral pressure, or other noxious stimuli.
  - Treatment starts with instructing the surgical team to stop and remove any stimulation.
  - The reflex can be fatigued with repeated action or blocked with local anesthetics.
  - Intravenous anticholinergics, such as glycopyrrolate or atropine, are also useful for prevention or treatment. Use caution as it is easy to give a larger then necessary dose since bradycardia will decrease circulation time and delay the onset time of medications given.
  - Chest compressions may be necessary to help to restart circulation if bradycardia is severe.
  - Pediatric patients often do not tolerate bradycardia hemodynamically because of decreased cardiac compliance.

    - Oculorespiratory reflexes have been described that resulted in dramatically reduced minute ventilation to similar stimuli as the OCR [17].

- Pediatric ophthalmologic procedures can be associated with certain defects and syndromes, which may or may not be diagnosed. Some of these syndromes may be associated with difficult airways and other potentially serious anesthetic issues [17].

  - Examples of syndromes that patients may have include: Down's syndrome, homocystinuria, mucopolysaccharidoses, craniosynostosis, craniofacial syndromes, neurofibromatosis and Marfan Syndrome.

- Ophthalmologic drugs

  - The convention in the United States is that drop containers with red tops dilate the pupil (sympamimetic or anticholinergic), while green tops constrict the pupil (cholinesterase inhibitors), and white tops do not affect the pupil.
  - Anticholinesterases, such as echothiophate iodide, may be given to patients with open angle glaucoma. It can have an effect that lasts for weeks [17]. Potential side effects include:

- Delaying the metabolism of ester local anesthetics
- Prolonging depolarizing relaxants
- Decreasing the duration of non-depolarizing anesthetics.

– Topical drugs, such as phenylephrine, can cause systemic toxicity in children despite small dosages [51].

- It has been described that phenylephrine solutions should be limited to 2.5%, but our experience is that 10% can be used successfully with limited complications.

– Avoid nitrous oxide if sulfur hexfluoride or air enters the globe, as it will diffuse into the space and cause potentially serious ophthalmic complications.

- Pain

  – Typically pain from pediatric ophthalmologic procedures is treatable with acetaminophen or non-steroidal analgesics.
  – Regional blocks, such as peribulbar or retrobulbar blocks, can be performed but can cause serious complications. They should only be performed by experienced providers [52].

GI Suite

- Gastrointestinal procedures are not as common for pediatric patients as with adults. Pediatric indications include foreign body removal, tracheoesophageal fistula, esophageal dysmotility, strictures, persistent vomiting or pain, and bleeding [53].
- Multiple anesthetics can be chosen. The decision of moderate, deep, or general anesthesia depends on the clinical factors involved.
- Common agents include midazolam, fentanyl, propofol, remifentanil, and volatile anesthetics.
- Propofol intravenous sedation has proven to be a reliably sound practice. Intravenous sedation for pediatric endoscopic procedures has been shown to be as safe and more cost effective in comparison to general anesthesia [54].
- Endoscopy is usually minimally painful and does not necessitate the use of opioids.
- Similar complications as in adults. Most commonly reported complication is respiratory related. These usually can be treated and resolved in the procedure room [55].
- The smaller pediatric anatomy may increase the risk of airway obstruction during endoscopy. It may be necessary to intubate and secure the airway for pediatric patients.
- Complications are highest in children younger than 6 months of age and are usually airway related. Young children may warrant a lower threshold for securing the airway [55].
- The overall immediate complication rate is 2.3% with hypoxia being the most common cause [56].

Procedures in In-patient Units

- At times, the anesthesiologist may be requested to sedate a pediatric patient undergoing minor procedures such as dressing changes, removal of sutures, removal of chest drains, and placement of nasogastric tubes.
- Intramuscular ketamine is a good choice to anesthetize these children for these quick procedures. It maintains spontaneous respiration, upper way reflexes and muscular tone but airway secretions may cause problems. Concomitant administration of an anticholinergic agent may be helpful in this regard.

Special Consideration: Intellectually Challenged Patient

- Some time should be spent to familiarize yourself with the child. Some patients with mental retardation are very friendly and respond positively to efforts to develop close and compassionate contact with them [57].
- Perform a careful airway examination. Have sound knowledge of airway difficulties associated with syndromes that also have mental retardation as a component.
- The major concern is obtaining intravenous access. If a patient is uncooperative and IV access is difficult, even short procedures may need a complete anesthesia set up with an anesthesia machine. The procedure either can be done under 50 % nitrous oxide/oxygen anesthesia or inhalational induction done to obtain an IV followed by propofol infusion, or other kind of sedation [58].
- If the airway is difficult, it is better to secure it up front. A safer approach is to secure the airway in the controlled environment of operating room and then transport the patient to the remote location for the procedure with intravenous propofol as the anesthetic of choice.
- Miyawaki et al. investigated the propofol dose needed for intravenous sedation in dental patients with Intellectual Disability. They found that they needed higher doses of sedatives to obtain an adequate level of sedation i.e. 4.74 mg/kg/h (2.63–10.33 mg/kg/h), vs. control (3.31, 1.72–4.80 mg/kg/h) [59].
- Another retrospective chart review of 260 developmentally disabled children showed similar requirement for the sedation medication (Pentobarbital and fentanyl) compared to control but three times higher risk of hypoxia (11.9 % versus 4.9 %) [60].
- A study by Enever et al. found no difference in post-operative morbidity after outpatient dental care under general anesthesia in 27 pediatric patients with disabilities compared to control [61].
- Be knowledgeable about associated anomalies in syndromes that have mental retardation as a component and incorporate the considerations related to these in the anesthetic plan.
- The prevalence of reflux esophagitis in the normal population is about 2 %, while in the intellectually disabled this condition has an estimated prevalence of 10 %

[62]. If gastroesophageal reflux is an associated syndrome, it is better to intubate these patients.

- Propofol is commonly used for sedating pediatric patients with neurologic conditions for diagnostic imaging, such as a CT scan or MRI. Propofol has anticonvulsant properties and reduces ICP, which can be advantageous in sedating a patient with epilepsy or a patient with concerns for obstructive hydrocephalus to obtain CT or MRI scan [63].

Special Consideration: Patient with Anatomical Abnormalities and Syndromes

- The volume of tonsillar tissue in the upper airway increases from about 6 months of age up to puberty and hypertrophic tonsils can significantly narrow oral and pharyngeal airways.

  - For children with a known severely bilateral **tonsillar hypertrophy**, inhalation induction with maintenance of spontaneous ventilation is preferred. Lateral positioning combined with jaw thrust significantly improves airway patency in these pediatric patients with tonsillar hypertrophy. If direct laryngoscopy fails, "*lightwand*" *guided intubation under laryngoscopy* can be used as rescue option [64].
  - For children with combined craniofacial anomalies and tonsillar hypertrophy, a laryngeal mask airway (LMA) is often employed to maintain airway patency during induction [64].
  - Fiberoptic nasotracheal intubation under inhaled anesthesia has been described to achieve an airway in a pediatric or uncooperative patient with **symptomatic lingual tonsillar hypertrophy** [65].

- Children with disabilities are a special group of pediatric patients, which require extra care in their anesthetic planning. Parents of children with disabilities are less satisfied with their anesthetic care when compared to children without disabilities [66]. It is a challenge providing kind and considerate anesthesia care and effective postoperative pain management for this patient population.

- **Down syndrome** occurs in 1/800 births. Several aspects of Down syndrome must be considered when planning safe anesthesia experience, including atlantoaxial instability, GERD, tracheal stenosis, bradyarrhythmias and chronic hypothyroidism.

  - Borland et al. studied 930 cases in patients with Down syndrome (DS) undergoing non-cardiac surgery. The most common anesthesia related complication were bradycardia (severe) (3.66%), natural airway obstruction (1.83%), difficult intubation (0.54%), and postintubation croup (1.83%) [67].
  - It is important for the anesthesiologist to exhibit calm and encouraging emotional behavior during pre-anesthetic periods of evaluation and preparation of

Table 21.5 Important anesthetic considerations in children with Down's syndrome [69]

Cardiovascular system	Children with DS are particularly prone to develop pulmonary hypertension, either in association with congenital heart disease (CHD) or as a result of chronic airway obstruction
	Ventricular septal defect (32%)
	Atrial septal defect (10%)
	Patent ductus arteriosus (4%)
Respiratory system	Midface hypoplasia causes nasal bone flattening, palate is short, tongue is large, possible tonsillar hypertrophy secondary to recurrent infections; all these factors makes for an airway prone to obstruction
Musculo-skeletal system	Upper cervical spine instability produced by ligamentous laxity, skeletal anomalies, or both
	If the history or physical examination reveals any signs or symptoms suspicious for cervical cord compression, elective surgery should be postponed
	For urgent surgeries, the patient should be treated with c-spine precautions [70]
Immunodeficiency	Strict asepsis is essential to reduce the risk of infections

DS patients. Most patients are warm, cheerful, and tolerant, but a few are stubborn and anxious. Patients with DS often have more receptive communication skills than expressive communication skills and establishing a rapport with the patient can help patients' anxiety and agitation [68].

 – Some of the important anesthetic considerations are enlisted in Table 21.5.

• **Williams Syndrome** is a rare neurodevelopmental disorder characterized by distinctive facial features, cognitive and developmental traits and multiple cardiac abnormalities including supravalvular and pulmonary aortic stenosis.

 – Patients with Williams syndrome are at an increased risk of adverse events during anesthesia and sedation, yet they are required to undergo several procedures that requires anesthesia during their lifetime. An anesthesiologist may be called upon to provide care for such patients in an off-site suite.

• A preoperative assessment of such a patient should be done to categorize anesthetic risk category and plan accordingly. The anesthetic goal in this case includes, preservation of sinus rhythm; maintenance of preload, contractility, and SVR; avoidance of anesthetic drugs that cause physiologic changes that may worsen ischemia; and avoidance of increased pulmonary vascular resistance [71].

• Similarly the anesthetic management of many other rare syndromes such as **Hamamy syndrome** [72] (craniofacial and cardiac abnormalities), **Job's syndrome** [73] (immunodeficiency, recurrent abscesses of staphylococcal origin) and **Jarcho Levin syndrome** [74] (abnormal fusion of ribs and vertebrae causing respiratory insufficiency) has been described in the literature as case-reports and should be reviewed if the anesthesiologist is taking care of a patient with such a syndrome.

The Role of Non-Pharmacological Interventions

- Non-pharmacological methods such as play therapy and presence of parents, for reducing anxiety and improving cooperation may avoid the adverse effects of preoperative sedation.
- A recent (2015) Cochrane review assessed the effectiveness of play therapy. 28 randomized-controlled trials (a total of 2681 children) investigating 17 interventions of interest were analyzed in a systemic way [75].
- In five trials (557 children), parental presence at induction of anesthesia did not reduce child anxiety compared with not having a parent present (standardized mean difference (SMD) 0.03, 95 % confidence interval (CI) −0.14 to 0.20).
- Other potentially helpful non pharmacological interventions *are clowns/clown doctors*; *playing videos of the child's choice during induction*; *low sensory stimulation*; *and hand-held video games*. There was equivocal result in various trials meaning these techniques should be further investigation in larger studies.

References

1. Couloures KG, Beach M, Cravero JP, Monroe KK, Hertzog JH. Impact of provider specialty on pediatric procedural sedation complication rates. Pediatrics. 2011;127(5):e1154–60. doi:10.1542/peds.2010-2960.
2. Coté CJ, Wilson S. Guidelines for monitoring and management of pediatric patients during and after sedation for diagnostic and therapeutic procedures: an update. Pediatrics. 2006;118(6):2587–602. doi:10.1542/peds.2006-2780.
3. Cravero JP, Beach ML, Blike GT, Gallagher SM, Hertzog JH. The incidence and nature of adverse events during pediatric sedation/anesthesia with propofol for procedures outside the operating room: a report from the Pediatric Sedation Research Consortium. Anesth Analg. 2009;108(3):795–804. doi:10.1213/ane.0b013e31818fc334.
4. Beach ML, Cohen DM, Gallagher SM, Cravero JP. Major adverse events and relationship to nil per Os status in pediatric sedation/anesthesia outside the operating room: a report of the pediatric sedation research consortium. Anesthesiology. 2016;124(1):80–88. doi: 10.1097/ALN.0000000000000933.
5. Skolnick ET, Vomvolakis MA. A prospective evaluation of children with upper respiratory infections undergoing a standardized anesthetic and the incidence of adverse respiratory events. Anesthesiology. 1998;89:A1309.
6. Tait AR, Shobha M, Voepel-Lewis T, Munro HM, Siewer M, Pandit UA. Risk factors for perioperative adverse respiratory events in children with upper respiratory tract infections. Anesthestiology. 2001;95(2):299–306.
7. Aquilina AT, Hall WJ, Douglas Jr RG, Utell MJ. Airway reactivity in subjects with viral upper respiratory tract infections: the effects of exercise and cold air. Am Rev Respir Dis. 1980;122(1):3–10.
8. Ghofaily LA, Simmons C, Chen L, Liu R. Negative pressure pulmonary edema after Laryngospasm: a revist with a case report. J Anesth Clin Res. 2013;3(10):252.
9. Raghavendran K, Nemzek J, Napolitano LM, Knight PR. Aspiration-induced lung injury. Crit Care Med. 2011;39(4):818–26.
10. Hudgetl DW. Mechanisms of obstructive sleep apnea. Chest. 1992;101(2):541–9.

11. Schwengel DA, Sterni LM, Tunkel DE, Heitmiller ES. Perioperative management of children with obstructive sleep apnea. Anesth Analg. 2009;109(1):60–75.
12. de Caen AR, Berg MD, Chameides L, Gooden CK, Hickey RW, Scott HF, Sutton RM, Tijsse JA, Topjian A, van der Jagt EW, Schexnayder SM, Samson RA. Part 12: pediatric advanced life support: 2015 American Heart Association Guidelines Update for Cardiopulmonary Resuscitation and Emergency Cardiovascular Care. Circulation. 2015;132(18 Suppl 2): S526–42.
13. Malignant Hyperthermia Association of the United States. http://www.mhaus.org/healthcare-professionals/be-prepared/associated-conditions.
14. Glahn KP, Ellis FR, Halsall PJ, Muller CR, Snoeck MM, Urwyler A, Wappler F. Recognizing and managing a malignant hyperthermia crisis: guidelines from European Malignant Hyperthermia Group. Br J Anaesth. 2010;105(4):417–20.
15. Hall SC, Santhanam S. Chapter 44. Neonatal anesthesia. In: Barash PG, Cullen BF, Stoelting RK, Cahalan MK, Stock MC, editors. Clinical anesthesia. 6th ed. Lippincott Williams & Wilkins; Philadelphia: 2009. p. 1171–205.
16. Kurth CD, Spitzer AR, Broennle AM, Downes JJ. Postoperative apnea in preterm infants. Anesthesiology. 1987;66:483.
17. Justice LT, Valley RD, Bailey AG, Hauser M. Chapter 27. Anesthesia for ophthalmic surgery. In Davis PJ, Cladis FP, Motoyama EK, editors. Smith's anesthesia for infants and children. 8th ed. 2011. p. 870–88. doi:10.1016/B978-0-323-06612-9.00044-4.
18. Martin T, Nicolson SC, Bargas MS. Propofol anesthesia reduces emesis and airway obstruction in pediatric outpatients. Anaesth Analg. 1993;76:144–8.
19. Apfelbaum JL, Caplan RA, Connis RT, Epstein BS, Nickinovich DG, Warner MA. Practice guidelines for preoperative fasting and the use of pharmacologic agents to reduce the risk of pulmonary aspiration: application to healthy patients undergoing elective procedures: an updated report by the American Society of Anesthesiologists Com. Anesthesiology. 2011;114(3):495–511. doi:10.1097/ALN.0b013e3181fcbfd9.
20. Engelhardt T, Wilson G, Horne L, Weiss M, Schmitz A. Are you hungry? Are you thirsty?–fasting times in elective outpatient pediatric patients. Paediatr Anaesth. 2011;21(9):964–8. doi:10.1111/j.1460-9592.2011.03573.x.
21. Brady M, Kinn S, Ness V, O'Rourke K, Randhawa N, Stuart P. Preoperative fasting for preventing perioperative complications in children. Cochrane Database Syst Rev. 2009;(4):CD005285. doi:10.1002/14651858.CD005285.pub2.
22. Krauss B. Procedural sedation and analgesia in children. Lancet. 2006;367:766–80. doi:10.1016/S0733-8627(02)00084-6.
23. Cravero JP, Blike GT. Review of pediatric sedation. Anesth Analg. 2004;99(5):1355–64.
24. Tobias JD. Dexmedetomidine: applications in pediatric critical care and pediatric anesthesiology. Pediatr Crit Care Med. 2007;8(2):115–31.
25. Duma A, Cartmill C, Blood J, Sharma A, Kharasch ED, Nagele P. The hematological effects of nitrous oxide anesthesia in pediatric patients. Anesth Analg. 2015;120(6):1325–30.
26. Patel RI, Davis PJ, Orr RJ, Ferrari LR, Rimar S, Hannallah RS, Cohen IT, Colingo K, Donlon JV, Haberkern CM, McGowan FX, Prillaman BA, Parasuraman TV, Creed MR. Single-dose Ondansetron prevents postoperative vomiting in pediatric outpatients. Anesth Analg. 1997;85:538–45.
27. Lim E, Rai E, Seow WT. Feasibility of anaesthetic provision for paediatric patients undergoing off-site intraoperative MRI-guided neurosurgery: the Singapore experience from 2009 to 2012. Anaesth Intensive Care. 2013;41(4):535–42. http://www.ncbi.nlm.nih.gov/pubmed/23808515. Accessed 3 Nov 2015.
28. Apfelbaum JL, Singleton MA, Ehrenwerth J, Bell C, Connis RT, Mason KP, McClain CD, Nickinovich DG, Sandberg WS. Practice advisory on anesthetic care for magnetic resonance imaging. An updated report by the American Society of Anesthesiologists Task Force on anesthetic care for magnetic resonance imaging. Anesthesiology. 2015;122:495–520.
29. Campbell K, Torres L, Stayer S. Anesthesia and sedation outside the operating room. Anesthesiol Clin. 2014;32(1):25–43. doi:10.1016/j.anclin.2013.10.010.

30. Thorp N. Basic principles of paediatric radiotherapy. Clin Oncol. 2013;25(1):3–10. doi:10.1016/j.clon.2012.08.006.
31. Merchant TE, Farr JB. Proton beam therapy. Curr Opin Pediatr. 2014;26(1):3–8. doi:10.1097/MOP.0000000000000048.
32. Scott L, Langton F, O'Donoghue J. Minimising the use of sedation/anaesthesia in young children receiving radiotherapy through an effective play preparation programme. Eur J Oncol Nurs Off J Eur Oncol Nurs Soc. 2002;6(1):15–22. doi:10.1054/ejon.2001.0162.
33. Fortney JT, Halperin EC, Hertz CM, Schulman SR. Anesthesia for pediatric external beam radiation therapy. Int J Radiat Oncol Biol Phys. 1999;44(3):587–91.
34. Saito T, Kaneko A, Muramatsu Y, et al. Difficult tracheal intubation in patients with retinoblastoma caused by 13q deficiency. Jpn J Clin Oncol. 1998;28(8):507–10. doi:10.1093/jjco/28.8.507.
35. Whyte SD, Mark AJ. Anesthetic considerations in the management of Wilms' tumor. Paediatr Anaesth. 2006;16(5):504–13. doi:10.1111/j.1460-9592.2006.01866.x.
36. Latham GJ, Greenberg RS. Anesthetic considerations for the pediatric oncology patient – part 3: pain, cognitive dysfunction, and preoperative evaluation. Paediatr Anaesth. 2010;20(6):479–89. doi:10.1111/j.1460-9592.2010.03261.x.
37. Evans P, Chisholm D. Anaesthesia and paediatric oncology. Curr Anaesth Crit Care. 2008;19(2):50–8. doi:10.1016/j.cacc.2007.07.012.
38. Buchsbaum JC, McMullen KP, Douglas JG, et al. Repetitive pediatric anesthesia in a non-hospital setting. Int J Radiat Oncol Biol Phys. 2013;85(5):1296–300. doi:10.1016/j.ijrobp.2012.10.006.
39. Anghelescu DL, Burgoyne LL, Liu W, et al. Safe anesthesia for radiotherapy in pediatric oncology: St. Jude Children's Research Hospital Experience, 2004–2006. Int J Radiat Oncol Biol Phys. 2008;71(2):491–7. doi:10.1016/j.ijrobp.2007.09.044.
40. Dagal A. Radiation safety for anesthesiologists. Curr Opin Anaesthesiol. 2011;24(4):445–50. doi:10.1097/ACO.0b013e328347f984.
41. Iravani M. Pediatric malignancies and anesthesia in out-of-or locations. Int Anesthesiol Clin. 2009;47(3):25–33. doi:10.1097/AIA.0b013e3181ab1271.
42. Pitetti RD, Singh S, Pierce MC. Safe and efficacious use of procedural sedation and analgesia by nonanesthesiologists in a pediatric emergency department. Arch Pediatr Adolesc Med. 2003;157(11):1090. doi:10.1001/archpedi.157.11.1090.
43. Shavit I, Hershman E. Management of children undergoing painful procedures in the emergency department by non-anesthesiologists. Israel Med Assoc J IMAJ. 2004;6(6):350–5. http://www.ncbi.nlm.nih.gov/pubmed/15214463.
44. Migita RT, Klein EJ, Garrison MM. Sedation and analgesia for pediatric fracture reduction in the emergency department. Arch Pediatr Adolesc Med. 2006;160(1):46. doi:10.1001/archpedi.160.1.46.
45. Kennedy RM, Luhmann JD, Luhmann SJ. Emergency department management of pain and anxiety related to orthopedic fracture care: a guide to analgesic techniques and procedural sedation in children. Paediatr Drugs. 2004;6(1):11–31. http://www.ncbi.nlm.nih.gov/pubmed/14969567. Accessed 15 Oct 2015.
46. Roback MG, Wathen JE, Bajaj L, Bothner JP. Adverse events associated with procedural sedation and analgesia in a pediatric emergency department: a comparison of common parenteral drugs. Acad Emerg Med Off J Soc Acad Emerg Med. 2005;12(6):508–13. doi:10.1197/j.aem.2004.12.009.
47. Kennedy RM, Porter FL, Miller JP, Jaffe DM. Comparison of fentanyl/midazolam with ketamine/midazolam for pediatric orthopedic emergencies. Pediatrics. 1998;102(4 Pt 1):956–63. http://www.ncbi.nlm.nih.gov/pubmed/9755272. Accessed 15 Oct 2015.
48. Lamond DW. Review article: safety profile of propofol for paediatric procedural sedation in the emergency department. Emerg Med Australas. 2010;22(4):265–86. doi:10.1111/j.1742-6723.2010.01298.x.
49. Mallory MD, Baxter AL, Yanosky DJ, Cravero JP. Emergency physician-administered propofol sedation: a report on 25,433 sedations from the pediatric sedation research consortium. Ann Emerg Med. 2011;57(5):462–468.e1. doi:10.1016/j.annemergmed.2011.03.008.

50. Lai YH, Hsu HT, Wang HZ, Cheng KI, Wu KY. The oculocardiac reflex during stabismus surgery: its relationship to preoperative clinical eye findings and subsequent postoperative emesis. J AAPOS. 2014;18(2):151–5.
51. Sbaraglia F, Mores N, Garra R, Giuratrabocchetta G, Lepore D, Molle F, Savino G, Piastra M, Pulitano S, Sammartino M. Phenylephrine eye drops in pediatric patients undergoing ophthalmic surgery: incidence, presentation, and management of complications during general anesthesia. Paediatr Anaesth. 2014;24(4):400–5.
52. McGoldrick KE. Complications of regional anesthesia for ophthalmic surgery. Yale J Biol Med. 1993;66(5):443–5.
53. Mason KP, Holzman RS. Chapter 33. Anesthesia and sedation for pediatric procedures outside the operating room. In: Davis PJ, Cladis FP, Motoyama EK, editors. Smith's anesthesia for infants and children. 8th ed. 2011. p. 1041–57. doi:10.1016/B978-0-323-06612-9.00044-4.
54. Squires R, Morriss F, Schluterman S, Drews B, Galyen L, Brown KO. Efficacy, safety, and cost of intravenous sedation versus general anesthesia in children undergoing endoscopic procedures. Gastrointest Endosc. 1995;41(2):99–104.
55. Koh JL, Black DD, LEatherman IK, Harrison RD, Schmitz ML. Experience with an anesthesiologist interventional model for endoscopy in a pediatric hospital. J Pediatr Gastroenterol Nutr. 2001;33:314–8.
56. Thakkar K, El-Serang HB, Mattek N, Gilger MA. Complications of pediatric EGD: a 4-year experience in PEDS-CORI. Gastrointest Endosc. 2007;65(2):213–21.
57. Stiles CM. Anesthesia for the mentally retarded patient. Orthop Clin North Am. 1981;12(1):45–56. http://www.ncbi.nlm.nih.gov/pubmed/7207992. Accessed 2 Nov 2015.
58. Macpherson A. Sevoflurane or halothane could be used for intellectually disabled children under day-stay general anaesthesia. Evid Based Dent. 2006;7(2):37. doi:10.1038/sj.ebd.6400408.
59. Miyawaki T, Kohjitani A, Maeda S, et al. Intravenous sedation for dental patients with intellectual disability. J Intellect Disabil Res JIDR. 2004;48(Pt 8):764–8. doi:10.1111/j.1365-2788.2004.00598.x.
60. Kannikeswaran N, Mahajan PV, Sethuraman U, Groebe A, Chen X. Sedation medication received and adverse events related to sedation for brain MRI in children with and without developmental disabilities. Paediatr Anaesth. 2009;19(3):250–6. doi:10.1111/j.1460-9592.2008.02900.x.
61. Enever GR, Nunn JH, Sheehan JK. A comparison of post-operative morbidity following outpatient dental care under general anaesthesia in paediatric patients with and without disabilities. Int J Paediatr Dent/British Paedodont Soc Int Assoc Dent Child. 2000;10(2):120–5. http://www.ncbi.nlm.nih.gov/pubmed/11310096. Accessed 2 Nov 2015.
62. Böhmer C, Niezen-de Boer M, Klinkenberg-Knol E, Nadorp J, Meuwissen S. Gastro-oesophageal reflux disease in institutionalised intellectually disabled individuals. Neth J Med. 1997;51(4):134–9. http://www.ncbi.nlm.nih.gov/pubmed/9643224.
63. Kilbaugh TJ, Friess SH, Raghupathi R, Huh JW. Sedation and analgesia in children with developmental disabilities and neurologic disorders. Int J Pediatr. 2010;2010. doi:10.1155/2010/189142.
64. Xue FS, Zhang YM, Liao X, Luo MP. Anesthesia and airway management for children with tonsillar hypertrophy. Paediatr Anaesth. 2009;19(6):642–3. doi:10.1111/j.1460-9592.2009.02950.x.
65. Nakazawa K, Ikeda D, Ishikawa S, Makita K. A case of difficult airway due to lingual tonsillar hypertrophy in a patient with Down's syndrome. Anesth Analg. 2003;97(3):704–5. http://www.ncbi.nlm.nih.gov/pubmed/12933389. Accessed 2 Nov 2015.
66. Schiff J-H, Russ N, Ihringer K, Heal C, Martin E, Walther A. Pediatric patients with disabilities – assessment of satisfaction with anesthesia. Paediatr Anaesth. 2012;22(11):1117–23. doi:10.1111/j.1460-9592.2012.03886.x.
67. Borland LM, Colligan J, Brandom BW. Frequency of anesthesia-related complications in children with Down syndrome under general anesthesia for noncardiac procedures. Paediatr Anaesth. 2004;14(9):733–8. doi:10.1111/j.1460-9592.2004.01329.x.
68. (NDSS) NDSS. National Down Syndrome Society. http://www.ndss.org/Resources/Health-Care/Associated-Conditions/Anesthesia-Down-Syndrome/#sthash.dcmRGqA0.dpuf.

69. Steward DJ. Anesthesia considerations in children with Down syndrome. Semin Anesth Perioperat Med Pain. 2006;25(3):136–41. doi:10.1053/j.sane.2006.05.001.

70. Hata T, Todd MM. Cervical spine considerations when anesthetizing patients with Down syndrome. Anesthesiology. 2005;102(3):680–5. http://anesthesiology.pubs.asahq.org/article. aspx?articleid=1942107. Accessed 3 Nov 2015.

71. Matisoff AJ, Olivieri L, Schwartz JM, Deutsch N. Risk assessment and anesthetic management of patients with Williams syndrome: a comprehensive review. Paediatr Anaesth. 2015;25(12):1207–15. doi:10.1111/pan.12775.

72. Buget MI, Canbolat N, Akgul T, Kucukay S. Anaesthesia and orphan disease: anaesthetic management of a child with Hamamy syndrome. Eur J Anaesthesiol. 2015;32(12):891–3. doi:10.1097/EJA.0000000000000263.

73. Kulkarni P, Shah R, Priyanka VN. Anesthetic management in a child with Job's syndrome. Anesth Essays Res. 2012;6(2):223–5. doi:10.4103/0259-1162.108342.

74. Geze S, Arslan U, Tusat M. Anaesthesia for infant with Jarcho Levin syndrome: case report. Braz J Anesthesiol (Elsevier). 2015;65(5):414–6. doi:10.1016/j.bjane.2012.12.005.

75. Manyande A, Cyna AM, Yip P, Chooi C, Middleton P. Non-pharmacological interventions for assisting the induction of anaesthesia in children. Cochrane Database Syst Rev. 2015;7:CD006447. doi:10.1002/14651858.CD006447.pub3.

Chapter 22
Procedural Sedation in the Emergency Department

Nancy Vinca, John Barrett, and Christopher J.D. Tems

Abstract Procedural sedation in the emergency department is performed success-fully across the country by many emergency medicine physicians. There are many varied styles of sedation in the ED that may vary from hospital to hospital. The required equipment, presences of additional providers, etc may vary slightly depending on the emergency department and its staffing complements. In addition, there are a variety of sedatives that may be used for sedation in the ED. Among the most common are ketamine and propofol, etomidate, and fentanyl/versed. Dexmedetomidine and remifentanyl remain on the horizon. Both the sedation prac-tice and the need for the ED physician to also perform the procedure himself/herself make the style and technique of procedural sedation in the ED unique. It many ways it is very different from elsewhere in the hospital. However, the emergency medi-cine physician still maintains a high standard of care and a high quality safety mar-gin. At all times there should be emergency airway equipment available. Also, an assessment of the urgency of the procedure is made by the ED physician. NPO sta-tus is less of a highlighted issue. In most all settings, it is also highly recommended that supplemental oxygen and capnography be used. The physician performing the sedation must be competent in emergency airway techniques.

Keywords Sedation • Emergency department • Emergency airway management • Ketamine • Propofol • Ketofol • Etomidate • Fentanyl/versed • Capnography • Providers

N. Vinca, MD (✉) • C.J.D. Tems, MD
Department of Anesthesiology, Hospital of the University of Pennsylvania,
3400 Spruce Street, Philadelphia, PA 19104, USA
e-mail: nancy.vinca@uphs.upenn.edu; chris.tems@gmail.com

J. Barrett, MD
Department of Emergency Medicine, Hospital of the University of Pennsylvania,
3400 Spruce Street, Philadelphia, PA 19104, USA
e-mail: john.barrett@uphs.upenn.edu

© Springer International Publishing Switzerland 2017
B.G. Goudra, P.M. Singh (eds.), *Out of Operating Room Anesthesia*,
DOI 10.1007/978-3-319-39150-2_22

Procedural sedation in the emergency department is a unique subset of sedation. First of all, many emergency departments throughout the country only have one physician staffing their department. This opportunity lends itself to the development of a unique skillset. An emergency medicine physician must be able to multi-task in the fullest possible way. While simultaneously directing the sedation plan, he/she must also be tasked with performing the procedure. There are a variety of practice models for this plan. In some hospitals, a physician assistant may be present to help with the procedure. In academic centers, there are residents who are available to help with both sedation practice and procedural practice. However, in many EDs, there is a single provider who needs to be able to "do it all." In addition to the physician, the American College of Emergency Physicians requires the presence of a certified provider to monitor the patient during sedation. In many EDs, this will be an emergency department nurse. Why is this unique? In virtually all other locations in the hospital, anesthesia staff are responsible for sedation practice. By the nature of the anesthesiologist's training and practice, which begins in the operating room, there are two providers present for surgical/operative procedures. One is the sedation provider and one is the proceduralist/surgeon. In the emergency department, it may be one physician and a nurse. Due to the inherent difference among the different specialties, this is a unique difference in practice. Due to staffing constraints number of physicians available in the ED may be limited. Both models serve to provide safe and excellent patient care in different settings.

Before the procedure begins the emergency physician examines the patient and has a sense of the patient's airway and potential airway complications. Although most emergency medicine physicians don't formally assess or score Mallampati exams, they are certainly aware of the patient's airway and its potential complications. Food intake is assessed and urgency of the procedure is addressed. Equipment is gathered prior to the start. The patient is placed on a cardiac monitor with telemetry, pulse oximetry, and in many places, capnography and/or respiratory rate monitoring. Suction is available and checked, intravenous access is obtained, airway equipment is made readily available, and the patient is consented both for the procedure and for the sedation.

What happens when the patient encounters complications during procedural sedation? Hypoxia and hypoventilation must be readily recognized. Often the patient is stimulated by voice, jaw thrust, or deep sternal rub. We believe that the best way to stimulate the patient is through jaw thrust. Not only is it a very stimulating maneuver, but it also serves to open the airway and help relieve any potential airway obstruction that may be occurring. If airway obstruction continues, a nasal trumpet can be placed. This too is a very stimulating maneuver and additionally serves to further open the airway and bypass any obstruction. Supplemental oxygen via nasal cannula (most often) serves to offer some buffer again the development of hypoxia during the sedation period. Based on available evidence we believe that capnography serves as the best gauge of depth of sedation and risk of the development of hypoxia. Hypoventilation will occur first, ahead of hypoxia, and if rapidly identified, adjustments can be made to prevent oxygen desaturation from occurring. In addition to cardiac monitor placement and capnography, the astute bedside physician is essential to the detection of hypoventilation and/or slowed minute ventilation. By simply watching the patient breathe, hypoventilation can easily be missed. Upper airway obstruction can be missed by only watching the rocking movements of the chest. While the chest may be moving in a rhythmic fashion consistent with breathing movements, upper airway obstruction may nonetheless be occurring. Most importantly, feeling the patient exhale onto the sedation providers gloved hand can rapidly detect or note the presence of exhaled gas flow due to the tactile stimulation of warm gas flow onto the provider. The sedation provider should use all senses to monitor depth and safety of sedation, including visual (capnography pattern, chest movements), auditory (pulse oximetry beeping, sonorous respirations), and tactile (warmth of exhaled gases on the clinician's hand) senses.

Emergency Airway Management

What happens if the sedation is too deep for the stimulation level of the procedure, or if the patient progresses to a deeper plane of sedation than initially intended? Obviously the above manipulations are first attempted, including voice, jaw thrust, and/or sternal rub. If this does not suffice, a nasal trumpet may be placed assuming there are no contraindications such as facial fractures, coagulopathy, etc. If the patient's breathing continues to decline, manual assisted ventilation must begin, often with a bag-valve-mask device or other circuit capable of delivering high flow oxygen. If the airway status continues to decline, on rare occasion, the patient may need to be intubated. The emergency medicine physician is skilled at emergency airway management and can quickly proceed with rapid sequence intubation. Preoxygenation is begun and suction is moved to the head of the bed. The most common drugs used for rapid sequence intubation in the ED are etomidate and succinylcholine. At times, rocuronium is also used. All ED patients are considered to have a full stomach and rapid sequence intubation is the safest method to secure the airway in the ED and prevent aspiration. Although it is rare to proceed with intubation during procedural sedation in the emergency department, it is essential to review the best means to perform it for the sake of completeness of the procedure and to fully review all aspects of procedural sedation in the ED [1].

There are many details essential to the performance of rapid sequence intubation in the emergency department. First of all, cricoid pressure was considered to be an essential part of the process for many years. An assistant places pressure over the mid trachea with two fingers in the hopes of closing the esophagus and preventing aspiration of stomach contents during the intubation process. Of late, there has been much discussion and debate as to the utility of this part of the procedure. Does cricoid pressure help? Does it prevent aspiration? The application of cricoid pressure developed in response to expert opinion. There was never a large body of evidence that prompted its use. It has recently been noted that indeed it may not prevent aspiration during rapid sequence intubation, but rather may worsen aspiration risk and cause harm. Cricoid pressure may increase peak inspiratory pressures during hand assisted ventilation, which may be necessary as a response to hypoxia. In turn, this may cause further gastric insufflation. Also, it may decrease lower esophageal pressure, thereby worsening aspiration risk. Often, it will worsen the view of the laryngoscopist during the intubation process. This can be extremely detrimental by delaying intubation. The best means to prevent aspiration during emergent intubation is to use rapidly acting induction anesthetics coupled with a rapidly acting neuromuscular blocking agent. With adequate pre-oxygenation, the goal is to avoid hand assisted ventilation whenever possible. This is the best way to prevent aspiration [2].

In addition, when rapid sequence intubation is performed in the ED, there is emerging evidence that success rates are higher with video laryngoscopy. Multiple studies have show that CMAC and/or GlideScope video laryngoscopy is more successful when compared to direct laryngoscopy in the ED. It is worth noting this prior to performing procedural sedation for many reasons. Where is the airway equipment? Is the suction being utilized? Are rapid sequence induction medications readily available? Are laryngoscope blades available? Is there a video laryngoscope available and if so where is it? All of the equipment should be checked and immediately available for use when performing procedural sedation in the ED.

Next we will discuss equipment needed for procedural sedation as well as the medications that are used for sedation.

Capnography, Supplemental Oxygen, and Ventilation Status During Procedural Sedation

As the use of procedural sedation continues to expand for painful and anxiety-provoking procedures in the emergency department, a well-controlled and monitored patient setting is of the utmost importance. Current guidelines from the American College of Emergency Physicians (ACEP) and the American Society of Anesthesiology (ASA) recommend continuous monitoring of respiratory and heart rate, blood pressure, and pulse oximetry during procedural sedation [3, 4]. New from previously published policy guidelines from both groups is a strong recommendation for capnography use from the American Society of Anesthesiology, and a Level B recommendation from the American College of Emergency Physicians (defined as reflecting moderate clinical certainty) that capnography may be used to monitor ventilation status as a means to detect apnea earlier than pulse oximetry alone. A 2009 randomized, controlled trial by Deitch et al. showed a 100% sensitivity of capnography identifying hypoxia before onset during propofol sedation, with the authors concluding that capnography provides advance warning for all hypoxic events [5]. The median onset of hypoxia after respiratory depression (defined as capnography reading >50 mmHg) was 60 s in their study, demonstrating obvious clinical utility for end tidal CO_2 monitoring. Advanced warning of hypoventilation or apnea can prompt the clinician to utilize airway adjuncts such as nasopharyngeal airways or bag valve masks if the need arises before oxygen desaturation occurs.

Supplemental oxygen is classically recommended as an adjunct to procedural sedation, however little data exists to date supporting a difference in significant outcomes with routine supplemental oxygen administration. Indeed, Deitch et al in 2008 did not show a significant decrease in hypoxia with supplemental oxygen via nasal cannula [6]. However, a 2011 randomized, controlled trial by the same group did show a clinically significant reduction in hypoxia during propofol sedation in a high-flow oxygen group (defined as 15 L/min via non-rebreather mask) when compared to 15 L/min flow of compressed air [7]. When choosing a sedative agent with apnea as a possible side effect, high-flow oxygen may be a useful supplement to procedural sedation.

Given the strong recommendations from both the ASA and ACEP on end-tidal CO_2 monitoring, we recommend consideration of high-flow oxygen supplementation along with routine use of both pulse oximetry and capnography as the safest approach for all procedural sedations.

Number of Providers Required

Competency and privilege credentialing is institution specific, with varying numbers of required physicians or other healthcare providers (nurses, physician assistants, nurse practitioners). All hospital staff should be aware of their own department's policies and guidelines for procedural sedation. The American College of Emergency Physicians provides a Level C recommendation (based on limited literature or expert consensus) for a "nurse or other qualified individual" to be present for monitoring the patient in addition to the medical provider performing the procedure [4]. The exact number and titles of providers necessary for procedural sedation is not specifically defined by either the ASA or ACEP, likely due to the void of evidence-based outcomes in the literature influenced by numbers and roles of providers. Two studies investigating single physician versus a two-physician procedural sedation team showed no statically significant difference in adverse events between the groups, where adverse events were defined as hypotension, hypoxia, apnea, or airway obstruction [8, 9]. Of note, the decision to staff each sedation with one or two physicians was made based on clinical judgment and not randomization, with no randomized trials existing to date comparing complication rates between single versus two-physician procedural sedation teams.

We recommend at least two healthcare providers (i.e. one physician and one nurse) be present for the entirety of the procedural sedation. Both providers should have experience with all drugs and monitoring equipment prior to the start of the procedure. Most importantly, any physician performing procedural sedation must be competent at both medical resuscitation and airway stabilization or intubation should the need arise.

Etomidate

Etomidate is an imidazole hypnotic that induces sedation via GABA receptors in the central nervous system. Etomidate is a common choice for induction of anesthesia or rapid sequence intubation, however a growing role for procedural sedation in the emergency department has been reported in the literature. The American College of Emergency Physicians currently gives a Level B recommendation (reflecting moderate clinical certainty) that etomidate can be administered safely to adults in the emergency department for procedural sedation [4]. Etomidate provides anxiolysis, sedation, and amnesia but has no analgesic properties. A short half-life makes etomidate ideal for brief but anxiety-provoking procedures in the emergency department.

Etomidate has similar pharmacological characteristics to propofol in regards to onset of action, clinical duration, and depth of sedation. Specifically, etomidate has an onset of action under 1 min, with a 5–10 min duration of moderate to deep sedation. The usual initial dose for procedural sedation with etomidate is 0.1–0.15 mg/kg intravenously [10, 11]. This dose may be repeated for clinical effect after 3–5 min. We recommend administering the intravenous dose over 30–45 s. A 2002 study by Vinson and Bradbury showed a mean cumulative dose of 0.2 mg/kg of intravenous etomidate for procedural sedation, with an additional 23 % of patient requiring additional medications (opiates and/or benzodiazepines) [12].

Etomidate is often praised as a sedation agent with minimal cardiovascular effects. Along with ketamine, etomidate is a good choice for sedation when hypotension is a concern. The clinical utility of etomidate for procedural sedation in the emergency department is broad, but etomidate is specifically useful for short procedures such as lumbar puncture, cardioversion, complicated laceration repairs, and abscess drainage. Additionally, etomidate use for procedural sedation has been shown to have good patient satisfaction and significant lack of procedure recall [12].

Etomidate has a few side effects and adverse reactions one should be aware of before utilization in procedural sedation. Relative adrenal sufficiency has been cited in the literature after a single dose of etomidate, which has been a concern when used as an induction agent prior to intubation in patients with sepsis or shock [4]. However, the clinical significance of transient adrenal suppression after routine procedural sedation is unknown and likely negligible. Myoclonus secondary to etomidate administration is also well described, possibly decreasing its utility in joint or fracture reductions, although it is certainly well established as a viable agent in those situations [10]. However, myoclonus can also lead to masseter muscle spasm, especially when administering the etomidate dose intravenously faster than the recommended 30–45 s, thus the clinician should be ready with airway adjuncts including nasopharyngeal airway and bag valve masks should the situation arise. Vomiting is also described with etomidate use, with a lower frequency of 2–5 % at doses less than 0.15 mg/kg IV, but up to 10 % when doses exceed 0.4 mg/kg IV [12]. Finally, etomidate can cause pain upon injection in a peripheral intravenous catheter.

Remifentanil

Remifentanil is a synthetic opiate similar to fentanyl in chemical structure, potency, and adverse effects. Onset of action is usually 1–3 min, with duration of clinical effect approximately 5 min. The usual starting dose for remifentanil intravenous administration alone is 0.5–3 mcg/kg, with additional doses of 0.25–1 mcg/kg given every 2 min to clinical effect [11]. When remifentanil is combined with other agents for procedural sedation, dose adjustments should be made. As a newer sedative and analgesic, remifentanil has no data published in the literature showing superiority over other sedative agents, such as propofol, or even compared to fentanyl. However, remifantanil is a viable option for procedural sedation if available.

Dexmedetomidine

Dexmedetomidine is an alpha two agonist with both sedative and analgesic effects. A 2010 case report of two patients illustrated success with dexmedetomidine for procedural sedation in shoulder reductions, however little additional literature has surfaced, and specifically no clinical trials exist using dexmedetomidine for procedural sedation in the emergency department. However, the popularity of dexmedetomidine in the operating room and intensive care units continues to increase, and further studies of dexmedetomidine for procedural sedation are expected. The main benefit of dexmedetomidine is its safety profile. It causes minimal if any respiratory depression and has few if any contraindications, making it an excellent choice for future study on ED patients.

Propofol

Propofol (2,6-diisopropylphenol) is a sedative/hypnotic agent which has no intrinsic analgesic effects but which does have potent amnestic and anxiolytic effects [3]. It is a commonly used agent to provide for moderate to deep procedural sedation. It rapidly equilibrates between plasma and the brain, resulting in a short time of onset of generally less than 1 min. Propofol distributes to tissues and is metabolized by the liver, and has a short duration of action of 5–15 min [4]. Propofol is given at an initial dose of 0.5–1 mg/kg IV (with 1 mg/kg being the most common dosing found in studies) followed by 0.5 mg/kg doses every 2–3 min as needed for additional sedation or for prolonged procedures [3].

Propofol has been shown to be as efficacious as other agents in providing adequate sedation and amnesia to perform procedures in both adults and children [3]. It is important to remember that propofol provides sedation without any analgesic effect, though studies have shown that reported procedural pain is low and satisfaction is high even when this agent is used alone. In one randomized controlled trial there was no difference in reported pain, procedural recall, or patient satisfaction when an opioid (alfentanil) was added to the sedation regimen [5]. Propofol has also been shown to have antiemetic properties which may decrease the incidence of vomiting as a complication of procedural sedation [6].

Multiple studies have shown that propofol can be safely administered to both adults and children for procedural sedation in the emergency department [13]. Propofol can cause respiratory depression and hypotension though trials have varied widely in rates of both [3]. One retrospective review of propofol use by emergency physicians in the emergency department (ED) showed adverse effects in 5% of sedations, due to hypotension in 2.33% and hypoxia in 1.4% [3]. Other studies have found rates of respiratory depression up to 49% when using propofol [14]. Due to differences in measured outcomes and confounding variables in many of the studies, an exact rate of respiratory depression is difficult to quantify. It has been suggested that slower administration rates likely decrease the incidence of respiratory depression [3]. Opioids in combination with propofol have been shown to significantly increase rates of respiratory depression and given a lack of demonstrated benefit should not be routinely co-administered [13]. Injection site pain is also a common side effect and can be mitigated with slower injections or with administration of a small dose of lidocaine prior to propofol. Propofol is contraindicated in those with egg or soy allergies. It should be used in caution with those with preexisting respiratory depression or hypotension.

Ketamine

Ketamine is a unique phencyclidine-derived dissociative agent which provides for analgesia, sedation, and amnesia during procedural sedation [7]. Its time to onset is 1 min when given IV and 3–5 min when given IM. Its duration of dissociation is 15 min for IV and 15–30 min for IM administration.

The effective dissociative dose of ketamine varies, but it is generally given in adults as an initial 0.25–0.5 mg/kg dose over 30–60 s with repeated dosing at 0.5–1 mg/kg if not fully dissociated or for prolonged procedures. In children, the initial dose is usually 0.5–1 mg/kg and repeated dosing remains the same as for adults. If given IM, the dose should be 4–5 mg/kg. IV dosing is preferred over IM given a higher risk of vomiting and longer time to recovery when the IM route is used [8]. At lower doses, ketamine will provide for analgesia but not dissociation. Ketamine exhibits a dosing threshold; after dissociation has occurred, further doses of ketamine may prolong the effects but do not deepen the level of sedation achieved [13].

Ketamine has benefits due to its properties of analgesia in addition to dissociation and amnesia. Patients maintain their airway reflexes and continue breathing spontaneously during sedation. It has been used safely around the world to facilitate everything from minor procedures to major surgery [15]. It has been shown to be safe for use when either the IV or IM routes are utilized [4]. Heart rate and blood pressure typically increase slightly with ketamine administration. When ketamine is given as a rapid IV push it can cause a transient respiratory depression or apnea, thus it should be given over 30–60 s. Laryngospasm is the most feared complication, but is seen mostly in pediatric patients, is rare (0.3 % in children) [7], and is most frequently transient. Laryngospasm should be treated with gentle positive pressure ventilation and oxygen, and almost always responds to these simple measures. If laryngospasm is persistent and unresponsive to the above, a paralytic should be given and endotracheal intubation performed. Clonus or rash may occur and are self-limited. Increased salivation is possible and may be treated with glycopyrrolate or atropine though these agents are no longer recommended for premedication [7]. There is a potential for increased intracranial pressure with ketamine, most notably if obstructive hydrocephalus is present. In cases of intracranial pathology or head trauma without obstructive hydrocephalus these increases are typically mild and newer studies have shown that ketamine may actually improve cerebral perfusion pressures [9]. There is some evidence that ketamine may increase intraocular pressure [7]. Emesis is possible though usually occurs in the late recovery phase when the patient is able to clear their own secretions. Emergence reactions with an agitated recovery may occur and are more frequent in adults with psychiatric comorbidities (especially schizophrenia) although are typically mild and of minimal clinical importance. Emergence reactions can be treated with a benzodiazepine. One study in adults showed that recovery agitation could be decreased by 17 % via pretreatment with midazolam (0.03 mg/kg IV), but while this approach could be adopted it is not considered mandatory [10].

Ketamine should not be used in patients younger than 3 months due to a potential increased risk of laryngospasm. It should not be used in those with hypertensive urgency or emergency due to effects on blood pressure. It should not be used in those with preexisting schizophrenia and should be used with caution in other psychotic diseases as it can exacerbate psychosis. It should not be used in those with obstructive hydrocephalus due to potential intracranial pressure changes. It should be used with caution in children with upper airway infections due to higher risk of laryngospasm, though this potential increased risk has not been seen in adults. It should be used with caution in those with known coronary artery disease due to its sympathomimetic effects [7].

Ketamine/Propofol (Ketofol)

A mixture of ketamine and propofol ("ketofol") is a relatively new addition to the procedural sedation armamentarium with the thought that the mixture of drugs may balance adverse effects of one with the beneficial effects of the other (e.g., respiratory depression, hypotension, and lack of analgesia seen with propofol are potentially mitigated by hemodynamic stability, lack of respiratory depression, and potent analgesic effects of ketamine; potential nausea/vomiting and recovery agitation of ketamine may be balanced by antiemetic and anxiolytic properties of propofol) [12]. Ketofol has been utilized in varying doses, but the most common combination in studies has been 1:1 dosing of ketamine to propofol, which is then usually given as a 1 mg/kg initial dose of ketofol (e.g., 0.5 mg/kg of ketamine and 0.5 mg/kg of propofol) followed by subsequent 0.5 mg/kg ketofol doses if needed. Different institutions may call for mixing of both drugs in the same syringe or separately giving 0.5 mg/kg aliquots of each medication. Mixing the drugs in the same syringe is not ideal. At one point one of the formulations of ketamine precipitated in the propofol. Also it is best to titrate single drugs so as not to inadvertently overdose a patient with mixtures of two medications [16].

Several studies have shown ketofol to be effective for procedural sedation in both adults and children. Despite giving lower doses of each medication and the use of generally sub-dissociative doses of ketamine, procedural amnesia, reported pain, recall, and patient satisfaction were similar in a trial that examined the use of propofol versus ketofol in varying ratios [12]. Some controversy remains as to its use due to several studies which have not shown a significant benefit over propofol use alone. There is some evidence that ketofol may provide a more consistent depth of sedation than propofol alone [16].

Ketofol has been safely used in both adults and children. Many studies have not shown significant differences in side effects between ketofol compared to propofol use alone. A recent meta-analysis did show decreased rates of respiratory depression (29 vs. 35.4 %) [16]. Contraindications are the same as for propofol and ketamine as listed above.

Fentanyl/Midazolam

Midazolam is a benzodiazepine sedative/anxiolytic with potent amnestic properties. Its effects are mediated by an increase of gamma-aminobutyric (GABA) receptors in the central nervous system [17]. As benzodiazepines lack any analgesic component, midazolam is usually given in combination with an opioid such as fentanyl to provide for pain control. Midazolam has a time of onset of 2–3 min when given IV and duration of action of 45–60 min. Fentanyl has a time of onset of 1–3 min and duration of action of 30–60 min. Midazolam is given in doses of 0.05–0.1 mg (to typical maximum of 5 mg) and fentanyl is given as 0.5 µg/kg/dose.

Midazolam/fentanyl generally provides adequate moderate sedation for procedures. Midazolam has significant amnestic properties as well. Compared to propofol, outpatient studies of sedation for endoscopy showed that midazolam/fentanyl had a longer time to onset, lesser sedation, longer time to recovery, and longer time to discharge [17, 18].

The main side effect of fentanyl/midazolam is respiratory depression, especially when benzodiazepines and opioids are used in combination. Several studies have found the rate of respiratory depression to be increased with the combination of midazolam/fentanyl compared to ketamine or midazolam alone [19]. Midazolam can be reversed with flumazenil, and fentanyl can be reversed with naloxone if needed. A very rare side effect of fentanyl may be chest wall rigidity which is generally seen at higher doses then those used for procedural sedation (e.g., 5 μg/kg/dose) and generally responds to positive pressure or naloxone. Midazolam/fentanyl should not be used in those with hemodynamic instability or preexisting respiratory depression.

Fasting Guidelines

Emesis with resultant aspiration is a rare risk with procedural sedation, thus anesthesia guidelines have historically suggested minimum fasting times prior to performing procedural sedation. These guidelines are based on data in an operating theater environment with general anesthesia [13]. Concerns have been raised about whether this data is applicable to urgent procedures done in the emergency department environment with procedural sedation being used, not general anesthesia. Several ED studies and review of the literature have now demonstrated no correlation between fasting time and incidence of emesis during procedural sedation [20–22]. Based on this data, the American College of Emergency Physicians' Clinical Policy on Procedural Sedation now recommends no delay in sedation based on fasting time. Also, of note, procedures performed in the ED are emergent by definition (and not elective) and thus unnecessary delays can be detrimental.

References

1. Sakles JC, et al. Comparison of the C-MAC video laryngoscope to the macintosh direct laryngoscope for intubation in the emergency department. Ann Emerg Med. 2012;60(6):739–48.
2. Ellis D, et al. Cricoid pressure in the emergency department rapid sequence tracheal intubations: a risk benefit. Ann Emerg Med. 2007;50(6):653–65.
3. American Society of Anesthesiology. Standards for basic anesthetic monitoring. Approved 21 Oct 1986 and last amended 20 Oct 2010.
4. American College of Emergency Physicians. Clinical policy: procedural sedation and analgesia in the emergency department. Ann Emerg Med. 2014;63:247–58.
5. Deitch K, Miner J, Chudnofsky CR, Dominici P, Latta D. Does end tidal CO_2 monitoring during emergency department procedural sedation and analgesia with propofol decrease the incidence of hypoxic events? a randomized, controlled trial. Ann Emerg Med. 2010;55(3): 258–64.
6. Deitch K, Chudnofsky CR, Dominici P. The utility of supplemental oxygen during emergency department procedural sedation and analgesia with propofol: a randomized, controlled trial. Ann Emerg Med. 2008;52:1–8.
7. Deitch K, Chudnofsky CR, Dominici P, Latta D, Salamanca Y. The utility of high-flow oxygen during emergency department procedural sedation and analgesia with propofol: a randomized controlled trial. Ann Emerg Med. 2011;58:360–4.
8. Sacchetti A, Senula G, Strickland J, et al. Procedural sedation in the community emergency department: initial results of the ProSCED registry. Acad Emerg Med. 2007;14:41–6.

9. Hogan K, Sacchetti A, Aman L, et al. The safety of single-physician procedural sedation in the emergency department. Emerg Med J. 2006;23:922–3.

10. Rosens. Emergency medicine, concepts and clinical practice.

11. http://www.uptodate.com/contents/sedative-analgesic-medications-in-critically-ill-adults-properties-dosage-regimens-and-adverse-effects.

12. Vinson D, Bradbury D. Etomidate for procedural sedation in emergency medicine. Ann Emerg Med. 2002;39:592–8.

13. Hayden RF. Procedural sedation and analgesia (conscious sedation). In: Reichman EF, Simon RR, editors. Emergency medicine procedures. New York: McGraw-Hill Medical Pub. Division; 2004. 1001–016. Print

14. Cohen L, Athaide V, Wickham ME, Doyle-Waters MM, Rose NGW, Hohl CM. The effect of ketamine on intracranial and cerebral perfusion pressure and health outcomes: a systematic review. Ann Emerg Med. 2015;65:43–51.

15. Green SM, Roback MG, Krauss B, et al. Predictors of emesis and recovery agitation with emergency department ketamine sedation: an individual-patient data meta-analysis of 8,282 children. Ann Emerg Med. 2009;54:171–80.

16. Dursteler BB, Wightman JM. Etomidate-facilitated hip reduction in the emergency department. Am J Emerg Med. 2000;18:204–8.

17. Black E, Campbell SG, Magee K, Zed P. Propofol for procedural sedation in the emergency department: a qualitative systematic review. Ann Pharmacother. 2011;47:856–68.

18. McGrane O, Hopkins G, Nielson A, Kang C. Procedural sedation with propofol: a retrospective review of the experiences of an emergency medicine residency program 2005–2010. Am J Emerg Med. 2011;30:706–11.

19. Miner JR, Gray RO, Stephens D, Biros MH. Randomized clinical trial of propofol with and without alfentanil for deep procedural sedation in the emergency department. Acad Emerg Med. 2009;16:825–34.

20. Godwin SA, Gerardo CJ, Hatten BW, Mace SE, Silvers SM, Fesmire FM. Clinical policy: procedural sedation and analgesia in the emergency department. Ann Emerg Med. 2014;63(2):247–58.

21. Borgeat A, Wilder-Smith OH, Saiah M, Rifat K. Subhypnotic doses of propofol possess direct antiemetic properties. Anesth Analg. 1992;74:539–41.

22. Green SM, Roback MG, Kennedy RM, Krauss B. Clinical practice guideline for emergency department ketamine dissociative sedation: 2011 update. Ann Emerg Med. 2011;57(5):449–61.

Further Reading

Andolfatto G, Abu-Laban RB, Zed PJ, Staniforth SM, Stackhouse S, Moadebi S. Ketamine-propofol combination (ketofol) versus propofol alone for emergency department procedural sedation and analgesia: a randomized double-blind trial. Ann Emerg Med. 2012;59:504–12.

Green SM, Roback MG, Miner JR, et al. Fasting and emergency department procedural sedation and analgesia: a consensus-based clinical practice advisory. Ann Emerg Med. 2007;49:454–61.

Havel CJ, Strait RT, Hennes H. A clinical trial of propofol vs. midazolam for procedural sedation in a pediatric emergency department. Acad Emerg Med. 1999;6(10):989–97.

Kurdi MS, Threeth KA, Deva RS. Ketamine: current applications in anesthesia, pain, and critical care. Anesth Essays Res. 2014;8(3):283–90.

Miner JR, Biros M, Krieg S, Johnson C, Heegaard W, Plummer D. Randomized clinical trial of propofol versus methohexital for procedural sedation during fracture and dislocation reduction in the emergency department. Acad Emerg Med. 2003;10:931–7.

Miner JR, Moore JC, Austad EJ, Plummer D, Hubbard L, Gray RO. Randomized, double-blinded clinical trial of propofol, 1:1 propofol/ketamine, and 4:1 propofol/ketamine for deep procedural sedation in the emergency department. Ann Emerg Med. 2015;65(5):479–88.

Molina JA, Lobo CA, Goh HK, et al. Review of studies and guidelines on fasting and procedural sedation at the emergency department. Int J Evid Based Healthc. 2010;8:75–8.

Roback MG, Walthen JE, Bajaj L, Bothner JP. Adverse events associated with procedural sedation and analgesia in a pediatric emergency department: a comparison of common parenteral drugs. Acad Emerg Med. 2005;12(6):508–13.

Sener S, Eken C, Schultz CH, et al. Ketamine with and without midazolam for emergency department sedation in adults: a randomized controlled trial. Ann Emerg Med. 2011;57:109–14.

Thorpe RJ, Benger J. Pre-procedural fasting in emergency sedation. Emerg Med J. 2010; 27:254–61.

Ulmer BJ, Hansen JJ, Overley CA, et al. Propofol versus midazolam/fentanyl for outpatient colonoscopy: administration by nurses supervised by endoscopists. Clin Gastroenterol Hepatol. 2003;1(6):425–32.

Yan JW, McLeod SL, Iansavitchene A. Ketamine-propofol versus propofol alone for procedural sedation in the emergency department: a systematic review and meta-analysis. Acad Emerg Med. 2015;22:1003–13.

Chapter 23
Cosmetic Procedures and Office Based Sedation

Basavana Goudra and Shubhangi Arora

Abstract Ageing population, stable economy and income, wider availability of cosmetic surgeons, improving safety are likely to increase the numbers of office based cosmetic surgery in the intermediate to long term.

Remote location, non-availability of sufficiently skilled manpower, increasing morbidity of the presenting patient population will add to the challenges.

Airway complications, sedation titration, effective resuscitation and total intravenous anesthesia will continue to stay relevant.

Availability of newer less toxic local anesthetics, video laryngoscopes, soft sedatives with better pharmacokinetic profile are likely decrease the sedation related adverse events during cosmetic office based surgeries

Training and regulation are some of the areas that should continue to receive attention, both from the safety stand point and reduction of litigation risks.

Keywords Office based cosmetic surgery • Local anesthetic toxicity • Liposuction • Airway management • Resuscitation

Introduction

The growth of office based cosmetic procedures is in line with similar growth in out of operating room anesthesia. The added patient safety and increasing procedural complexity have increased the use of monitored anesthesia care, regional anesthesia and general anesthesia in this field. As some of the issues are unique, it is deemed that a separate chapter is necessary to discuss the specific concerns.

B. Goudra, MD, FRCA, FCARCSI (✉)
Department of Anesthesiology and Critical Care Medicine, Hospital of the University of Pennsylvania, 3400 Spruce Street, 5042 Silverstein Building, Philadelphia, PA 19104, USA
e-mail: goudrab@uphs.upenn.edu

S. Arora, MBBS, MD
Department of Anesthesia, Brigham and Women's Hospital,
75, Francis Street, Boston, MA 02115, USA
e-mail: shubhangikkr@gmail.com

© Springer International Publishing Switzerland 2017
B.G. Goudra, P.M. Singh (eds.), *Out of Operating Room Anesthesia*,
DOI 10.1007/978-3-319-39150-2_23

History and Physical Findings

Patients presenting for cosmetic surgery in an office based setting are likely to be elderly. It is generally presumed that these procedures are of low risk As a result, the patients might not have undergone the same structured preoperative evaluation and optimization as those presenting for a major surgery. It should be borne in mind that here might be "minor surgeries" but there is no such thing as "minor anesthetic".

Elderly patients are one of the growing groups of patients presenting for office based cosmetic procedures including facelift. Typically, they present on the morning of the procedure and as a result, less time is available for a comprehensive evaluation.

The prevalence of atrial fibrillation increases with age and is more prevalent in men than in women. The estimated prevalence in the general population is 1–2 % [1, 2]. The prevalence increases from 1 % in individuals aged >60 years to 7.2 % in individuals aged >65 years and 10 % in individuals aged >75 years [3]. The estimated number of individuals with AF globally in 2010 was 33.5 million (20.9 million males and 12.6 million) [4]. Patients may not report paroxysmal atrial fibrillation unless specifically sought. Anticoagulation, antiarrhythmic medications, and rate control are the cornerstone of contemporary management. Atrial fibrillation is recognized as a major risk factor for cognitive decline [5]. A ventricular rate of over 100 or a significant pulse deficit (difference between the pulse rate and he EKG derived heart rate) are traditionally regarded as markers of poor heart rate control.

Along with atrial fibrillation, patients with uncontrolled hypertension and diabetes present frequently for office based cosmetic procedures. The Society of ambulatory anesthesia has published guidelines for perioperative blood glucose management in diabetic patients undergoing ambulatory surgery [6]. However, it fails to provide any specific levels of either blood glucose or hemoglobin A1c. As a result, the anesthesiologist should use their discretion.

Considering that local anesthesia is used generously and the presence of heart disease increases the risk of cardiac toxicity of local anesthetics, extra vigilance is taken in the preoperative evaluation. A history of congestive heart failure is frequent and assessment based on effort intolerance is insufficient and unreliable. A review of the previous investigations is mandatory and failure might be a ground for litigation in the event of a major adverse outcome.

Pharmacokinetic/pharmacodynamic (Pk/Pd) variability is significant with all central nervous system depressants in the elderly [7, 8]. In general, the Pk/Pd variability of propofol is 300–400 % [9, 10]. Additionally, elderly are very sensitive to the effects of sedatives. Associated cardiovascular or (and) respiratory diseases might have additional impact on both the distribution and the clinical effects of sedative/hypnotics.

Many patients with chronic obstructive disease may present for office based procedures. The degree of the disease will affect the choice of anesthesia. Modern anesthetics-local, regional and Pk/Pd friendly general anesthesia have allowed more flexibility in terms of patient selection. Yet, symptomatic patients and patient using oxygen at home are best referred to a hospital based practice.

Patients who were morbidly obese present for frequent office based cosmetic procedures. Studies assessing the prevalence of post-operative gastro-esophageal reflux disease (GERD) show that sleeve gastrectomy may provoke de novo new reflux symptoms or might worsen pre-existing GERD [11]. Worsening or newly developed reflux symptoms and esophagitis are found in a subset of patients during longer follow-up after gastric banding [12]. Risk of aspiration needs to be taken into consideration. An appropriate discussion of the risks of aspiration with both the surgeon and the patient along with justification for the choice of anesthesia should be documented.

Fasting guidelines are published by various national and regional societies [13–15]. Inadvertent gum chewing poses frequent difficulties [16]. Although prospective randomized controlled studies have demonstrated absence of any additional risk, these findings are not incorporated in American Society of Anesthesiology (ASA) guidelines

The patient with a current or former history of substance use might pose challenges in an office setting [17]. Importance of the assessment of the effects of the substance abuse, associated diseases, end-organ damage is obvious. Even patients on prescription sedatives/narcotics are a separate group when it comes to pre-procedure evaluation. The implications might be increased intraoperative anesthetic requirements, unpredictable postoperative recovery and choice of postoperative pain relief.

Procedures

The following table lists the common cosmetic procedures performed in an office based setting. It is clear that anesthesia provider's involvement is minimal in many of these however, the requirements approach those of major surgery in others (Table 23.1).

Table 23.1 List of common cosmetic procedures performed in an office based setting

Surgery for the face	Rest of the body
Botox injections	Wrinkle treatment
Cheek lift	Abdomen reduction (Tummy tuck)
Chemical peel	Arm lift
Chin surgery	Body liposuction
Dermabrasion	Breast augmentation
Eyebrow/forehead rejuvenation (Brow lift)	Breast lift
Eyelid surgery (Blepharoplasty)	Breast reduction
Face-lift	Buttock lift (Belt lipectomy)
Facial contouring	Circumferential body lift
Facial fillers	Inner thigh lift
Laser hair removal	Laser hair removal
Laser resurfacing	
Neck lift and neck liposuction	
Otoplasty (Alterations of the ears)	
Rhinoplasty (Alterations of the nose)	
Skin problems (Blemishes, spider veins, scar revisions, tattoo removal)	

Choice of Anesthesia Technique and Anticipated Adverse Events

Monitored Anesthesia Care

The majority of the aforementioned procedures can be performed with monitored anesthesia care (MAC). Although the ASA recently revised the definitions of sedation and anesthesia, the term monitored anesthesia care continues to be used [18]. Of note, the ASA statement mandates exhaled end-tidal carbon dioxide (E_tCO_2) monitoring during both moderate and deep sedation with effect from July 2011. Even though it is of questionable utility in some situations, failure to adhere is a problem in case of litigation [19, 20]. It has been recently demonstrated that majority of patients thought to be receiving moderate sedation are frequently under general anesthesia and even deep general anesthesia [21]. Sedation related adverse events are in fact more frequent in patients receiving MAC [22, 23]. The majority of the adverse events are airway related. The importance of appropriate preparation in terms of drugs and equipment cannot be overstated [24].

The use of airway adjuncts like nasal airway is described in the chapter on airway management for gastrointestinal endoscopic procedures. Some of these techniques reduce the incidence of hypoxemia and its associated complications. In fact, such a management is demonstrated to improve the safety and increase the efficiency in many endoscopic procedures [25, 26] including obese patients.

The choice of drugs and their administration are no different than in any other care setting. Pk/Pd variability is a major concern. Propofol is best administered as a regulated bolus (titrated to the effect) followed by an infusion. Although addition of opioid decreases the propofol requirement, the practice also increases the Pk/Pd variability.

Patients with a history of sleep apnea pose additional challenges. If the airway is not accessible (for example surgeries involving face), these patients are best intubated, even for short procedures. Disturbance of the surgical field (with face surgery) and rapid desaturation in the event of apnea can be eliminated by a secure airway. Intubation difficulties present in this subset of patients create additional problems in an emergency and are best avoided. A STOP-BANG questionnaire might be suitable as a screening tool, both in self-reported and observer evaluated model [27].

Morbidly obese patients have slightly different pharmacokinetics and dosing of both propofol and opioids should take this into consideration [28–30]. However, no system can predict the behavior of these drugs with accuracy. As a result, factors such as the patient's clinical condition, comorbidity, and the response of various physiological variables to anesthetic drugs should dictate the dosing of intravenous anesthetic agents, rather than any calculated or actual body weight.

Newer sedatives like dexmedetomidine can be employed for some of the office based cosmetic procedures. Absence of significant respiratory depression is a major advantage. Similarly, ketamine is a good choice in selected patients and has additional benefits in decreasing the incidence of respiratory depression. It is popular as "ketofol," a mixture of ketamine and propofol for an infusion. However, such a mixture is not Food and Drug Administration (FDA) approved. Moreover, the stability of the mixture and its effect on the pharmacokinetics is unknown.

Remimazolam is likely to overcome many of the drawbacks of both propofol and midazolam. It combines the properties of two unique and established drugs in anesthesia, namely midazolam and remiefentanil. It produces hypnosis by binding to GABA receptors (like midazolam) and has organ-independent metabolism (like remifentanil). It is likely to be the sedative/hypnotic of the future, as evidence by the published studies [31, 32]. It has potential to be used as a sedative for procedural sedation. Unlike many rapidly acting intravenous sedatives presently available, the propensity to cause apnea is very low. Availability of a specific antagonist (flumazenil) is a major safety benefit [33].

Tumescent Anesthesia

Tumescent anesthesia is the practice of injecting a very dilute solution of local anesthetic reconstituted with epinephrine and sodium bicarbonate into a tissue, until it becomes firm and tense (tumescent) [34]. Although the practice started with liposuction, it is presently used across vascular surgery, breast surgery, plastic surgery and ENT procedures. Even though it can be used as a sole anesthetic technique, it is used with MAC in the office based setting. Addition of epinephrine reduces the blood loss and addition of bicarbonate reduces pain associated with local anesthetic injection. Tumescent lidocaine is absorbed very slowly from subcutaneous tissues, thereby producing lower, and more delayed, peak blood levels compared to other routes, along with prolonged postoperative analgesia.

Doses of up to 40 mg/Kg have been injected safety along with MAC [35], although the recommended safe dose is 35 mg/Kg. In this study involving ten patients, lidocaine was injected in two segments after an interval of time. Eight hundred-milligram lidocaine (40 mL 2% lidocaine), 125 mL 5% sodium bicarbonate, and 5 mL 1:1000 epinephrine were added into each bag of 3-L normal saline solution as 1 set of tumescent anesthesia solution. For infiltration volumes greater than 3 sets (9510 mL), the additional infiltration solution was made without sodium bicarbonate (8 mL 2% lidocaine and 1 mL 1:1000 epinephrine in each bottle of 500 mL saline solution). The infusion rate was set at a speed around 160 mL/min. Patients also received MAC with propofol and remifentanil. Serum levels of lidocaine were measured every 4 h during the first 24 h after the second infiltration. The peak lidocaine levels [2.18 (0.63)μg/mL] occurred after 12–20 h [16.4 (2.27) h]. Moreover, there was no significant correlation between dose per kilogram body weight or total dose of lidocaine infiltrated and its peak levels or time.

Although this study demonstrates the safety of tumescent anesthesia, there are always factors like hepatic dysfunction, low cardiac output states, high cardiac output states, reduced plasma proteins and concomitant use of beta-blockers and calcium antagonists that can increase the risk of toxicity [36].

General Anesthesia

The issues with general anesthesia are no different than those encountered during many similar procedures performed in a hospital based setting. The need for early and uncomplicated discharge necessitates more reliance on total intravenous anesthesia. Use of short acting opioids with fixed context sensitive half-life like remifentanil can archive many of the objectives of an office based service. However, preparedness for any unanticipated adverse events including laryngospasm, malignant hyperthermia and failed intubation is essential. Use of video laryngoscopes for intubation and intravenous infusion pumps to deliver anesthesia is common and does not need any further discussion.

Regional Anesthesia

In relation to cosmetic surgery, few procedures are amenable for sole regional anesthesia. The regional blockade is typically used in conjunction with other methods [37]. For example, as a supplement to field block and MAC in an abdominoplasty, bilateral posterior intercostal nerve block is used safely. It requires injecting from T-5 or T-6 through T-12, using 3 mL/block of a local anesthetic mixture of lidocaine 0.5 %/bupivacaine 0.125 %/with epinephrine 1:200,000 [38]. However, most anesthesia providers will be averse to the idea of a bilateral intercostal nerve block for the fear of bilateral pneumothorax. Moreover, the safety and efficacy of such a technique has not been demonstrated in a scientific study.

Most of the nerve blocks are performed by the surgeons for facial and rhinological procedures. With the increase in ultrasound regional anesthesia has made a resurgence.

Specific Procedure Related Complications

Liposuction

Hypoxia during or after surgeries involving liposuction can be caused by fat embolism [39–41]. Fat embolism is primarily a mechanical blockage of the vascular lumen by circulating fat globules. It typically presents with symptoms referable to the respiratory system. However, fat globules can also block the circulation to the central nervous system, retina, and skin. With regards to its occurrence during liposuction, most of the reported evidence is in the form of case reports. As it is an uncommon complication, a certain degree of suspicion is necessary. The clinical signs and symptoms can manifest even 2–3 days after the procedure. The obvious other diagnoses that need to be considered are pulmonary infection, pulmonary embolism and aspiration of gastric contents.

The classic fat embolism syndrome is defined by the presence of two of three clinical findings including petechial rash, pulmonary distress, and mental disturbances within the first 48 h after the inciting event. Common signs include hypoxia, fever, tachycardia, and tachypnea with bilateral radiographic changes and urinary changes. The presentation is very similar to acute respiratory distress syndrome and the condition carries a high mortality of approximately 10–15% [42, 43]. The treatment is largely supportive.

Facial Cosmetic Surgery

As briefly discussed above, surgeries involving the face carry a higher risk of hypoxemia [44]. The challenges are related to the anesthetic requirements- a quiet and clear surgical field, absence of patient movement, no stimulation during emergence from anesthesia, a rapid return of consciousness and protective airway reflexes, prevention of postoperative nausea and vomiting, and fast-tracking for discharge. Frequently, the surgeons do not understand the airway issues that can arise when attempts are made to meet these intraoperative expectations. It is not uncommon for some surgeons to promise MAC to the patients (who are convinced that MAC is less dangerous than general anesthesia) and make request for what is essentially "a general anesthesia with an unprotected airway". An honest explanation is normally sufficient to overcome the hurdle. The implications of hypopnea or apnea and the associated oxygen desaturation are different in facial cosmetic surgery. Delayed recovery and discharge are the main reasons for both patients and surgeons to request MAC. Use of total intravenous anesthesia with short acting opioids like remifentanil and propofol can achieve the goals of the surgeon and the patient and make it safer.

Conclusions

We have discussed issues considered relevant in the practice of office based anesthesia for cosmetic procedures. Matters like post-operative nausea, vomiting, pain, admission and discharge criteria are deliberately left out, as they are considered basic to the practice of any anesthesia. The future is likely to be dictated by migration of surgeries from hospital based to office based practice. Developments in the field of total intravenous anesthesia and soft pharmacology might have significant influence in the years to come.

References

1. Miyasaka Y, Barnes ME, Gersh BJ, Cha SS, Bailey KR, Abhayaratna WP, et al. Secular trends in incidence of atrial fibrillation in Olmsted County, Minnesota, 1980 to 2000, and implications on the projections for future prevalence. Circulation. 2006;114(2):119–25.

2. Camm AJ, Lip GYH, De Caterina R, Savelieva I, Atar D, Hohnloser SH, et al. 2012 focused update of the ESC Guidelines for the management of atrial fibrillation: an update of the 2010 ESC Guidelines for the management of atrial fibrillation – developed with the special contribution of the European Heart Rhythm Association. Eur Pacing Arrhythm Card Electrophysiol J Work Groups Card Pacing Arrhythm Card Cell Electrophysiol Eur Soc Cardiol. 2012;14(10):1385–413.

3. Liao H-R, Poon K-S, Chen K-B. Atrial fibrillation: an anesthesiologist's perspective. Acta Anaesthesiol Taiwan. 2013;51(1):34–6.

4. Chugh SS, Havmoeller R, Narayanan K, Singh D, Rienstra M, Benjamin EJ, et al. Worldwide epidemiology of atrial fibrillation: a Global Burden of Disease 2010 Study. Circulation. 2014;129(8):837–47.

5. Hui DS, Morley JE, Mikolajczak PC, Lee R. Atrial fibrillation: a major risk factor for cognitive decline. Am Heart J. 2015;169(4):448–56.

6. Joshi GP, Chung F, Vann MA, Ahmad S, Gan TJ, Goulson DT, et al. Society for ambulatory anesthesia consensus statement on perioperative blood glucose management in diabetic patients undergoing ambulatory surgery. Anesth Analg. 2010;111(6):1378–87.

7. Albrecht S, Ihmsen H, Hering W, Geisslinger G, Dingemanse J, Schwilden H, et al. The effect of age on the pharmacokinetics and pharmacodynamics of midazolam. Clin Pharmacol Ther. 1999;65(6):630–9.

8. Platten HP, Schweizer E, Dilger K, Mikus G, Klotz U. Pharmacokinetics and the pharmacodynamic action of midazolam in young and elderly patients undergoing tooth extraction. Clin Pharmacol Ther. 1998;63(5):552–60.

9. Vuyk J. Pharmacokinetic and pharmacodynamic interactions between opioids and propofol. J Clin Anesth. 1997;9(6 Suppl):23S–6.

10. Vuyk J. TCI: supplementation and drug interactions. Anaesthesia. 1998;53 Suppl 1:35–41.

11. Hayat JO, Wan A. The effects of sleeve gastectomy on gastro-esophageal reflux and gastro-esophageal motility. Expert Rev Gastroenterol Hepatol. 2014;8(4):445–52.

12. de Jong JR, Besselink MGH, van Ramshorst B, Gooszen HG, Smout AJPM. Effects of adjustable gastric banding on gastroesophageal reflux and esophageal motility: a systematic review. Obes Rev Off J Int Assoc Study Obes. 2010;11(4):297–305.

13. Lambert E, Carey S. Practice guideline recommendations on perioperative fasting: a systematic review. JPEN J Parenter Enteral Nutr. 2015. pii: 0148607114567713. [Epub ahead of print].

14. American Society of Anesthesiologists Committee. Practice guidelines for preoperative fasting and the use of pharmacologic agents to reduce the risk of pulmonary aspiration: application to healthy patients undergoing elective procedures: an updated report by the American Society of Anesthesiologists Committee on Standards and Practice Parameters. Anesthesiology. 2011;114(3):495–511.

15. Smith I, Kranke P, Murat I, Smith A, O'Sullivan G, Søreide E, et al. Perioperative fasting in adults and children: guidelines from the European Society of Anaesthesiology. Eur J Anaesthesiol. 2011;28(8):556–69.

16. Goudra BG, Singh PM, Carlin A, Manjunath AK, Reihmer J, Gouda GB, et al. Effect of gum chewing on the volume and pH of gastric contents: a prospective randomized study. Dig Dis Sci. 2014;60:979–83.

17. Pulley DD. Preoperative evaluation of the patient with substance use disorder and perioperative considerations. Anesthesiol Clin. 2016;34(1):201–11.

18. Continuum of Depth of Sedation: Definition of General Anesthesia and Levels of Sedation/Analgesia* Committee of origin: quality management and departmental administration (Approved by the ASA House of Delegates on October 13, 1999, and last amended on October 15, 2014).

19. Goudra BG. Comparison of acoustic respiration rate, impedance pneumography and capnometry monitors for respiration rate accuracy and apnea detection during GI endoscopy anesthesia. Open J Anesthesiol. 2013;03(02):74–9.

20. Weaver J. The latest ASA mandate: CO2 monitoring for moderate and deep sedation. Anesth Prog. 2011;58(3):111–2.

21. Goudra B, Singh PM, Gouda G, Borle A, Carlin A, Yadwad A. Propofol and non-propofol based sedation for outpatient colonoscopy-prospective comparison of depth of sedation using an EEG based SEDLine monitor. J Clin Monit Comput. 2015. [Epub ahead of print]. PMID: 26364193.

22. Goudra B, Nuzat A, Singh PM, Borle A, Carlin A, Gouda G. Association between type of sedation and the adverse events associated with gastrointestinal endoscopy: an analysis of 5 years' data from a tertiary center in the USA. Clin Endosc. 2016. doi:10.5946/ce.2016.019.

23. Goudra B, Nuzat A, Singh PM, Gouda GB, Carlin A, Manjunath AK. Cardiac arrests in patients undergoing gastrointestinal endoscopy: a retrospective analysis of 73,029 procedures. Saudi J Gastroenterol Off J Saudi Gastroenterol Assoc. 2015. doi:10.4103/1319-3767.164202.

24. Goudra B, Alvarez A, Singh PM. Practical considerations in the development of a non-operating room anesthesia practice.Curr Opin Anaesthesiol. 2016;29(4):526–30.

25. Goudra BG, Singh PM, Sinha AC. Anesthesia for ERCP: impact of anesthesiologist's experience on outcome and cost. Anesthesiol Res Pract. 2013;2013:570518.

26. Goudra B, Singh P, Sinha A. Outpatient endoscopic retrograde cholangiopancreatography: safety and efficacy of anesthetic management with a natural airway in 653 consecutive procedures. Saudi J Anaesth. 2013;7(3):259.

27. Boynton G, Vahabzadeh A, Hammoud S, Ruzicka DL, Chervin RD. Validation of the STOP-BANG questionnaire among patients referred for suspected obstructive sleep apnea. J Sleep Disord Treat Care [Internet]. 23 Sept 2013 [Cited 25 Mar 2016];2(4). Available from: http://www.ncbi.nlm.nih.gov/pmc/articles/PMC4008971/.

28. Goudra BG, Ortego A, Selassie M, Sinha AC. Lessons from providing total intravenous anesthesia (TIVA) to a morbidly obese patient (294 kg [648 lbs], body mass index 85.5 kg/m2). J Clin Anesth. 2013;25(5):428–9.

29. Ingrande J, Lemmens HJM. Dose adjustment of anaesthetics in the morbidly obese. Br J Anaesth. 2010;105 Suppl 1:i16–23.

30. Coetzee JF. Allometric or lean body mass scaling of propofol pharmacokinetics: towards simplifying parameter sets for target-controlled infusions. Clin Pharmacokinet. 2012;51(3):137–45.

31. Borkett KM, Riff DS, Schwartz HI, Winkle PJ, Pambianco DJ, Lees JP, et al. A Phase IIa, randomized, double-blind study of remimazolam (CNS 7056) versus midazolam for sedation in upper gastrointestinal endoscopy. Anesth Analg. 2015;120(4):771–80.

32. Pambianco DJ, Borkett KM, Riff DS, Winkle PJ, Schwartz HI, Melson TI, et al. A phase IIb study comparing the safety and efficacy of remimazolam and midazolam in patients undergoing colonoscopy. Gastrointest Endosc. 2016;83(5):984–92.

33. Goudra B, Singh P. Remimazolam: the future of its sedative potential. Saudi J Anaesth. 2014;8(3):388.

34. Conroy PH, O'Rourke J. Tumescent anaesthesia. Surg J R Coll Surg Edinb Irel. 2013;11(4):210–21.

35. Wang G, Cao W-G, Li S-L, Liu L-N, Jiang Z-H. Safe extensive tumescent liposuction with segmental infiltration of lower concentration lidocaine under monitored anesthesia care. Ann Plast Surg. 2015;74(1):6–11.

36. Dickerson DM, Apfelbaum JL. Local anesthetic systemic toxicity. Aesthet Surg J. 2014;34(7):1111–9.

37. Hausman LM, Dickstein EJ, Rosenblatt MA. Types of office-based anesthetics. Mt Sinai J Med NY. 2012;79(1):107–15.

38. Blake DR. Office-based anesthesia: dispelling common myths. Aesthetic Surg J Am Soc Aesthetic Plast Surg. 2008;28(5):564–70; discussion 571–2.

39. Cohen L, Engdahl R, Latrenta G. Hypoxia after abdominal and thigh liposuction: pulmonary embolism or fat embolism? Eplasty. 2014;14:ic19.

40. Wang H-D, Zheng J-H, Deng C-L, Liu Q-Y, Yang S-L. Fat embolism syndromes following liposuction. Aesthetic Plast Surg. 2008;32(5):731–6.

41. Costa AN, Mendes DM, Toufen C, Arrunátegui G, Caruso P, de Carvalho CRR. Adult respiratory distress syndrome due to fat embolism in the postoperative period following liposuction and fat grafting. J Bras Pneumol Publicação Soc Bras Pneumol E Tisilogia. 2008;34(8): 622–5.
42. Fulde GW, Harrison P. Fat embolism – a review. Arch Emerg Med. 1991;8(4):233–9.
43. Newbigin K, Souza CA, Torres C, Marchiori E, Gupta A, Inacio J, et al. Fat embolism syndrome: state-of-the-art review focused on pulmonary imaging findings. Respir Med. 2016;113:93–100.
44. Nekhendzy V, Ramaiah VK. Prevention of perioperative and anesthesia-related complications in facial cosmetic surgery. Facial Plast Surg Clin N Am. 2013;21(4):559–77.

Chapter 24
Anesthesia for Ophthalmologic Surgery

Julie Mani and Melissa Ann Brodsky

Abstract This chapter takes a look at the special challenges of conducting an anesthetic for ophthalmologic procedures. These cases carry the important responsibility of preserving patient vision and maintaining patient comfort and safety. It is no easy task performing these procedures under minimal sedation in a uniquely challenging patient population where extremes of age, multiple comorbidities, traumas, and communication deficits are rampant. The anesthesiologist has to continually balance the ability to control intraocular pressure, prevent arrhythmias, control gas bubble expansion and maintain adequate analgesia and akinesia. Various surgeries can be carried out by a variety of regional techniques with supplementation from topical, local or general anesthesia. It answers the difficult question of whether retrobulbar, peribulbar, or sub-Tenon's blocks individually carry any distinct advantages as well as examine their various side effects and complications. It will examine ocular anatomy, the physiology of anesthetic drugs, and sometimes-dangerous consequences of ocular medications these patients may be taking. It will prepare any provider for adequate vigilance during monitoring, detection of the oculocardiac reflex, and prompt treatment and resolution of such arrhythmias.

Keywords Intraocular pressure • Aqueous humor • Oculocardiac reflex • Open globe injury • Succinylcholine • Echothiophate • Retrobulbar block • Peribulbar block • Sub-Tenon's block • Strabismus repair • Cataract surgery

J. Mani, MD (✉)
Department of Anesthesiology and Perioperative Medicine, Drexel University College of Medicine, Hahnemann University Hospital, 245 North 15th Street Mail Stop 310, Philadelphia, PA 19102, USA
e-mail: Julie.m.mani@gmail.com

M.A. Brodsky, MD
Department of Anesthesiology and Perioperative Medicine, Drexel University College of Medicine, Hahnemann University Hospital, 245 North 15th Street Mail Stop 310, Philadelphia, PA 19102, USA
e-mail: melissa.brodsky@drexelmed.edu

© Springer International Publishing Switzerland 2017
B.G. Goudra, P.M. Singh (eds.), *Out of Operating Room Anesthesia*,
DOI 10.1007/978-3-319-39150-2_24

Introduction

There are unique challenges in ophthalmologic surgeries especially when accounting for the unique anxiety a patient experiences facing possible vision loss. These operations are often performed on the elderly and in children, where issues of dementia, delirium and preoperative agitation can present even greater challenges to navigating an anesthetic plan. In the case of trauma and open eye injuries, the issue of controlling intraocular pressure comes to the forefront. When procedures are performed instead on extraocular muscles, dangerous arrhythmias and prevention of the oculocardiac reflex becomes the primary concern. The many checks and balances of these procedures include control of intraocular pressure, prevention of gas bubble expansion, careful recognition of the oculocardiac reflex and other arrhythmias whilst achieving adequate akinesia and analgesia. Most often these competing requirements are done under minimal to moderate sedation, making these goals all the more challenging. The anesthesiologist should feel comfortable with regional, topical anesthesia, sedation, and general anesthesia techniques that can be used to facilitate these surgeries safely and do what is best for the patient.

Ocular Anatomy and Its Relevance

Understanding basics of ocular anatomy will help in understanding the surgical repairs, the various regional techniques that can be employed, as well as the physiological effects of certain ophthalmologic medications the patient may be taking and how it may alter the anesthetic plan and the patient's response to anesthesia.

- The human **orbit** is formed by a series of rigid bones that enclose the globe and related structures.
- The intraocular content produces a given intraocular pressure.
- The **subchoroidal space** is a potential space important in surgical bleeding or ocular trauma. It is a potential space between the sclera and uveal tract that can fill up with blood [1].
- The **ciliary body** is the component responsible for forming and draining the aqueous humor.
- The **retina** is a ten-layer membrane that converts light into neurosensory data for the brain.
- The **vitreous humor** covers the anterior retina. If the vitreous tugs on the retina, the result can range from retinal tearing to complete retinal detachment [1].
- There are a total of six **extraocular muscles** that move the eye: the superior and inferior oblique, the superior, medial, lateral, and inferior rectus muscles. Traction on these muscles can elicit the oculocardiac reflex that will be discussed later in this chapter.
- The **lacrimal duct** and drainage system is responsible for processing nasal drainage.

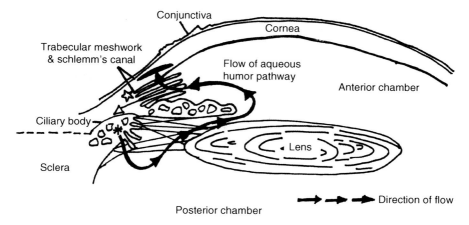

Fig. 24.1 Aqueous humor flow pathway. The aqueous humor is formed by the ciliary body. It then passes from the posterior into the anterior chamber and then eventually drains out of the trabecular meshwork into Schlemm's canal where it exits. Any blockage along this pathway, particularly in the trabecular pathway or canal, leads to accumulation of this highly osmotic fluid and increases IOP, which can lead to glaucoma

- The **aqueous humor** is formed in the posterior chamber by the ciliary body in a metabolic process that utilizes both enzymes carbonic anhydrase and cytochrome oxidase making it an ATP-requiring process [1]. Vessels on the iris surface form the remaining aqueous humor (See Fig. 24.1).
- The **conjunctiva** covers both the surface of the globe and eyelids. The surgeon can deploy various local anesthetics to these areas, and it is important for the anesthesiologist to tally those volumes along with any induction doses of lidocaine to prevent local anesthetic toxicity.
- *NOTE: when a local anesthetic such as lidocaine is applied topically to the conjunctiva, its absorption falls in between intravenous and subcutaneous administration [2].*
- **Blood supply** to the eye is primarily via the internal and external carotid arteries and the drainage is chiefly through the interwoven bridges between the superior and inferior ophthalmic veins which merge in one outflow tract from the central retinal vein [1].

The Physiology of Intraocular Pressure

What is the function of intraocular pressure? It maintains the spherical shape of the eye and that facilitates our vision. For most patients, small changes in intraocular pressure are of no major concern but for patients who have arteriosclerotic disease from diabetes, peripheral vascular disease, or other chronic conditions, small increases in IOP may be the nidus to retinal ischemia [2].

Normal intraocular pressure lies in the range of 10–22 mmHg, but if the contents inside the eye increase then so will intraocular pressure [3]. In fact, ocular hypertension is defined as any pressure reading higher than 21 mmHg [4]. The net difference between ciliary body production of aqueous humor and its elimination via Schlemm's canal, the ebb and flow of choroid volume, extraocular muscle contraction, and volume of vitreous humor create a constant change of IOP flux [5]. If there is bleeding within the eye or if there is an obstruction in the trabecular network that allows aqueous humor to accumulate in this space, there can be an increase in total content in the eye and intraocular pressure. Other changes associated with anesthesia can directly affect intraocular pressure including arterial blood pressure, ventilation [6], oxygenation, and medications [2]. At all times, it is best to prevent coughing and gagging that can dramatically increase eye pressure (See Table 24.1).

What cases most greatly threaten this balance? Patients with open globe traumas where the globe may need to be opened in surgery inevitably causing intraocular pressure to equilibrate with atmospheric pressure. These types of injuries may lead to vitreous humor extrusion or aqueous humor travelling through an open wound. In cases where the posterior segment may be involved, the result can be permanent blindness [2].

Table 24.1 Factors affecting intraocular pressure (IOP)

Causes of increased IOP	Causes of decreased IOP
Increased production of aqueous humor (or decreased drainage of aqueous humor)	Inhalational anesthetics
Medications (*e.g. steroid medications for asthma*)	Decreased production aqueous humor
Eye trauma	Increased flow/drainage aqueous humor
Glaucoma	
Factors that may be controllable under anesthesia	
Succinycholine	
Ketamine (+/−)	
Increased CVP	Low CVP
Increased arterial BP	Low arterial BP
Increased $PaCO_2$ (*hypoventilation*)	Decreased $PaCO_2$ (*hyperventilation*)
Decreased PaO_2 (*hypoxia*)	Adequate PaO_2

Preoperative Evaluation

Patients presenting for ophthalmologic surgery are often at the extremes of age and have a high incidence of concomitant systemic disease, so a careful preoperative exam and assessment is a must.

- Ophthalmologic surgery is considered low-risk, as there are no major physiologic changes and no significant blood losses or fluid shifts.
- A large multi-center trial showed that patients presenting for cataract surgery under local anesthetic with no acute medical conditions, no preoperative labs or EKGs are required [7].
- If local/Monitored anesthesia care (MAC) is to be used the patient must be evaluated for their ability to lie flat, have no symptomatic gastroesophageal reflux, have no neuropsychiatric disturbances, no tremor of the head and neck, no uncontrollable cough, and be able to follow commands [8]
- If general anesthesia (GA) is to be performed on patients with >4 METS, they require no further cardiac workup [9].
- Lab tests and EKG should be obtained if indicated by history [8].
- For cataract surgery, vitreoretinal surgery and oculoplastic surgery, patients may continue to take their aspirin, antiplatelet agents, and warfarin without increased risk for ocular hemorrhage [10, 11].
- Special attention should be paid to ophthalmologic medications patients may be taking preoperatively, because adverse side effects may be observed under anesthesia. Such medications can be found in Table 24.2

Table 24.2 Ophthalmologic medications and their effects under anesthesia

Medication	Mechanism of action	Adverse effects under anesthesia
Timolol	Antagonizes beta receptors on the ciliary body which decreases aqueous humor production	Bradycardia, heart failure, asthma attacks, arrhythmia
Acetazolamide	Inhibits carbonic anhydrase which reduces aqueous humor production	Diuresis, hypokalemic hyperchloremic metabolic acidosis
Echothiophate	Irreversibly binds to & inhibits plasma cholinesterase (12)	Prolongation of action of succinylcholine & mivacurium, pupil dilation, bronchospasm
Phenylephrine (drops)	Induces mydriasis	Although possibility of HTN, tachycardia, and arrhythmia exist, a 2015 JAMA meta-analysis demonstrated no significant change in HR or BP & when changes were seen, they were short-lived (13)
Epinephrine (drops)	Induces mydriasis, can potentially decrease IOP	HTN, tachycardia, arrhythmias
Atropine/scopolamine	Induces mydriasis	Tachycardia, agitation, apnea, hypertension

Choice of Anesthetic Technique: Local Versus General for Ophthalmic Surgery

- Local anesthesia has been associated with fewer complications than general anesthesia for ophthalmic surgery [8].
- In one study comprising 81 patients with 2 or more risk factors for heart disease having cataract surgery under general or local anesthesia, there were significantly less intraoperative events in the local anesthesia group [14].
- Many patients presenting for ophthalmic surgery are elderly, putting them at increased risk for cognitive dysfunction following general anesthesia [15].
- There is significant reduction in incidence of nausea, sore throat and time to eat and drink with local/MAC vs. general anesthesia [16].

General Anesthesia

In certain cases, e.g., full stomach, open globe injuries, or in cases where patients have multiple comorbidities general anesthesia may be the desired anesthesia technique. Children, adults with psychiatric or mental deficits or those whose are unable to cooperate and communicate, individuals who have physiologic tremors or who cannot tolerate being supine may need general anesthesia [8]. In addition, if the procedure exceeds 3 hr or if the surgical field cannot be covered by local/regional techniques, then general anesthesia may be the only option. Relative indications for GA would include surgeon preference or concern for coagulopathy and bleeding. Even if one's initial plan is to conduct the surgery under MAC/local, the potential to convert to general always exists. Whether elective or emergent, here are the goals for induction, maintenance, monitoring, and emergence to execute a successful anesthetic for ophthalmologic procedures.

Induction

- During induction, do not place any extra pressure on the eye e.g., from mask during pre-oxygenation.
- A smooth induction is of paramount importance especially for open globe injuries. The anesthesiologist must minimize coughing, gagging and therefore, escalation of already increased IOP during induction. This can be abated preemptively with premedication: IV lidocaine or opiates e.g., fentanyl, remifentanyl, or alfentanil [2].
- In a randomized control trial which compared propofol 2 mg/kg with remifentanil 4 mcg/kg induction versus succinylcholine 1.5 mg/kg for induction, remifentanil was able to reduce IOP by 39 %, reduce MAP by 24–31 % and was effective in blocking the hemodynamic response to direct laryngoscopy and

intubation [17]. Other studies have also shown that a combination of propofol with alfentanil has also counteracted the increase in IOP associated with airway manipulation [18]. These cases highlight the importance of adequate narcotic for smooth induction.

- Make sure that enough time has passed from the time the narcotic and paralytic were administered to intubation in order to reduce the chance of coughing against the tube.
- The question of profound paralysis with a modified rapid sequence induction via a nondepolarizing agent such as rocuronium or true rapid sequence with succinylcholine is at the discretion of the anesthesiologist. In the patient with a full stomach and open globe injury, the debate is whether the risk of aspiration or the risk of increasing IOP to the point of ocular expulsion is the priority. Most anesthesia providers carry a sense of relative or absolute contraindication to succinylcholine in these cases. However, the cases that reported increased IOP after succinylcholine administration in the 1950s are based on physiologic studies and not on any specific or documented case reports of vitreal extrusion [19].
- Currently, the main school of thought is that where prompt securing of the airway is important, succinylcholine can be used judiciously. The advantages of using succinylcholine are not trivial: It has an incredibly rapid onset, reliably hastens apnea and achieves dense muscle relaxation with an equally rapid recovery [19].
- *How much has succinylcholine been estimated to increase IOP?*
- Succinylcholine follows a "5–10" rule. It raises IOP an estimated 5–10 mmHg for duration of 5–10 min [2]. Is this clinically significant for us as providers? As stated earlier, the clinical outcomes have not proven it should always be avoided and its deleterious effect on IOP pales in comparison to airway manipulation [20].
- The mechanism by which succinylcholine increases IOP has to do with its site of action on the extraocular muscles. The extraocular muscles have copious neuromuscular junctions. When those numerous junctions are activated by succinylcholine, the repeated depolarization leads to prolonged contraction and therefore higher IOP [2]. It has also been postulated that fasciculation of the orbicularis oculi, ocular venous congestion, and changes in venous return from abdominal fasciculation may also contribute to the rise in IOP [8].

Maintenance

- One goal is to maintain a motionless surgical field whether the patient is under MAC or GA.
- Most anesthetics, volatile and IV, reduce IOP with the exception of ketamine.
- In a study performed by Wadia [21] that looked at IOP changes after administration of ketamine in sample size of 60 children, only mild increases in IOP were

observed ranging from 0 to 8 mmHg with a median change of 3 mmHg. Only 15 children experienced a brief increase of 5 mmHg or greater increase in IOP. Antal's study of the effect of ketamine on intraocular pressure demonstrated that on average ketamine increases IOP about 7% [22].

- If performing MAC/Local, small boluses of versed, fentanyl, or propofol may be necessary if the patient is uncomfortable and there is risk for movement.
- However, the provider should avoid excess narcotic that can cause hypercarbia-induced intraocular hypertension.
- If the patient is intubated, maintenance on volatile anesthetics or TIVA with propofol/remifentanyl is suitable.
- There are three main physiologic changes created by anesthetic agents:

  1. Reduced MAP = less choroid volume
  2. Relaxation of extraocular muscles = less wall tension
  3. Pupil constriction = better flow of the aqueous humor

The net effect is either no change or a decrease in IOP.

- Nitrous is dangerous if the surgeon plans to administer intravitreal gas. In retinal detachments, the surgeon can employ a gas bubble (air, sulfur hexafluoride SF_6, or octafluoropropane C_3F_8) to replace vitreous that has leaked out. N_2O is 117 times more soluble than SF_6 and therefore, if the patient is breathing it after gas bubble placement, the injected gas volume can as much as triple from its original size. Once, the nitrous is discontinued, the bubble will rapidly decrease, and this rapid rise and decline of IOP can culminate in complete retinal detachment [8].
- As a rule, one should not use N_2O less than 20 min from the time the surgeon plans to instill any intravitreal gas. If the patient is to have any other surgical procedures following intravitreal gas injection, they should avoid N_2O for another 3–4 weeks [8]. Furthermore, patients should avoid flying or any activities with rapid pressurization above sea level for the same 3–4 week duration.
- If there is any concern for choroid hemorrhage, MAP should be monitored closely to avoid hypertension and increased bleeding [8].

Monitoring

- These cases usually involve field avoidance with the patient's face turned towards the ophthalmologist and away from the anesthesiologist. Capnography and pulse oximetry can provide early signals of hypoxia, circuit disconnects, and airway obstruction when direct visualization of the head and neck may not be possible.
- Tachycardia and hypertension may be harbingers of patient movement secondary to discomfort. Therefore, pain medications and anxiolytics should carefully be titrated to avoid any disastrous consequences of a patient moving amidst fine procedures performed on the eye.
- EKG monitoring is of utmost importance to detect cardiac arrhythmias.

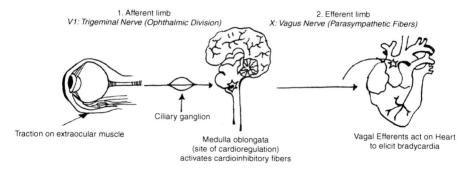

Fig. 24.2 The oculocardiac reflex

The Oculocardiac Reflex

- The oculocardiac reflex is a key physiologic response we want to avoid in these surgeries. The reflex may be elicited by a number of things: pressure on the globe, surgical traction on the extraocular muscles, conjunctiva, or structures of the orbit, retrobulbar blocks, or the initial eye trauma itself [2].
- The cardiac manifestations can range from bradycardia to ventricular arrhythmias or even cardiac arrest. Which patients are most vulnerable? The reflex is most often seen in the pediatric population undergoing strabismus repairs because they employ intermittent surgical traction. However, this risk remains present for any age population and for many different types of eye surgeries.
- *To pre-treat or not to pre-treat?*
- There is not a consensus whether medical prophylaxis against the oculocardiac reflex is the standard of care, and a look at the specific comorbidities of each individual patient becomes paramount. Most pediatric patients receive intravenous anticholinergic such as glycopyrrolate or atropine to try and prevent this reflex from occurring. However, it behooves the anesthesia provider to avoid any anticholinergic in the adult patient with diagnosed or high risk for coronary artery disease as the elicited tachycardia can cause cardiac ischemia.
- Treatment is to stop surgical traction & increase depth of anesthesia if patient is light.
- If the bradycardia still remains, administer anticholinergic. 10 mcg/kg of atropine has been shown to be effective [23].
- Eventually, the rectus muscles will fatigue and no longer elicit this reflex. The anatomy of the pathway is shown in Fig. 24.2.

Extubation and Emergence

- The primary goals of emergence are to wake up smoothly and avoid postoperative nausea and vomiting which may increase IOP and stand in the way of proper wound healing.
- Deep extubation may be indicated in the case of a severe globe injury or if there has been injection of intravitreal gas [8].

- IV Lidocaine 1.5 mg/kg can be administered to decrease the risk of airway irritation and coughing against the ETT. 1–2 min should be allowed after administration before extubation [2].
- Ophthalmologic surgery is in and of itself a risk factor for PONV. Valsalva maneuvers at the end of the surgery and their equivalents such as vomiting increase IOP and put the patient at higher risk for aspiration.
- The Massachusetts Eye and Ear Infirmary has a standard practice for high risk PONV patients to transition from inhalational induction to TIVA maintenance with propofol and remifentanyl, as well as administer a weight-based dose of odensetron and decadron [8].

Regional Blocks

- For open eye procedures, eye blocks can be performed to allow for analgesia, akinesia of the eye and hypotonia of the eyeball.

Retrobulbar Block

- Retrobulbar block requires injection of 3–5 mL local anesthetic behind the eye within the cone formed by the extraocular muscles See Fig. 24.3.
- Complications include globe rupture, optic nerve injection, retinal artery hemorrhage, and brain stem anesthesia which can present as apnea, hypotension, cardiac arrest, and potentially seizure from retrograde injection of local [24].

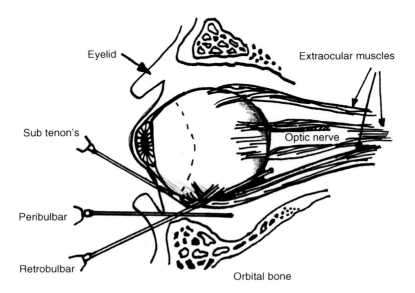

Fig. 24.3 Retrobulbar, peribulbar, and sub-tenon's blocks in their various needle orientations

Peribulbar Block

- Injection of 10–12 mL local anesthetic outside of the muscle cone, see Fig. 24.3. The larger volume of injectate allows inraconal spread [25].
- Theoretically, the peribulbar block should have fewer complications due to the needle position being further from the structures of the globe.
- A Cochrane review showed no difference between these two blocks in terms of pain, akinesia, ocular and systemic complications [6].

Sub Tenon's Block

- A hole is made in the conjunctiva and Tenon's capsule and a blunt cannula is inserted into the episcleral space, see Fig. 24.3. Local spreads around the whole globe to provide analgesia and, with sufficient volume, can also spread to the extraocular muscles to provide akinesia.
- If the cannula is blunt enough, there is virtually no risk of penetrating the globe or optic nerve.
- Injectate does not reach the brainstem.
- It is associated with fewer complications than retrobulbar or peribulbar block.
- Chemosis and subconjunctival hemorrhage are very common [26].

Topical

- 61 % of cataracts in the United States are repaired using topical anesthesia [27].
- Local anesthetics can be applied directly to the cornea via eye drops avoiding many complications of the injection techniques.
- Topical anesthesia does not provide akinesia or hypotonia. This can be overcome by directing the patient to look up into the operating microscope light, therefore patient cooperation is necessary [25].
- Topical drops provide limited analgesia so surgery is limited to repairs of the cornea. If needed, the eye drops can be supplemented with intracameral injection of local anesthetic.

Sedation for Block Techniques

The performance of a retrobulbar or peribulbar block can be painful and short-acting anesthetics are often given to minimize patient discomfort. No block/sedation technique has been shown to be superior to the next. The choice of technique should be based on surgeon's skill and preference, anesthesiologist's comfort with the technique, and patient's expectations.

Propofol

- A single bolus dose of propofol is often used.
- Using the formula of Hockings and Balmer [56 + {0.25 × weight in kg} − {0.53 × age in years}] to dose the propofol. 88 % of patients receiving this dosing did not experience recall, systemic side effects, or require airway support.
- Grimacing and verbal response did not correlate with actual recall [28].

Remifentanil

- Patients move less when given 0.3 mcg/kg of reminfentanil as compared to propofol 0.5 mg/kg [29].
- Higher incidence of recall.
- Minimal discomfort reported.
- More nausea and vomiting than with propofol.

Dexmedetomidine

- The limited studies that have been done have shown dexmedetomidine at 1 mcg/kg followed by an infusion yeilds good patient and surgeon satisfaction scores [29, 30].

Cataract Surgery (Phacoemulsification with Intraocular Lens Insertion)

- A cataract is an opacification of the lens that causes lack of transparency in the eye. It is treated by removing the lens and placing an artificial lens.
- Cataract extraction is the most common surgery performed on Medicare patients in the United States [31].
- A small incision is made in the cornea, then the anterior capsule of the lens is removed and the nucleus is emulsified with ultrasonic fragmentation and then vacuumed out. The cortex is then aspirated and a plastic intraocular lens is placed behind the iris. The incision is then closed.

Anesthesia Techniques for Cataract Surgery

- In the 1990s, large incision cataract surgery was replaced by modern small incision phacoemulsification procedures and akinesia was no longer necessary [26].
- The majority of cataract surgeries are performed with topical drops and little to no sedation.

Glaucoma Surgery

- Glaucoma is a group of eye conditions that can injure the optic nerve and cause vision loss. A major risk factor is increased intraocular pressure (IOP).
- Glaucoma is the 2nd leading cause of blindness worldwide and the leading cause of blindness in African Americans [32].
- IOP is dependent on the rate of production and the rate of drainage of aqueous humor. Therefore, reducing the secretion or improving the drainage of aqueous humor can lower IOP.
- The most common type of glaucoma is open angle glaucoma where there is increased resistance to the flow of aqueous humor and, therefore, IOP is elevated. It is usually painless and develops gradually over time.
- Closed angle glaucoma is more rare. It is caused by an acute rise in IOP, is usually painful and considered a medical emergency. It can be treated with medication or laser iridectomy in the ophthalmologist's office [33].

Common Procedures for Patients with Glaucoma

- Trabeculectomy: A small hole is made in the sclera to allow aqueous fluid to drain from the anterior chamber to the subconjunctival space and thus, lowers IOP. This is the most common procedure to lower IOP in patients with glaucoma [33].
- Tubes and valves: The conjunctiva is dissected away from the sclera and a small tube is inserted into the anterior chamber to aid in aqueous humor drainage.

Anesthetic Techniques for Glaucoma Surgery

- Patients with glaucoma often have associated medical problems and need careful preoperative assessment.
- There is no difference in surgical outcome related to anesthetic technique [33].
- General anesthesia avoids the risks of regional blocks and provides good operating conditions, but it requires more resources and time.
- A small bolus of propofol can be given to facilitate performing the regional block and once the effect wears off, the patient can be allowed to wake up and the team can proceed with surgery.

Vitreo-Retinal Surgery

- The vitreous cavity occupies >80% of the volume of the globe and is important for the metabolism of intraocular tissue.

- The separation of the vitreous from the retina occurs with age and is the most common form of retinal detachment requiring vitrectomy. Scarring, bleeding, or opacification of the vitreous are also treated by vitrectomy.
- Vitrectomy is the removal of vitreous contents from the eye and it can be replaced by many solutions including air, air-gas mixtures such as sulfahexafluoride (SF_6) and perfluoropropane (C_3F_8), and silicone oils.
- These gases can expand precluding the use of nitrous oxide before placement and for several weeks after surgery.
- Flying is also prohibited for a period of time post operatively because of cabin pressure changes and the possibility of gas bubble expansion and increased intraocular pressure [34].

Anesthetic technique for Vitreo-Retinal Surgery

- These cases can be done with GA or regional/MAC.
- Regional/MAC allows for rapid recovery and immediate prone positioning post-operatively if necessary.

Anesthesia for Strabismus Surgery

- The majority of patients presenting for strabismus surgery are pediatric and will require general anesthesia.
- Patients presenting for strabismus surgery will often have concomitant neurological disorders or congenital syndromes such as cerebral palsy, hydrocephalus, myotonic dystrophy, and Marfan syndrome amongst others [35].
- A careful physical exam and history should be performed to look for associated problems such as congenital heart disease or possible airway anomalies that can create difficulty with intubation.
- Previous concerns about increased risk for malignant hyperthermia in patients with strabismus appear to be unfounded [35].
- There is increased propensity for the OCR to occur in strabismus surgery due to the pulling on extraocular muscles and increased vagal tone in children. Incidence has been shown to be as high as 40 % in this age group.
- Glycopyrrolate or atropine can be effective in preventing the OCR.
- OCR occurs twice as often with surgical traction on the medial rectus versus the lateral rectus [36].
- OCR is elicited more readily when abrupt stimulation occurs and "gentle" surgery is advocated.

Anesthetic Technique for Strabismus Surgery (Pediatric)

- LMA is an acceptable airway to use and allows for smoother emergence [35].
- Opioid-sparing medications such as ketorolac or acetaminophen should be utilized.

- Postoperative prophylaxis for vomiting should be given since strabismus surgery can provoke emesis.
- Multiple studies have shown that combination therapy with dexamethasone and ondansetron is superior to either agent alone [37].
- Deeper planes of anesthesia can protect against the OCR [38].
- There is no difference in incidence of OCR with either desflurane or sevoflurane [39].

Anesthetic Technique for Strabismus Surgery (Adult)

- Adult patients presenting for strabismus surgery can undergo regional/MAC or GA.
- Patient satisfaction, out of operating room time, and discharge time have been shown to be superior with sedation and sub-Tenon's block [40, 41].
- Usually requires deep sedation.

Oculoplastics

- Many oculoplastic surgical procedures such as blepharoplasties and ptosis surgeries are done in an office setting under local anesthesia with oral sedatives such as diazepam or zolpidem and utilizes both topical and subcutaneous injection without the need for anesthesia personnel [42].
- For patients who do not meet requirements for office-based anesthesia, a dose of propofol or other sedative for comfortable block placement is acceptable.
- These cases often use electrocautery, which precludes a deep sedation with supplemental oxygen due to the risk of fire hazard.

Summary Points

1. The human eye is essentially a bony orbit filled with the eye and its related structures. When the intraocular content increases in size due to bleeding or accumulation of aqueous humor there can be an increase in IOP.
2. Any increase in aqueous humor production by the ciliary body or decreased drainage via the trabecular meshwork and Schlemm's canal will lead to an increase in this highly osmotic fluid and therefore IOP.
3. If a patient has been taking echothiophate chronically for their glaucoma, they can have a very prolonged duration of muscle relaxation if succinylcholine is administered.
4. Normal IOP is 10–22 mmHg. Ocular hypertension is defined as any pressure higher than 21 mmHg.
5. "The 5–10 Rule:" Succinylcholine increases intraocular pressure 5–10 mmHg for 5–10 min. Many studies have looked at patients with open eye injuries who

have been administered succinylcholine, and there has been no proven case of extrusion of eye contents related to this drug. As such, it can be used judiciously where there is a need to quickly establish an airway, full stomach, or other emergent situation.

6. The use of nitrous oxide should be completely avoided for at least 20 min before the ophthalmologist injects intravitreal air of any type. Furthermore, nitrous should be avoided in any other procedures falling within 4 weeks of intravitreal gas insertion.

7. Patients with no acute medical conditions presenting for cataract surgery require no preoperative labs or EKG.

8. Patients who cannot tolerate lying supine, have significant tremor, young children or adults with mental or psychological deficits, have severe hearing loss or who cannot cooperate or communicate may require general anesthesia.

9. The goals of general anesthesia are smooth induction with minimal coughing, adequate analgesia and akinesia, and a smooth emergence with adequate premedication to prevent the occurrence of PONV.

10. Most anesthetic agents decrease or maintain IOP, with the exception of ketamine. The explanation for this is that they decrease MAP creating a decrease in choroid volume, relax extraocular muscles, and constrict the pupil, facilitating flow of aqueous humor.

11. Careful monitoring of the capnogram and pulse oximetry, heart rate and blood pressure can alert one early to hypoxia, circuit disconnects, airway obstruction, or early signals of patient movement.

12. One must carefully observe the EKG pattern intraoperatively as surgical traction on extraocular muscles or pressure on the globe can lead to a myriad of cardiac arrhythmias ranging from bradycardia to ventricular fibrillation or complete cardiac arrest.

13. Pretreatment with IV glycopyrrolate or IV atropine, as long as the patient does not have CAD, can safely reduce the risk of the oculocardiac reflex.

14. Complications of retrobulbar blocks include globe rupture, injection of the optic nerve, retinal artery hemorrhage, and total spinal anesthesia which can lead to respiratory arrest, hypotension, seizures, and potentially cardiac arrest from retrograde spread of local anesthetic.

15. Peribulbar blocks are performed outside the cone with larger volumes of local anesthetic, and theoretically should have fewer complications. However, studies have not shown any superiority of peribulbar to retrobulbar blocks in analgesia, akinesia, or complications.

16. Sub Tenon's block is performed in the episcleral space and can provide local anesthesia to the entire globe with sufficient volume as well as some akinesia of the surrounding extraocular muscles. It is associated with fewer complications than retrobulbar and peribulbar blocks, but carries the risk of chemosis and subconjunctival hemorrhage.

17. Patients undergoing strabismus repairs are more susceptible to the oculocardiac reflex due to surgical traction on the extraocular muscles.

Bibliography

1. Barash PG, Bruce FC, Stoelting RK, Cahalan MK, Stock MC, Ortega, R. Clinical anesthesia. 7th ed. Lipincott, Williams and Wilkins Philadelphia. 2013. p. 1373–97.
2. Butterworth JF, Mackey DC, Wasnick JD. Morgan & Mikhail's clinical anesthesiology. Mcgraw-Hill, New York. 2013. p. 759–77.
3. Chidiac EJ, Raiskin AO. Succinylcholine and the open eye. Ophthalmol Clin North Am. 2006;19(2):279–85.
4. Tuulonen A. Treatment of ocular hypertension: is it cost effective? Curr Opin Ophthalmol. 2016;27(2):89–93.
5. Cunningham AJ, Barry P. Intraocular pressure – physiology and implications for anaesthetic management. Can Anaesth Soc J. 1986;33(2):195–208.
6. Alhassan MB, Kyari F, Ejere HO. Peribulbar versus retrobulbar anaesthesia for cataract surgery. Cochrane Database Syst Rev. 2015;(7):CD004083.
7. Schein OD, Katz J, Bass EB, Tielsch JM, Lubomski LH, Feldman MA, et al. The value of routine preoperative medical testing before cataract surgery. Study of Medical Testing for Cataract Surgery. N Engl J Med. 2000;342(3):168–75.
8. Longnecker DE. Chapter 65. Anesthesia for ophthalmic surgery. In: Anesthesiology. 2nd ed. EBSCO Publishing; Mcgraw-Hill, New York. 2012. p. 1558–80.
9. Fleisher LA, Fleischmann KE, Auerbach AD, Barnason SA, Beckman JA, Bozkurt B, et al. 2014 ACC/AHA guideline on perioperative cardiovascular evaluation and management of patients undergoing noncardiac surgery: a report of the American College of Cardiology/American Heart Association Task Force on Practice Guidelines. Circulation. 2014; 130(24):e278–333.
10. Katz J, Feldman MA, Bass EB, Lubomski LH, Tielsch JM, Petty BG, et al. Risks and benefits of anticoagulant and antiplatelet medication use before cataract surgery. Ophthalmology. 2003;110(9):1784–8.
11. Kong KL, Khan J. Ophthalmic patients on antithrombotic drugs: a review and guide to perioperative management. Br J Ophthalmol. 2015;99(8):1025–30.
12. Gabelt BT, Hennes EA, Seeman JL, Tian B, Kaufman PL. H-7 effect on outflow facility after trabecular obstruction following long-term echothiophate treatment in monkeys. Invest Ophthalmol Vis Sci. 2004;45(8):2732–6.
13. Stavert B, McGuinness MB, Harper CA, Guymer RH, Finger RP. Cardiovascular adverse effects of phenylephrine eyedrops: a systematic review and meta-analysis. JAMA Ophthalmol. 2015;133(6):647–52.
14. Glantz L, Drenger B, Gozal Y. Perioperative myocardial ischemia in cataract surgery patients: general versus local anesthesia. Anesth Analg. 2000;91(6):1415–9.
15. Rasmussen LS, Johnson T, Kuipers HM, Kristensen D, Siersma VD, Vila P, et al. Does anaesthesia cause postoperative cognitive dysfunction? A randomised study of regional versus general anaesthesia in 438 elderly patients. Acta Anaesthesiol Scand. 2003;47(3):260–6.
16. Barker JP, Vafidis GC, Hall GM. Postoperative morbidity following cataract surgery. A comparison of local and general anaesthesia. Anaesthesia. 1996;51(5):435–7.
17. Hanna SF, Ahmad F, Pappas AL, Mikat-Stevens M, Jellish WS, Kleinman B, et al. The effect of propofol/remifentanil rapid-induction technique without muscle relaxants on intraocular pressure. J Clin Anesth. 2010;22(6):437–42.
18. Zimmerman AA, Funk KJ, Tidwell JL. Propofol and alfentanil prevent the increase in intraocular pressure caused by succinylcholine and endotracheal intubation during a rapid sequence induction of anesthesia. Anesth Analg. 1996;83(4):814–7.
19. Vachon CA, Warner DO, Bacon DR. Succinylcholine and the open globe. Tracing the teaching. Anesthesiol. 2003;99(1):220–3.
20. Duncalf D, Foldes FF. Effect of anesthetic drugs and muscle relaxants on intraocular pressure. Int Ophthalmol Clin. 1973;13(2):21–33.

21. Wadia S, Bhola R, Lorenz D, Padmanabhan P, Gross J, Stevenson M. Ketamine and intraocular pressure in children. Ann Emerg Med. 2014;64(4):385–8.e1.
22. Antal M, Mucsi G, Faludi A. Ketamine anesthesia and intraocular pressure. Ann Ophthalmol. 1978;10(9):1281–4, 9.
23. Alexander JP. Reflex disturbances of cardiac rhythm during ophthalmic surgery. Br J Ophthalmol. 1975;59(9):518–24.
24. Wong DH, Koehrer E, Sutton HF, Merrick P. A modified retrobulbar block for eye surgery. Can J Anaesthesia J canadien d'anesthesie. 1993;40(6):547–53.
25. Nouvellon E, Cuvillon P, Ripart J. Regional anesthesia and eye surgery. Anesthesiology. 2010;113(5):1236–42.
26. Spaeth GL, Danesh-Meyer HV, Goldberg I, Kampik A. Opthalmic surgery principles and practice. 4th ed. Elsevier, Edinburgh. 2012. p. 40–4.
27. Ezra DG, Allan BD. Topical anaesthesia alone versus topical anaesthesia with intracameral lidocaine for phacoemulsification. Cochrane Database Syst Rev. 2007;(3):CD005276.
28. Habib NE, Balmer HG, Hocking G. Efficacy and safety of sedation with propofol in peribulbar anaesthesia. Eye (Lond). 2002;16(1):60–2.
29. Vann MA, Ogunnaike BO, Joshi GP. Sedation and anesthesia care for ophthalmologic surgery during local/regional anesthesia. Anesthesiology. 2007;107(3):502–8.
30. Ghali AM, Shabana AM, El Btarny AM. The effect of low-dose dexmedetomidine as an adjuvant to levobupivacaine in patients undergoing vitreoretinal surgery under sub-tenon's block anesthesia. Anesth Analg. 2015;121(5):1378–82.
31. Schein OD, Cassard SD, Tielsch JM, Gower EW. Cataract surgery among medicare beneficiaries. Ophthalmic Epidemiol. 2012;19(5):257–64.
32. Tian K, Shibata-Germanos S, Pahlitzsch M, Cordeiro MF. Current perspective of neuroprotection and glaucoma. Clini Ophthalmol (Auckland NZ). 2015;9:2109–18.
33. Eke T. Anesthesia for glaucoma surgery. Ophthalmol Clin North Am. 2006;19(2):245–55.
34. Dieckert JP, O'Connor PS, Schacklett DE, Tredici TJ, Lambert HM, Fanton JW, et al. Air travel and intraocular gas. Ophthalmology. 1986;93(5):642–5.
35. Rodgers A, Cox RG. Anesthetic management for pediatric strabismus surgery: continuing professional development. Can J Anaesthesia J canadien d'anesthesie. 2010;57(6):602–17.
36. Karaman T, Demir S, Dogru S, Sahin A, Tapar H, Karaman S, et al. The effect of anesthesia depth on the oculocardiac reflex in strabismus surgery. J Clin Monit Comput. 2015.
37. Shen YD, Chen CY, Wu CH, Cherng YG, Tam KW. Dexamethasone, ondansetron, and their combination and postoperative nausea and vomiting in children undergoing strabismus surgery: a meta-analysis of randomized controlled trials. Paediatr Anaesth. 2014;24(5):490–8.
38. Yi C, Jee D. Influence of the anaesthetic depth on the inhibition of the oculocardiac reflex during sevoflurane anaesthesia for paediatric strabismus surgery. Br J Anaesth. 2008;101(2):234–8.
39. Oh AY, Yun MJ, Kim HJ, Kim HS. Comparison of desflurane with sevoflurane for the incidence of oculocardiac reflex in children undergoing strabismus surgery. Br J Anaesth. 2007;99(2):262–5.
40. Snir M, Bachar M, Katz J, Friling R, Weinberger D, Axer-Siegel R. Combined propofol sedation with sub-tenon's lidocaine/mercaine infusion for strabismus surgery in adults. Eye (Lond). 2007;21(9):1155–61.
41. Greenberg MF, Pollard ZF. Adult strabismus surgery under propofol sedation with local versus general anesthesia. J AAPOS Off Pub Am Asso Pediatric Ophthalmol Strabismus Am Asso Pediatric Ophthalmol Strabismus. 2003;7(2):116–20.
42. Moody BR, Holds JB. Anesthesia for office-based oculoplastic surgery. Dermatol Surg Off Pub Am Soc Dermatol Surg. 2005;31(7 Pt 1):766–9.

Chapter 25
Anesthesia and Radiotherapy Suite

Kara M. Barnett, Amy Catherine Lu, and Luis E. Tollinche

Abstract Radiotherapy is an important treatment modality for several cancers. Brachytherapy involves the placement of radioactive material inside of the body. External Beam Radiation uses a machine to deliver radiation from outside of the body. The anesthesia technique for brachytherapy will depend on several factors including the area of the body, length of case and anesthesia provider availability. It may further be complicated by the need to transport the patient to an MRI or CT scanner. External Beam Radiation in adults does not usually require anesthesia. However, if it is required, usually sedation with propofol is adequate.

Keywords Brachytherapy • External beam radiation • Radiotherapy • Radiation • Applicator • Low-dose implants • High-dose implants • Immobilizers • Radiation Simulation • Radiation Treatment • Mask • Sedation • Local • General anesthesia • Regional anesthesia • Spinal • Epidural

Introduction

- Radiotherapy is the treatment of cancer cells with radiation.
- Radiotherapy requires immobility so that treatments can be accurate [1, 2].
- Brachytherapy involves the placement of radioactive material inside of the body.

K.M. Barnett, MD (✉)
Department of Anesthesiology and Critical Care Medicine, Memorial Sloan Kettering Cancer Center, 1275 York Avenue, New York, NY 10065, USA
e-mail: barnettk@mskcc.org

A.C. Lu, MD, MPH
Department of Anesthesiology, Perioperative, and Pain Medicine, Stanford University, 300 Pasteur Drive, Room H-3580, MC 5640, Stanford, CA 94305, USA
e-mail: aclu@stanford.edu

L.E. Tollinche, MD
Anesthesia and Critical Care Medicine, Memorial Sloan Kettering Cancer Center, 1275 York Avenue #C330F, New York, NY 10065, USA
e-mail: tollincl@mskcc.org

© Springer International Publishing Switzerland 2017   347
B.G. Goudra, P.M. Singh (eds.), *Out of Operating Room Anesthesia*,
DOI 10.1007/978-3-319-39150-2_25

Table 25.1 Types of brachytherapy

Low-dose rate implants	High-dose rate implants
Lower dose of radiation requiring more treatments	Higher dose of radiation requiring a shorter period of treatment (e.g., 5–10 min). Newer method that has the advantage that staff does not get exposed to radiation
May be permanent seeds or involve temporary applicator placement for a period of time	Implantation and treatment done in several sessions and involves temporary placement of an applicator. The applicator may be implanted over a period of days for daily treatments or removed and replaced weekly for weekly treatments

- Implantation can be painful and often requires anesthesia.
- Brachytherapy is often treatment for gastrointestinal, urologic, gynecologic, esophageal, breast, thoracic, and retinal cancer [1].
- Radiation oncologists use applicators for the placement of the radioactive substance. Anesthesia providers may be involved when applications are placed intracavitary (inside a cavity) or interstitial (inside tissue) [1].
- If applicators are left in the patient, it can involve a hospital stay. Removal can be painful and the patient may benefit from additional anesthesia.
- See Table 25.1 for a summary of the two commonly performed types of brachytherapy.

- External Beam Radiation uses a machine to deliver radiation from outside of the body.

  - Usually several treatments are required.
  - Treatments are not painful.

- The anesthesia provider should formulate the anesthetic plan after discussing the needs of the procedure and patient.

Brachytherapy

- Applicator placement and removal may be painful [3].
- There is a wide range of options of anesthetic techniques for brachytherapy procedures. See Table 25.2 for a summary of advantages and disadvantages. Considerations for choosing a technique include:

  - Patient specific, such as a patient who is morbidly obese, has risk factors for aspiration, or a known or suspected difficult airway. Non-breast patients undergoing brachytherapy are usually older and sicker and may not be candidates for major surgery [1, 4].
  - Body region of brachytherapy [1, 4].
  - Length of procedure. Brachytherapy can be lengthy because of the need to confirm placement of the applicator and perform calculations prior to treatment [4].

Table 25.2 Advantages and disadvantages of anesthetic techniques

Type of anesthesia	Advantages	Disadvantages
Local	• May be done by the radiotherapist if anesthesia staff unavailable	• Analgesia may be inadequate • Patient immobility may be inadequate
Sedation	• May be done by the radiotherapist if anesthesia staff unavailable • Sedation may be useful for applicator removal	• Analgesia may be inadequate • If performed by a radiotherapist, may need assistance if the patient has respiratory depression
Regional	• Useful for procedures of the lower body • In a functioning epidural or spinal block, provides adequate analgesia • Easy to safely transport especially if the anesthesia provider needs to bring the patient immobilized to a scanner or treatment room • Few complications • Epidural catheters left in place allow for use during applicator removal	• Patient must be an appropriate candidate (e.g., not coagulopathic) for a spinal or and epidural • Lengthy procedures may outlast a spinal or one shot epidural block
General	• Immobility and analgesia requirements easily met • Must be done for certain cases such as upper body • Few complications	• Requires full anesthetic equipment/ventilator, which may be unavailable if scans in other areas of the hospital must be performed

- Immobility to ensure proper placement of the applicator and whether the patient will need to remain immobile after the procedure.
- Whether the patient will need to be transported to a scanner or radiation room while anesthetized [1].

  - If a patient is under general anesthesia, ensure that a ventilator and full monitoring are available in these other areas.
  - Use of a camera on the patient and monitors or use of slave monitor during treatments. Rooms are shielded and should be fully equipped with anesthesia equipment.

- Minimize post-operative nausea and vomiting.
- Operating/procedural room environment and infrastructure.
- Possible influence of anesthetic technique on outcome of brachytherapy, although few randomized controlled trials exist.

• Local anesthesia for Brachytherapy

  - Used widely by radiotherapists. Although more effective than placebo, pain has been found to exist after this technique, as it is often performed without anesthesia staff present [1, 5].
  - Also likely to result in inferior applicator placement because the patient may move from insufficient analgesia [1].

- Sedation for Brachytherapy

  – Considered as an alternative to general anesthesia in less painful brachytherapy cases [1].
  – Radiotherapists have administered sedation when anesthesia providers are not available [1].
  – Options include:

    • Nitrous oxide for inhalation analgesia during applicator placement or removal [6].
    • Intravenous medications like opioids, midazolam, and/or propofol [3, 7].

  – If possible, patient discomfort can be alleviated during applicator removal in patients without an epidural catheter. Consider a small dose of propofol. Once the applicator is removed, the pain will cease so beware of over sedating [1, 4].

- Regional anesthesia for Brachytherapy

  – Used mainly for brachytherapy of the lower body, including patients with urological, lower rectal, and gynecologic cancers.
  – Advantages of regional anesthesia include sufficient analgesia and immobilization, high degree of patient satisfaction, and safer transfer of patients between different sites of care [1].
  – Options for regional anesthesia include spinal, lumbar epidural, caudal, and combined spinal-epidural techniques [1].

    • Spinal anesthesia represents high proportion of patients receiving regional anesthesia for brachytherapy [4]. Advantages of spinal anesthesia include rapid onset and known duration of anesthesia [1].
    • Combined spinal-epidural or solely an epidural may be a better choice for longer procedures.
    • Caudal epidural blocks have been described for gynecological brachytherapy. Its disadvantages include its technical difficulty in placing the block especially in obese patients, its limited duration and insufficient analgesia for applicator placement [8].
    • Lumbar epidural catheter technique is popular for gynecological, urological and rectal cases. When compared to epidural patient-controlled analgesia in patients who underwent HDR of the prostate, it was shown to be significantly superior [1, 9]. It may also offer the advantage of providing analgesia during applicator removal when bolused [1].

  – A retrospective review of over 5000 brachytherapy cases found regional anesthesia performed in 30 % of lower body brachytherapy cases and in the majority of pelvic brachytherapy cases [4].

- General anesthesia for Brachytherapy

  – Indications for general anesthesia include brachytherapy for malignancies of upper body (e.g., oropharyngeal cancer, bronchus carcinoma), patient choice, and patients with contraindications to regional anesthesia [1, 4].

- Some institutions like ours prefer general anesthesia for all brachytherapy cases. An MRI and CT scanner equipped with our anesthetic monitors, ventilator and equipment are readily available allowing for easy and safe transport. Our patients are transported and recovered in the PACU.
- General anesthesia requires more preparation and equipment. For example, if a patient is to have a CT or MRI, a ventilator will be necessary in both the brachytherapy suite and scanner.

- When selecting an anesthetic technique, it is important to keep in mind that many brachytherapy patients are considered ASA III or IV and are over the age of 60 years [4].
- Overall, complications from both regional and general anesthesia techniques are minor and include hypotension, bradycardia, and postoperative nausea and vomiting [4].
- Studies in this area show no significant difference between general and regional anesthesia techniques in postoperative complications or satisfaction [1, 10]. A prospective trial in this area compared patients receiving four different anesthetic techniques: general anesthesia with TIVA, general anesthesia with isoflurane, small dose spinal block, or large dose spinal block. The TIVA technique was found to have earliest voiding and fastest discharge of all techniques, although there was no difference in any choice on the outcome of postoperative nausea or vomiting, pain score, return to normal function at home, or overall patient satisfaction [10].
- Retrospective review of general anesthesia versus regional anesthesia in prostate brachytherapy showed no correlation between anesthetic technique and postoperative prostate gland swelling, acute toxicity, or implant dosimetric quality [11].
- In patients without an epidural catheter, acetaminophen, morphine, codeine, and NSAIDS may be considered for postoperative analgesia [1].
- If applicators remain in the patient, the patient may experience discomfort and may need to be immobilized while in the hospital.

External Beam Radiation

- Radiation therapy is typically once or twice daily doses for up to 6 weeks of treatment [12].
- Precise positioning is paramount for repeat procedures. Must replicate exact beam direction prescribed by the radiation oncologist [13].
- Good preanesthesia evaluation and a collaborative team approach optimize patient safety [12].
- Unlike young children, few adults require anesthesia for external beam radiation. Adult patients may need sedation for reasons such as severe pain, claustrophobia, altered mental status, or mental retardation. For example, radiation to the brain may require a tight fitting mask that a claustrophobic patient may not tolerate.
- Simulation allows for precise prescribing by the radiation oncologist [13].

- Simulates exact conditions.
- Skin sites are marked with tattoos to facilitate repeat treatment positioning.
- Plaster immobilizers are created.
- Blocks are obtained to protect organs near radiation beam (e.g., genitals, other vital organs).
- Offers an opportunity to gauge patient cooperation and ability to tolerate treatment without anesthesia.
- Tend to be longer then the actual treatment (30–60 min). More sedation may be necessary than what is needed during actual treatments.
- Because treatment is not given, the anesthesia provider is able to remain with the patient except during times of CT scanning.

• Three types of immobilizers/positioning: [13]

- Mask (aquaplast) for brain/head treatments.
- Body mold (aquacradle) for body/extremity treatments.
- Floor positioning for Total Body Irradiation (TBI).

• MAC is usually well tolerated and adequate for treatment [2, 13].

- Treatments are painless.
- If muscle paralysis is not necessary, it allows for spontaneous ventilation.
- The use of a nasal cannula with the ability to monitor end tidal $CO2$. The nasal cannula may need to be taped to the mask if one is needed during treatments.
- Short duration lasting 5–20 min, depending on the number of sites being irradiated.
- Fasting guidelines must be maintained. Extend guidelines and consider general anesthesia with an endotracheal tube in the event of outflow obstruction by tumor [13].
- Midazolam 0.05 mg/kg IV anxiolysis may be used [14].
- Propofol 0.5 mg/kg IV bolus followed by an infusion 10 mg/kg/hields spontaneous eye opening within 4 minutes after stopping the infusion [14].

• General anesthesia considerations

- If there are patient indications (airway protection necessary, etc.).
- If muscle paralysis is required (e.g., treating globe as in Retinoblastoma RT, extraocular muscles must be paralyzed) [13, 15].
- Patient positioning [15].
- Circuit hose extension required for general anesthetics [13]. Ensure that the IV line, monitors and supplemental oxygen are long enough and do not interfere with the radiation equipment.
- The anesthesia ventilator and equipment cannot interfere with lateral x-ray beam [13].
- Vaporizers and ventilator are more cumbersome and difficult to transport. [14]
- Slower to induce a patient than administering MAC.
- More difficult to titrate to an optimal anesthetic level [14].

- Monitoring requires the use of two cameras (closed circuit television) in order to visualize:
    - Patient for breathing and movement.
    - Monitor (ASA monitors-NIBP, ECG, SpO2, ETCO2. Also able to monitor ventilator during general anesthesia) [2, 13].
- The microphone in the room will allow the anesthesia provider to transmit the tones of the pulse oximeter [13].
- The anesthesia provider will need a mobile work cart and emergency drugs [2, 16].
- If a ventilator is unavailable, emergency airway equipment including an ambu bag should be readily available [16].
- Ensure that there is suction available and functioning.
- XRT can exacerbate nausea/vomiting more than chemotherapy alone. Consider the addition of antiemetics such as intravenous ondansetron 0.1 mg/kg [13].

Challenges

- Radiotherapy is challenging because of the remoteness of the treatment room and periods of monitoring the patient from a distance [1].
    - The anesthesia provider must leave the room during treatment [13].
    - Help may not be readily available.
    - Transportation of the patient to the recovery area may be challenging.
- Quick emergence required because most RT and brachy suites lack a dedicated PACU [13].
- Brachytherapy
    - During brachytherapy, the anesthesia provider may need to transport the patient to the MRI or CT scanner for applicator placement confirmation or a treatment room. The transportation of an anesthetized patient is challenging [1].
    - MRI scans will necessitate the use of MRI compatible equipment. If the patient is under general anesthesia, MRI compatible ventilator and monitoring are necessary.
    - Brachytherapy can be lengthy because of the need to confirm placement of the applicator and do calculations [1].
- External Beam Radiation
    - Mask immobilizers used during external beam radiation can impede air exchange or lead to upper airway obstruction. Suggest jaw extension during mask creation [13].
    - Access to patient is limited during treatments and providers must consider time delay to attend to patient in emergency (e.g., heavy lead door opening, etc.) [13].

- Repeat access of mediport, etc. demands aseptic technique—many patients are neutropenic [13].
- Common acute side effects with potential anesthetic implications [12].

  • Fatigue
  • Redness/blistering of skin and hair loss
  • Mucositis and xerostomia
  • Neurocognitive changes and leukoencephalopathy
  • Neuroendocrine dysfunction
  • Nausea/vomiting and diarrhea
  • Survivors of cancer (radiation) are at increased risk of a second malignant neoplasm

- Weight gain secondary to steroids can result in ill-fitting immobilizers requiring new simulation [12].
- If the patient has vomiting or an upper respiratory infection, the risks of proceeding with anesthesia may outweigh benefit and treatment may be cancelled. It is important to have a dialogue with the patient and radiation oncologist in order to assist with decision-making [12].
- There is controversy regarding tachyphylaxis and the need for escalating propofol dosages. It is the authors' opinion that most patients require increased doses over the course of radiation therapy [12].

References

1. Roessler B, Lucia S, Gustorff B. Anaesthesia for brachytherapy. Curr Opin Anaesthesiol. 2008;21(4):514–8.
2. Katrin C, Laura T, Stephen S. Anesthesia and sedation outside the operating room. Anesthesiol Clin. 2014;32(1):25–43.
3. Hurd C. A comparison of acute effects and patient acceptability of high dose rate with low dose rate after-loading in intra-vaginal radiotherapy. Radiogr Today. 1991;57:25–8.
4. Benrath J, Kozek-Langenecker S, Hupfl M, Lierz P, Gustoff B. Anaesthesia for brachytherapy—5 ½ yr of experience in 1622 procedures. Br J Anaesth. 2006;96(2):195–200.
5. Lim KH, Lu JJ, Wynne CJ, et al. A study of complications arising from different methods of anesthesia used in high-dose-rate BT for cervical cancer. Am J Clin Oncol. 2004;27:449–51.
6. Tyrie LK, Hoskin PJ. Intrauterine high dose rate afterloading BT: experience of fractionated therapy using a cervical sleeve technique. Clin Oncol (R Coll Radiol). 1996;8:376–9.
7. Nguyen TV, Petereit DG. High-dose-rate BT for medically inoperable stage I endometrial cancer. Gynecol Oncol. 1998;71:196–203.
8. Smith MD, Todd JG, Symonds RP. Analgesia for pelivic brachytherapy. Br J Anaesth. 2002;88(2):270–6.
9. Colella J, Scrofine S, Galli B, et al. Prostate HDR radiation therapy: a comparative study evaluating the effectiveness of pain management with peripheral PCA vs. PCEA. Urol Nurs. 2006;26:57–61.
10. Flaishon R, Ekstein P, Matzkin H, Weinbroum AA. An evaluation of general and spinal anesthesia techniques for prostate BT in a day surgery setting. Anesth Analg. 2005;101:1656–8.
11. Aronowitz J, Follette J, Moran MJ. Does anesthesia method affect implant induced prostate swelling? Urology. 2005;65:513–6.

12. McFadyen J, Pelly N, Orr R. Sedation and anesthesia for the pediatric patient undergoing radiation therapy. Curr Opin Anaesthesiol. 2011;24:433–8.
13. Harris E. Sedation and anesthesia options for pediatric patients in the radiation oncology suite. Int J Pediatr. 2010;Article ID 870921:9.
14. Buehrer S, Immoos S, Frei M, Timmermann B, Weiss M. Evaluation of propofol for repeated prolonged deep sedation in children undergoing proton radiation therapy. Br J Anaesth. 2007;99(4):556–60.
15. Chalabi J, Patel S. Radiation therapy in children. Int Anesthesiol Clin. 2009;47:45–53.
16. Galvagno SM, Kodali BS. Critical monitoring issues outside the operating room. Anesthesiol Clin. 2009;27:141–56.

Chapter 26
Infertility Treatment: The Role of Anesthesia Techniques

John Fitzgerald, Nikki Higgins, and John P.R. Loughrey

Abstract The rise in numbers of couples attempting to conceive later in life and the success of fertility procedures has led to a worldwide increase in assisted reproduction. The retrieval of oocytes from the ovaries under ultrasound guidance is painful and requires anesthesia or sedation. Any technique adopted must be safe, and deemed to cause minimal detrimental effect on the retrieved oocyte, the subsequent embryo, and successful pregnancy rates. The early focus of different anesthesia techniques was centred on pregnancy outcomes but so many other factors influence outcomes including laboratory techniques and parental age. A lack of willingness exists in this group of patients to submit to randomisation of treatments. This largely resides in patient fear over impact on outcomes, so large quality randomised trials of anesthesia techniques are rare.

Anesthesiologists may be called upon to provide anesthesia or sedation in in-vitro fertilisation (IVF) units, which may be in standalone units or part of a main hospital complex. These procedures are rarely performed in main operating rooms as adjacency to the fertilization laboratory confers advantages in minimising oocyte transport and processing.

The aims of this chapter are to give the anesthesia providers who may not be familiar with the options a good overview and a sound knowledge on which to provide a service.

Keywords Fertility • Anesthesia • Assisted Reproduction • IVF

Introduction

The rise in numbers of couples attempting to conceive later in life and the success of fertility procedures has led to a worldwide increase in assisted reproduction. The retrieval of oocytes from the ovaries under ultrasound guidance is painful and

J. Fitzgerald, MB, FRCA, FCAI, EDIC • N. Higgins, MB, BSc, FCAI, FJFICMI
J.P.R. Loughrey, MB, FCAI, FFPMCAI (✉)
Department of Anesthesia, The Rotunda Hospital, Parnell Street West, Dublin, Ireland
e-mail: jloughrey@rotunda.ie

© Springer International Publishing Switzerland 2017
B.G. Goudra, P.M. Singh (eds.), *Out of Operating Room Anesthesia*,
DOI 10.1007/978-3-319-39150-2_26

357

requires anesthesia or sedation. Any technique adopted must be safe, and deemed to cause minimal detrimental effect on the retrieved oocyte, the subsequent embryo, and successful pregnancy rates. The early focus of different anesthesia techniques was centred on pregnancy outcomes but so many other factors influence outcomes including laboratory techniques and parental age. A lack of willingness exists in this group of patients to submit to randomisation of treatments. This largely resides in patient fear over impact on outcomes, so large quality randomised trials of anesthesia techniques are rare.

Anesthesiologists may be called upon to provide anesthesia or sedation in in-vitro fertilisation (IVF) units, which may be in standalone units or part of a main hospital complex. These procedures are rarely performed in main operating rooms as adjacency to the fertilization laboratory confers advantages in minimising oocyte transport and processing.

The aims of this chapter are to give the anesthesia providers who may not be familiar with the options a good overview and a sound knowledge on which to provide a service.

In-Vitro Fertilization Overview

Assisted Reproductive Technology (ART) encompasses a number of fertility treatments whereby the sperm, the oocyte, or both are manipulated in order to achieve pregnancy. It includes a spectrum of procedures that may include one or more of the following:

In-vitro fertilization (IVF)
Intra-cytoplasmic sperm injection (ICSI)
Intra-uterine insemination (IUI)
Gamete intrafallopian transfer (GIFT)
Zygote intrafallopian transfer (ZIFT)

IVF was initially developed as a treatment option for patients with fallopian tube disease. However since it's introduction, the number of indications have broadened. Current indications for this developing specialty include:

- Tubal Disease
- Male factor subfertility. This accounts for 35 % of cases of sub fertile couples [1]. Male subfertility is most commonly associated with semen abnormalities resulting in azoospermia (no sperm in ejaculate) or oligozoospermia (reduced number of sperm in ejaculate)
- Endometriosis
- Anovulation which can be due to primary or secondary ovarian disorders
- Reduced fertility observed with increased maternal age
- Unexplained infertility for more than 2 years.

Despite the growing indications and utilization for IVF across a wide range of different pathologies the success rates have improved over the years. Over 33 % of

ART cycles result in either single or multiple fetus pregnancy [2]. The etiology of these improved success rates is likely multifactorial suggesting a combination of improved retrieval and transfer techniques, laboratory methods & hormonal therapy. It is important to analyse the effect of anesthesia techniques on patient satisfaction and also any potential discrete role on outcomes in assisted reproduction.

An understanding of the IVF process is also important in order to make well-informed decisions regarding the anesthesia techniques these patients should receive.

Broadly, the IVF process involves the following steps

1. Hormonal stimulation. Typically a cycle is initiated with gonadotropin-releasing hormone agonist (GnRH-a), which acts to induce pituitary and ovarian suppression. This is then followed by follicle-stimulating hormone (FSH) and human menopausal gonadotropin (hMG), which supports the development and growth of multiple ovarian follicles. The response may be monitored by serial trans-vaginal ultrasound. Follicular maturation is then induced with the introduction of Human chorionic gonadotropin (hCG) These regimens can generate up to 10–15 oocytes per cycle [3] whereby each follicle usually contains a single oocyte.
2. Oocyte retrieval: this generally occurs by needle-guided aspiration around 36 h following hCG administration. It is this retrieval process that requires anesthesia support.
3. In-vitro fertilisation: the retrieved oocyte is fertilised with a sperm sample previously collected. If there are issues with sperm mobility or penetration, the process of intra-cytoplasmic sperm injection (ICSI) with previously prepared spermatozoa may be considered.
4. Embryo transfer. A zygote is the earliest developmental stage in multicellular organisms. A collection of cells with an outer layer is termed a blastocyst. Further cell division results in an embryo. The embryo is usually directly transferred into the uterine cavity at a later stage after monitored cellular development. The injection into the uterine cavity via a catheter is relatively painless and does not require anesthesia. This occurs sometime in the days following oocyte retrieval. Sometimes the zygote may be transferred directly into the fallopian tube in a procedure known as zygote intrafallopian transfer (ZIFT). This latter technique, which requires general anesthesia has reduced in popularity due to concerns about ectopic pregnancy.

Role of Anesthesia and the Anesthesiologist

Although there are a number of procedures associated with IVF such as ovarian cyst drainage, anesthesiology involvement is primarily requested in the oocyte retrieval process of IVF. Ovarian cyst drainage is performed when large ovarian cysts can impede ovarian follicle development in adjacent ovarian tissue. This is still performed trans-vaginally but with usually a single needle pass.

In the early years of IVF, retrieval of oocytes was sometimes conducted via laparoscopy whereby the ovary could be directly visualized. Consequently, this meant that patients received general anesthesia with endotracheal intubation during oocyte retrieval. Oocyte retrieval may occasionally require laparoscopic retrieval if prior surgery has resulted in a high ovarian position in the pelvis rendering the ovaries inaccessible by the trans-vaginal route.

Laparoscopy is rarely reserved for scenarios where tubal transfer of gamete or zygote is planned during the same procedure, namely gamete intra-fallopian transfer (GIFT) or zygote intra-fallopian transfer (ZIFT). Gamete refers to the haploid sex cell, an oocyte in females and the sperm in males.

Presently, oocyte retrievals are predominantly done with ultrasound guidance via a trans-vaginal approach. The trans-vaginal method of oocyte retrieval compared with laparoscopy is associated with higher pregnancy rates [4].

However, despite this less invasive approach, the oocyte retrieval process is still perceived by many patients as one of the most stressful and possibly painful components of the entire assisted reproductive treatment.

Patients may find discomfort during insertion of the trans-vaginal probe. Pain occurs during advancement of the aspirating needle through the vaginal fornix into the ovary. Figure 26.1. Manipulation of the ovary during this procedure can also be a significant source of visceral discomfort for the patient. The procedure duration is usually 20–30 min.

The goal is provision of intravenous analgesia, sedation or anesthesia, which relieves pain, but also allows the patient to remain relatively motionless. By keeping

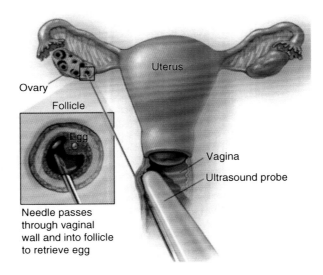

Fig. 26.1 O™ocyte-retrieval procedure. A needle is passed through the vaginal fornix into the ovary (under ultrasound guidance) to enter and aspirate multiple follicles (By permission of Mayo Foundation for Medical Education and Research. All Rights Reserved) (Source: Mayo foundation for Medical Education

the patient comfortable, retrieval of the oocyte form the ovarian follicles is easier for the operator. Once the needle enters the ovary, minor redirections within the ovary are not as stimulating so bolus agents should be timed in anticipation of initial needle placement into the ovary on each side. Some units flush and aspirate each follicle necessitating a wider needle and prolonging total procedure time.

Complications such as bleeding should be suspected in any patient who becomes hypotensive following the procedure. The anesthesia technique must clearly be outlined to the patient to prevent a complaint of awareness when sedation only was the technique utilized.

Pre-assessments/Timing/Facility Location

The patient population undergoing IVF are mainly ASA 1 or II women with few co-morbidities. However the increase in utilization of these techniques for a number of other pathologies places more of an emphasis on the need for adequate pre-operative assessment and investigations. If the stimulation of oocytes has already begun, deferring a case can lead to complications such as ovarian hyperstimulation syndrome. Therefore fitness for anesthesia should be determined prior to this, and an avenue for anesthesia assessment or consultation should exist for the referring fertility specialist.

Infertility may be a consequence of certain co-morbidities that also have implications for anesthesia:

1. Morbid obesity. These patients require assessment of their cardiovascular risk as well as suitability for sedation and ambulatory surgery. Many centers, 84 % in the US, have policies on a maximum body mass index (BMI) for IVF procedures, citing anesthesia concerns as a main reason for this [5].
2. Hypo or hyperthyroidism as a cause of infertility is often considered and will likely have been screened for and treated prior to IVF.
3. Patients with a diagnosis of cancer may be undergoing oocyte retrieval prior to receiving treatment with chemotherapy or radiotherapy. These particular patients can have organ specific dysfunction such as pleural effusions. Appropriate clinical history and examination would guide further investigations or interventions in these patients.

Timing of oocyte retrieval is important for oocyte number and embryo quality. The optimum time frame for oocyte retrieval is 24–36 h after hCG administration. The consequence of not adhering to this time window has the potential for spontaneous ovulation and resultant loss of oocytes. Every effort must be made to optimize a patient prior to surgery so that there are no undue delays or cancelations. Once hormonal preparation is commenced these cases are no longer as deferrable as elective general surgical cases without adverse impact on outcomes.

Routine fasting guidelines for patients should be mandatory as would be expected in other forms of day-case surgery. 6 h for solid foods and 2 h for clear liquids are appropriate in this population. Consider an anti-reflux agent in patients who have symptomatic gastroesophageal reflux disease. Some units consider spinal anesthesia in patients that have not adhered to fasting guidelines. Policies should exist for the management of postoperative nausea and vomiting (PONV). Prophylactic antiemetics are generally not utilized even with a prior history of PONV. Metoclopramide can have an impact on prolactin causing increased plasma concentration. This occurs via inhibition of gonadotrophin-releasing hormone [6]. Concerns around unknown effects of antiemetics on the IVF process are the reasons cited for withholding antiemetics although there is no good evidence that other agents such as ondansetron are contraindicated. Intravenous fluids can enhance the patients' feeling of wellbeing and further reduce PONV incidence [7]. Appropriate discharge analgesia should be standard and usually consists of acetaminophen, while avoiding NSAIDs. Use of anti-inflammatory drugs are avoided as certain prostaglandins in the embryo and endometrium are important for implantation [8]. However, as embryo transfer usually does not occur for a further 48 h a single dose short acting agent may be appropriate for patients with problematic postprocedural pain.

Pre-medication with benzodiazepine anxiolytics should not be considered routine practice for day case procedures however they should be considered on a patient with high levels of anxiety.

The location or facility used to perform sedation for IVF must conform to the appropriate standards expected of an anesthesia suite. These include:

- Appropriate monitors including continuous ECG, non-invasive blood pressure monitoring, pulse oximetry and continuous CO2 Capnography.
- A reliable oxygen source, airway equipment and suction.
- Appropriate anesthesia pharmacological agents including reversal agents.
- Resuscitation equipment including a defibrillator and drugs.
- A post-anesthesia care unit where the patient can be appropriately monitored while they recover from their anesthesia agents until discharge criteria are met.
- Transportation solutions to an appropriate centre in the event of prolonged recovery or other complications such as anaphylaxis or bleeding.

Anesthesia Techniques

Intravenous sedation/anesthesia are currently the most commonly used techniques for patients undergoing oocyte retrieval via the trans-vaginal route. Other options for analgesia include spinal anesthesia. Para-cervical nerve block administered by the gynaecologist can reduce the requirement for intravenous agents. Some unusual methods employed for patient comfort include hypnosis, electro-acupuncture, and even no pain relief whatsoever. Application of topical local anesthetic creams have also been utilized to reduce sedation requirements.

Conscious Sedation

Conscious sedation, defined as a 'minimally depressed level of consciousness that retains the ability of the patient to maintain a patent airway independently and continuously and to respond to verbal commands' is recommended by the UK National Institute for Clinical Excellence (NICE) to be offered to all women undergoing trans-vaginal retrieval of oocytes [9]. The institute proposes adhering to the Academy of Medical Royal Colleges (AOMRC) UK's safe sedation practice guideline when administering sedative drugs [10].

Conscious sedation is usually achieved by administration of intravenous benzodiazepines and/or opioids. Patients can self-administer from a timed pump in the form of patient controlled analgesia (PCA), or more traditionally a care provider can administer the drugs. Patient satisfaction is high with both methods of delivery, but pain scores in one study were typically higher in the PCA group [11].

As conscious sedation by definition does not require an anesthetist to secure the airway, it is normally delivered by non-anesthesia personnel. Practice surveys in the UK have confirmed that a great deal of variation in personnel delivering care exists [12]. Non-utilisation of anesthesia physicians confers inherent economic benefit, as IVF is costly and mainly carried out in privately funded clinics. This must be balanced with consideration of patient safety, particularly in those with serious medical conditions such as obesity, obstructive sleep apnoea and cancer. The latter group are increasingly presenting for oocyte harvesting for use after cessation of chemotherapy. All of these patient groups should be attended to in larger centres with an available anesthetist.

According to the AOMRC's safe sedation practice guideline monitoring must be applied in all cases of conscious sedation. This includes an oxygen saturation probe and non-invasive blood pressure monitor set to cycle automatically. The use of electrocardiogram and available end tidal carbon dioxide monitoring are minimal standards. All drugs used for sedation have the danger of causing respiratory arrest and the AOMRC mandates assessment of verbal responsiveness of the patient throughout the procedure.

Intravenous Anesthesia

Propofol is the favoured drug for anesthetists for provision of conscious sedation. It is short acting, titratable to clinical effect, cost effective, and provides good hypnosis. It may be administered via a target controlled infusion (TCI) pump. Here the patient's age and weight are stored, and a target plasma concentration is chosen. Various pharmacokinetic models are incorporated into the infusion pump technology. This results in fewer interventions in dosing being required, and lends itself more easily to conscious sedation being delivered by non-anesthetists in one study [13]. Usually a second agent would be required for bolusing at the more stimulating parts of the procedure. Undesirable side-effects of propofol include respiratory depression with oxygen desaturation, airway obstruction requiring manipulation such as jaw thrust or airway insertion (more common in the obese), hypotension and some reduction in cardiac output. It has a narrow therapeutic index, and thus administration by personnel who are not confident in managing airway obstruction is not recommended. For this reason midazolam or diazepam are preferred by non-anesthetists. They are also chosen for their anxiolytic and amnesic effects. Benzodiazepines cause less cardiac instability than propofol. As with propofol, benzodiazepines may also cause respiratory depression and a resulting airway obstruction. Follicular fluid level ratios of 1:20 have been reported for midazolam and these low levels do not appear to impact on implantation or pregnancy rates [14]. The detection of drugs in ovarian follicular fluid is dependent on timing of administration.

Opioids are frequently co-administered with anxiolytics for the painful parts of the procedure, such as puncturing of the fornix by the aspirating needle for each ovary. Analgesia attenuates distress and movement of the patient at these crucial moments, thus lessening the chance of damaging adjacent organs, nerves and vessels. Common analgesic choices are; morphine, meperidine, fentanyl, alfentanyl and remifentanil- listed in order of decreasing length of duration of effect. No one agent has been shown to be superior over another with regard to successful pregnancy rate, or intra-operative or post-operative pain relief. Patients with obstructive sleep apnoea may be particularly susceptible to respiratory depression, hypercapnia and desaturation with opioids, and this class of drug should be used with extreme caution in this group.

The concentration of opioid agent in follicular fluid is small with follicular to plasma ratios of 1:10 for fentanyl [14]. Remifentanil is ultra-short acting, and is suitable to be given as a target controlled infusion, or in a patient controlled pump. Additional side effects of remifentanil include bradycardia, hypotension, apnoea and muscle rigidity. Other agents such as ketamine have also been used in low doses to supplement analgesia.

Spinal Anesthesia

Spinal anesthesia techniques are well described methods of providing analgesia for patients undergoing oocyte retrieval [15]. As these are ambulatory patients, delayed discharge, post dural puncture headache and radicular irritation or neurological syndrome with short-acting drugs such as lidocaine are unwanted side effects. Other risks with neuraxial techniques include hypotension with associated nausea and vomiting, delay in voiding post-procedure, nerve damage, haematoma, infection, insufficient anesthesia, and high spinal block with subsequent respiratory and/or cardiovascular collapse. Local anesthetic drugs in different doses and volumes can seek to provide sensory anesthesia to T10 with short acting agents such as lidocaine producing patients that are fit to ambulate after their short procedure. The use of neuraxial techniques necessitates oocyte retrieval being performed in a hospital setting with trained personnel present to administer the injection, monitor the result and assess the patient in recovery.

Commonly used drugs for spinal injection for IVF procedures include bupivacaine, lidocaine and mepivacaine. These local anesthetic agents may be combined with small doses of fentanyl to improve efficacy. While spinal anesthesia is successful epidural anesthesia has also been described for oocyte retrieval [16].

Para-Cervical Block

Gynaecologists may perform a para-cervical block (PCB) before commencement of the oocyte retrieval process. This typically involves injection of up to 150 mg of lidocaine at two to six sites around the cervix. Lower doses of 50 mgs have also been shown to be effective. This block anesthetises the vaginal mucosa, the uterosacral ligaments and also the peritoneal membrane involving the pouch of Douglas. Higher doses of lidocaine have been used, but there is no additional analgesic effect, and side effects become more common at higher doses [17]. Lidocaine has been found at varying amounts within the follicular fluid after PCB, but human studies have not shown a detrimental effect on cleavage rates, implantation numbers or live births [18]. PCBs can be used with conscious sedation to provide enhanced pain relief for patients.

Male Patients

IVF units may also provide services such as testicular biopsies for males with low sperm counts to isolate spermatozoa for fertilization. Anesthesiologists may be required to provide care for this group of patients. The commonest techniques are general anesthesia or sedation with local anesthesia including spermatic cord block and skin infiltration. Other block options are genitofemoral nerve block.

Conclusion

Anesthesia for Assisted Reproduction is an increasing activity for patients who have an increasing incidence of co- morbidity. Intravenous sedation or anesthesia is the most common technique for transvaginal oocyte retrieval, although other techniques including para-cervical block and neuraxial block are used. The potential impact of anesthesia technique on resulting embryos should be considered. However, no robust clinical evidence on any adverse effect of current anesthesia drugs on pregnancy outcome exists [19, 20].

References

1. Arulkumaran S, Collins S, Hayes K, Impey L, Jackson S. Oxford handbook of obstetrics and gynaecology. 3rd ed. Oxford Univ Press; 2013. ISBN-13:978019968400.
2. U.S. Department of Health and Human Services, Centers for Disease Control and Prevention, Division of Reproductive Health. 2013, Assisted Reproductive Technology (ART) Report. Atlanta: CDC. www.cdc.gov/art/.
3. Chapter 5. In vitro fertilisation and other assisted reproductive technology. In: Chestnut DH, Wong CA, Tsen LC, Ngan Kee WD, Beilin Y, Mhyre J. Chestnut's obstetric anesthesia: principles and practice. 5th ed. Elsevier. ISBN:9781455748662.
4. Tanbo T, Henriksen T, Magnus O, Abyholm T. Oocyte retrieval in an IVF program. A comparison of laparoscopic and vaginal ultrasound guided follicular puncture. Acta Obstet Gynecol Scand. 1988;67:243–6.
5. Kaye L, Sueldo C, Engmann L, Nulsen J, Benadiva C. Survey assessing obesity policies for assisted reproductive technology in the United States. Fertil Steril. 2016;105(3):703–6.
6. Kaupppila A, Leionenon P, Vihko R, et al. Metoclopramide-induced hyperprolactinaemia impairs ovarian follicle maturation and corpus luteum function in women. J Clin Endocrinol Metab. 1982;54:955–60.
7. Yogendran S, Asokumar B, Cheng DCH, Chung F. A prospective randomized double-blind study of the effect of intravenous fluid therapy on adverse outcomes on outpatient surgery. Anesth Analg. 1995;80:682–6.
8. Van der Weiden RM, Helmerhorst FM, Keirse MJ. Influence of prostaglandins and platelet activating factor on implantation. Hum Reprod. 1991;6:436–42.
9. NICE. Fertility: assessment and treatment for people with fertility problems. London: National Collaborating Centre for Women's and Children's Heath for the National Institute of Clinical Excellence; 2016. www.nice.org.uk/guidance/cg156. Accessed Feb 2016.
10. Safe sedation practice for Healthcare Procedures. Standards and Guidance. Academy of Royal Medical Colleges. 2013. www.aomrc.org.uk/index.php/publications/reports-a-guidance. Accessed Feb 2016.
11. Lok IH, Chan DL, Cheung LP, Haines CJ, Yeun PM. A prospective randomized trial comparing patient-controlled sedation using propofol and alfentanil and physician-administered sedation using diazepam and pethidine during transvaginal ultrasound-guided oocyte retrieval. Hum Reprod. 2002;17(8):2101–6.
12. Elkington NM, Kehoe J, Acharya U. Intravenous sedation in assisted conception units: a UK survey. Hum Fertil. 2003;6(2):74–6.
13. Edwards JA, Kinsella J, Shaw A, Evans S, Anderson KJ. Sedation for oocyte retrieval using target controlled infusion of propofol and incremental alfentanil delivered by non-anaesthetists. Anaesthesia. 2010;65:453–61.
14. Soussis I, Boyd O, Paraschos T, Duffy S, Bower S, Troughton P, et al. Follicular fluid levels of midazolam, fentanyl, and alfentanil during transvaginal oocyte retrieval. Fertil Steril. 1995;64(5):1003–7.
15. Tsen LT, Schultz R, Martin R, et al. Intrathecal low dose bupivacaine vs lidocaine for in vitro fertilization procedures. Reg Anesth Pain Med. 2001;26:52–6.
16. Kogosowski A, Lessing JB, Amit A, Rudick V, Peyser MR, David MP. Epidural block: a preferred method of anaesthesia for ultrasonically guided oocyte retrieval. Fertil Steril. 1987;47(1):166–8.
17. Ng EH, Miao B, Ho PC. A randomized double-blind study to compare the effectiveness of three different doses of lignocaine used in paracervical block during oocyte retrieval. J Assist Reprod Genet. 2003;20:8–12.
18. Wikland M, Evers H, Jakobsson AH, et al. The concentration of lidocaine in follicular fluid when used for paracervical block in a human IVF-ET programme. Hum Reprod. 1990;5:920–3.

19. Gonen O, Shulman A, Ghetler Y, Shapiro A, Judeiken R, Beyth Y, Ben-Nun I. The impact of different types of anesthesia on in vitro fertilization-embryo transfer treatment outcome. J Assist Reprod Genet. 1995;12(10):678–82.
20. Piroli A, Marci R, Marinangeli F, Paladini A, Di Emidio G, Giovanni Artini P, Caserta D, Tatone C. Comparison of different anaesthetic methodologies for sedation during in vitro fertilization procedures: effects on patient physiology and oocyte competence. Gynecol Endocrinol. 2012;28(10):796–9.

Chapter 27
Challenges of Performing Out of Operating Room Anesthesia on the Morbidly Obese

Mansoor M. Aman and Ashish C. Sinha

Abstract Out of operating room anesthesia continues to evolve as we see a change in the healthcare paradigm that once was process driven, to one that emphasizes measured outcomes. While providing anesthetic care outside the traditional operative can be advantageous for the patient, hospital, and physicians alike, it comes with numerous challenges that must be recognized and planned for. One of these concerns is the prevalence of morbid obesity in the patients we anesthetize in a suboptimal location. Body weight is commonly indirectly quantified using the body mass index (BMI), which is weight in kilograms divided by height in meters squared (kg/m^2). A patient is considered obese with a BMI of greater than 30 kg/m^2, and morbidly obese when the BMI is greater than 40 kg/m^2. The prevalence of morbid obesity in the United States over the last three decades has grown at an alarming rate, far greater than that of obesity. This chapter will provide a review of various prudent patient and procedural aspects involved in the delivery of a safe anesthetic care outside the operating room.

Keywords Obesity • Morbidly obese • Adipose • BMI • Endoscopy • Colonoscopy • ERCP • Bronchoscopy • Radiology • MRI • Obstructive sleep apnea • Sedation

Introduction

It is estimated that obesity affects one third of the United States population [1–3] and presents many unique concerns when preparing to deliver anesthetic care. Clinically, obesity is defined as an increase in body fat content that leads to an array of obesity associated comorbidities, and is most often indirectly quantified via the body mass index (BMI). This measurement serves a surrogate to the more accurate,

M.M. Aman, MD (✉) • A.C. Sinha, MD, PhD, DABA, MBA
Department of Anesthesiology and Perioperative Medicine,
Drexel University College of Medicine/Hahnemann University Hospital,
245 N. 15TH St, New College Building, MS 310, Philadelphia, PA 19102, USA
e-mail: mansoor.aman@drexelmed.edu; ashish.sinha@drexelmed.edu

© Springer International Publishing Switzerland 2017
B.G. Goudra, P.M. Singh (eds.), *Out of Operating Room Anesthesia*,
DOI 10.1007/978-3-319-39150-2_27

Table 27.1 Table stratifying co-morbidity risk based upon increasing BMI in male and females

	BMI (kg/m²)	Obesity class	Disease risk[a] relative to normal weight and waist circumference	
			Men 102 cm (40 in) or less Women 88 cm (35 in) or less	Men > 102 cm (40 in) Women > 88 cm (35 in)
Underweight	<18.5		–	–
Normal	18.5–24.9		–	–
Overweight	25.0–29.9		Increased	High
Obesity	30.0–34.9	I	High	Very high
	35.0–39.9	II	Very high	Very high
Morbid obesity	40.0[b]	III	Extremely high	Extremely high

Source: National Heart, Lung, and Blood Institute, National Institutes of Health
[a]Disease risk for type 2 diabetes, hypertension, and CVD
[b]Increased waist circumference also can be a marker for increased risk, even in persons of normal weight

yet tedious determination of body fat content. A BMI of greater than 30 kg/m² constitutes obesity and has many subsets as shown in (Table 27.1). Morbid obesity starts at a BMI of greater than 40 kg/m² and directly correlates with an increase in hypoxemia and all cause mortality in the perioperative period [4, 5]. The incidence and prevalence of morbid obesity is challenging to enumerate. Studies in the past have used various methods of collecting this data, with the most common being self- reporting tools with adjustments made for bias. Interestingly, between 1986 and 2000 the prevalence obesity doubled, while patients with reported BMI >40 kg/m² quadrupled, and those with a BMI >50 kg/m² quintupled [6]. Current data suggests that the incidence has decreased since 2005, but a staggering 15.5 million adult Americans are estimated to be morbidly obese [7]. Not only is morbid obesity deleterious to health, but also owing to its associated comorbidities imposes a great financial burden on the healthcare system [8].

While providing an anesthetic in a familiar operating room (OR) environment to morbidly obese patients is challenging enough, we are now increasingly required to anesthetize these patients outside of the OR for various procedures. Large portions of these cases are done under monitored anesthesia care, and the patients can range from clinically stable to critically ill [9]. Common out of OR locations are shown in Table 27.2. Performing procedures outside the traditional OR environment provides the benefit of quicker turn over time at a lower overhead cost. In other instances, these procedures are performed off-site due to specialized equipment, or patient needs. Surgeons, other proceduralists and post anesthesia care unit nurses alike, depend on the use of agents with quick onset, and offset in order to best utilize limited resources. Furthermore, this out of traditional OR model is less than optimized to handle any clinical crisis given limited support staff. This chapter will aim to present an in depth review of various challenges that can be anticipated, and prepared for, in order to ensure a safe anesthetic delivery to morbidly obese patients undergoing various procedures.

Table 27.2 Common locations for procedures outside the OR

Endoscopy suite
Gastroenterology procedures
Bronchoscopy
Cardiac lab
Electrophysiology
Catheterization lab
Radiology
CT/MRI
Neurointerventional and vascular
ICU
Tracheostomy, percutaneous gastrostomy
Various other procedural sedation

Patient Selection

Patient selection takes into consideration the extent of surgical stress, anesthetic concerns [10], and post-operative recovery. The procedure should have nominal expectant blood loss and minimal derangements in physiology. The American Society of Anesthesia (ASA) patient stratification score is often used when selecting patients for elective procedures in remote settings. ASA class 1 and 2 are considered safe to be performed, while class 3 is relatively safe if comorbid systemic diseases are well controlled. If at all possible, performing procedures on ASA classification four and five patients should be done in a well-equipped environment such as the OR. Unfortunately, the clinical decision-making is not always that simple. Clinical judgment must be exercised as the patient may require an urgent procedure in and out of OR setting. For example, you are asked to perform a bedside Esophagogastroduodenoscopy (EGD), and Colonoscopy in the Critical Care Unit for a patient with a BMI of 56 kg/m². Of note, his past medical history includes ischemic cardiomyopathy and he is status post a biventricular assist device 8 years ago. He now presents with hematochezia and hemoglobin of 6.4 g/dl. At the time of his BiVAD placement his BMI was 42 kg/m², meeting inclusion criteria. There are numerous challenges in this anesthetic. Is it safe to perform this bedside, outside of the operating room given associated risks with his obesity, and comorbidities? Should this patient receive a general anesthetic with an assisted airway in order to avoid obstruction, and hypoxemia? If over sedated bedside, are resources available to treat the expected drop in systemic vascular resistance and subsequent reduced pulse index on his BiVAD? There are numerous ways to perform this anesthetic, but it's important to identify such concerns in this high-risk patient population. Although obesity alone is not this patient's most concerning medical problem; the physiologic differences in this patient, compared to the normal BMI patient make him more susceptible to anesthetic induced morbidity.

Environment

The basic requirements of equipment and personnel resources, as defined by the ASA practice guidelines [11] for out of operating room anesthesia must be met for every procedure. The position of the patient should allow for quick access to the patient, have adequate lighting, sufficient power sources (and back up sources), gas supply, oxygen cylinders and hand resuscitation bags capable of 90% oxygen delivery. Access to emergency drugs and more personnel should be readily available. Monitoring should at minimum include oxygenation, ventilation, circulation and temperature. Airway equipment, suction, and emergency drugs should be readily available. Trained staff under the supervision of an Anesthesiologist should provide post anesthesia management.

Physiology in the Morbidly Obese

It is well established that excess adipose tissue increases the risk of metabolic syndrome (MetS), diabetes, cardiovascular disease, cancer, and premature death [12–16]. The presence of metabolic syndrome is implicated in the increased all-cause mortality seen in morbidly obese patients [17]. Broadly, MetS is characterized by an imbalance between glucose and insulin homeostasis, dyslipidemia, obesity (in particular abdominal fat distribution), and hypertension. The postulated pathogenesis of this condition takes into account possible genetic susceptibility, however living a sedentary lifestyle and obesity is widely accepted as the predominant contributing factors [18, 19]. Studies have identified a direct correlation between waist size and incidence of coronary artery disease, independent of morbid obesity. That is to say, a male that has a BMI of <30, with a waist of greater than 40 in. also is at risk of coronary artery disease (CAD). Body fat content, not BMI, is the primary determinant that leads to the cascade of physiologic changes commonly present in the morbidly obese population [20]. The high vascularity of fat creates an elevation in both cardiovascular and metabolic demand. Adipose tissue also serves as a powerhouse for numerous endocrine and paracrine cytokines that trigger physiologic change [21, 22]. Accelerated atherosclerosis, insulin resistance, alterations in lipid levels, coagulation, and elevation c-reactive protein (CRP) is all seen secondary to the various bioactive markers present in adipose tissue [23–25]. Many of these processes are reversible with optimization of diet, and weight loss. Given the physiologic changes that result from an elevated body fat content in combination with the limited mobility owing to an increase in musculoskeletal disorders [26], surgical intervention is often explored by these patients for weight loss.

Preoperative Assessment

As with any good anesthetic, it is crucial to obtain an in depth history and focused physical examination. If available, it is helpful to review past anesthetic records, as any concerning information gathered may lead to an alteration in the planned

Table 27.3 Table showing system based comorbidies associated with morbid obesity

Cardiovascular	Congestive heart failure, ischemic heart disease, atrial fibrillation, dysrhythmias
Endocrine	Diabetes Type II, metabolic syndrome, hypothyroidism
Respiratory	Pulmonary hypertension, OSA
Cancer	Endometrial cancer, esophageal adenocarcinoma
Musculoskeletal	Osteoarthritis, spondylolisthesis
Hepatic	NASH, cholelithiasis
Reproductive	Infertility

anesthetic. A detailed history must include an assessment of obstructive sleep apnea, cardiopulmonary and other common systemic diseased associated with morbid obesity (Table 27.3).

Obstructive Sleep Apnea

Morbid obesity has a direct correlation with obstructive sleep apnea (OSA) [27, 28], however this is often undiagnosed [29]. The diagnosis is made on polysomnography by measuring the apnea- hypopnea index (AHI)- a measure of complete cessation and partial obstructions during an hour of sleep. Each event must be at least 10 s in duration and accompanied by a desaturation as measured by pulse oximetry. OSA is considered to be mild with an AHI of 5–15, moderate if 15–30, and severe when >30. There is data to suggest that having moderate to severe OSA increases all cause mortality [3, 30]. It is prudent to have a high level of clinical suspicion when conducting the pre-anesthetic evaluation. When inquired, patients will report fatigue, daytime sleepiness, loud snoring and possibly witnessed apnea episodes by their family. Screening for OSA can quickly be performed using one of the many existing questionnaires including STOP-BANG [31, 32]. Non-invasive therapy for diagnosed patients consists of providing continuous positive airway pressure (CPAP) at night during sleep [33]. Current data available on the correlation between OSA and the rate of perioperative complication shows varying results [34–38]. It is still useful to know if the patient is being treated at home, and their settings for CPAP, which can be made available for the post operative course if needed. Once identified, it is important to strategize a plan that will optimize ventilation and oxygenation [39, 40].

Furthermore, the diagnosis of OSA carries with it additional criteria that must me met prior to discharge. The ASA practice guidelines on the perioperative management of patients with OSA, has set forth supplementary guidelines for discharge. They recommend that OSA patients should be:

- Monitored for 3 h longer compared to healthy patients
- Not have hypoxemic episodes or airway obstruction when left alone
- Return to their baseline oxygen saturation on room air
- Monitored for an additional 7 h after an episode of airway obstruction or hypoxemia while breathing room air in an un-stimulating environment.

Position

Morbidly obese patients have a lower threshold for desaturation due to dramatic changes in their physiologic reserves, increased oxygen consumption, and anatomical obstruction. Positioning the head of the bed at a 30° elevation helps maintain functional residual capacity (FRC) and limits redundant tissue from obstructing the airway [41]. If the patient is to be supine for the procedure, it is helpful to construct a ramp elevating the chest and allowing for better alignment of the oropharyngeal and laryngeal axis'. This is accomplished when the external auditory meatus is parallel with the level of the chest. It is advantageous to have the patient in lateral or prone position, as these positions are less associated with airway obstruction when compared to being supine [42].

Intravenous Access

Starting an intravenous line (IV) can be a laborious task in this patient population. Redundant adipose tissue often impairs direct visualization on commonly sought after cannulation sites such as the hands, forearms, and antecubital fossa. Tactile sensation sometimes used to find veins is also diminished for the same reason. Unfortunately, there is no secret strategy to better identifying veins. The method of applying heat using a warm towel to facilitate vasodilation of the vessel in question is helpful. If available, ultrasound can facilitate cannulation in the antecubital fossa, however its success is dependent on user proficiency. It is important to realize that when encountering this problem in a situation where image guidance is not available, more unconventional sites for IVs can be explored. A small 22–24-guage in the volar surface of the hand, fingers, abdomen and chest wall may suffice. Larger peripheral access is more easily obtained with the resultant vasodilatory effects of anesthetic agents. If an adequately functional peripheral IV cannot be obtained for the procedure, central access, with ultra sound guidance should be considered.

Airway

The airway assessment should focus on both the predictors of difficult mask ventilation and intubation. Morbidly obese patients by definition meet at least one of the predetermined risks for difficult ventilation, a $BMI > 26$ Kg/m^2. Other factors that are known to impede ventilation include age >55 years, edentulous, presence of a beard, and a history of snoring [43]. The sensitivity and specificity, if two factors are present is 72 % and 73 % respectively. Predictors of having a challenging laryngoscopy include having a history of difficult intubation, Mallampati 3–4 classification, short thyromental distance, inter-incisor gap of less than 3 cm, limited Atlanto-Occipital extension, limited mandibular protrusion, prominent incisors, or a high arched palate [44]. There is conflicting data regarding the correlation amongst elevated BMI and difficult/failed intubation [45, 46]. Traditionally, it has been taught to control a difficult or questionable airway at the start of the case in order to avoid complications during the procedure. When performing out of OR anesthesia, invariably all morbidly obese patients present with numerous risk factors identified above. The length of the procedure, need for paralysis, and patient specific concerns are often the driving variables whether to perform sedation or general anesthesia with a supraglottic or endotracheal airway.

General Anesthesia

Appropriate pre-oxygenation is of the utmost importance in these patients. It should be conducted in head up position (reverse Trendelenburg) to minimize the profound reduction in functional residual capacity that occurs in the supine position. Owning to a higher metabolic demand, obese patients have increased oxygen consumption per kg of body weight at approximately 4–6 ml/kg. An increase in airway resistance also makes these patients prone to quickly becoming hypoxemic. There may be some benefit in using low pressure CPAP while pre-oxygenating in effort to further reduce atelectasis [47]. Routine airway equipment such as oropharyngeal airways, and nasal trumpets must be available to assist with ventilation. Although an elevated BMI in itself is not a determinant of difficult laryngoscopy, it is advisable to have access to an intubating bougie, and video laryngoscopes should an unanticipated airway be encountered. While on mechanical ventilation, the use of vital capacity maneuvers in addition to positive end-expiratory pressure (PEEP) helps to improve oxygenation [48].

Sedation

When providing sedation in an out of OR setting, the guidelines for monitoring must be adhered to as outlined earlier. The depth of unconsciousness required varies by the procedure being performed. The patient should be kept spontaneously breathing, as entering deep sedation or general anesthesia without a protected airway increases the risk of complications resulting from hypoxia. The spectrum of sedation to general anesthesia is best examined by assessing patient response to verbal or painful stimuli, need for assistance with airway, ability to ventilate, and cardiovascular stability (Table 27.4).

Spectrum of Sedation

Table 27.4 Table showing spectrum of increasing sedation (Adapted from Practice Guidelines for Sedation and Analgesia by Non-Anesthesiologist, developed by American Society of Anesthesiologists)

	Minimal sedation (anxiolysis)	Moderate sedation/analgesia (conscious sedation)	Deep sedation/ analgesia	General anesthesia
Responsiveness	Normal response to verbal stimulation	Purposeful[a] response to verbal or tactile stimulation	Purposeful[a] response after repeated or painful stimulation	Unarousable, even with painful stimulus
Airway	Unaffected	No intervention required	Intervention may be required	Intervention often required
Spontaneous ventilation	Unaffected	Adequate	May be inadequate	Frequently inadequate
Cardiovascular function	Unaffected	Usually maintained	Usually maintained	May be impaired

With permission Wolters Kluwer Health, Inc, American Society of Anesthesiologists Task Force on Sedation and Analgesia by Non-Anesthesiologists [67], Table 1

Minimal Sedation (Anxiolysis) = a drug-induced state during which patients respond normally to verbal commands. Although cognitive function and coordination may be impaired, ventilatory and cardiovascular functions are unaffected

Moderate Sedation/Analgesia (Conscious Sedation) = a drug-induced depression of consciousness during which patients respond purposefully[a] to verbal commands, either alone or accompanied by light tactile stimulation. No interventions are required to maintain a patent airway, and spontaneous ventilation is adequate. Cardiovascular function is usually maintained

Deep Sedation/Analgesia = a drug-induced depression of consciousness during which patients cannot be easily aroused but respond purposefully[a] following repeated or painful stimulation. The ability to independently maintain ventilatory function may be impaired. Patients may require assistance in maintaining a patent airway, and spontaneous ventilation may be inadequate. Cardiovascular function is usually maintained

General Anesthesia = a drug-induced loss of consciousness during which patients are not arousable, even by painful stimulation. The ability to independently maintain ventilatory function is often impaired. Patients often require assistance in maintaining a patent airway, and positive pressure ventilation may be required because of depressed spontaneous ventilation or drug-induced depression of neuromuscular function. Cardiovascular function may be impaired

Because sedation is a continuum, it is not always possible to predict how an individual patient will respond. Hence, practitioners intending to produce a given level of sedation should be able to rescue patients whose level of sedation becomes deeper than initially intended. Individuals administering *Moderate Sedation/Analgesia (Conscious Sedation)* should be able to rescue patients who enter a state of *Deep Sedation/Analgesia,* while those administering *Deep Sedation/Analgesia* Should be able to rescue patients who enter a state of general anesthesia

Developed by the American Society of Anesthesiologists; approved by the ASA House of Delegates October 13, 1999

[a]Reflex withdrawal from a painful stimulus is not considered a purposeful response

Gastroenterology Suite

The use of monitored anesthesia care has seen a rapid rise over the years in the ambulatory setting [49]. The ASA closed claims database identified that out of OR anesthesia care is associated with increased morbidity when compared to closed claims examined for anesthetics delivered in the OR [50]. A large proportion of these were related to over sedation and inadequate oxygenation/ventilation in the GI suite [51].

EGD-Esophagogastroduodenoscopy

The combination of a shared airway, increased risk of aspiration, need for spontaneous ventilation, and ability to safely turnover dozens of cases a day are some of the concerns in the GI suite. The later is the primary reason why Gastroenterologists prefer anesthesia providers monitor sedation. Procedural sedation was routinely delivered by nurses under the supervision of the gastroenterologist, with the drug of choice being Midazolam and Fentanyl. However the synergistic effects of benzodiazepine's and opioids was shown to prolong recovery and reduce efficiency in the GI suite. This combination must be used with caution in morbidly obese patients with OSA as it can quickly compromise the airway. For similar reasons, Propofol has found its way as being the drug of choice due to its fast onset and rapid redistribution [52]. Careful weight adjusted titration is essential, as morbidly obese patients can easily become apneic and hypoxemic with Propofol sedation as well. Many providers prefer to use small boluses throughout the procedure while others maintain an infusion. There is no evidence to suggest one is superior to the other in the morbidly obese patients. The bolus technique offers the advantage of providing depth during the stimulating insertion of the scope, while allowing for lighter sedation throughout in effort to limit airway obstruction. The routine use of capnography during upper endoscopy can help recognize and limit these events [53]. The use of innovative advanced airways that serve as a bite block for insertion of the endoscope and allow for oxygenation, and end tidal monitoring show promise in the world of off-site anesthesia. Another technique we suggest is the insertion of a nasal trumpet with CPAP after achieving adequate depth to suppress the gag reflex. CPAP can be maintained throughout the procedure to improve ventilation [54].

Colonoscopy

Over the last few decades there has been an increased effort in patient education on primary prevention of colon cancer. Subsequently, we see a dramatic rise in the number of colonoscopies being performed annually. These procedures are less challenging given the airway is not stimulated and the patient is usually in lateral decubitus. Should over sedation become a concern, a simple chin lift or jaw thrust might suffice. Further basic airway management techniques such an insertion of an oropharyngeal airway, nasal trumpet, with a facemask might improve oxygenation/ventilation. The implementation of CPAP is also useful. Among available benzodiazepines, midazolam is the most commonly used in the GI suite. While it is effective in inducing sedation, it comes with its disadvantages- it does not provide analgesia, and has a profoundly longer residual effect than procedure duration. Furthermore, in patients with renal impairment the predictability of sedation duration is reduced due to its active metabolite [55].

Blunting noxious stimuli with narcotics during midazolam sedation can lead to inadequate ventilation. This has led to the development of newer agents that are currently being studied for their efficacy and safety during GI procedures. Remimazolam is an ultra short acting analgesic/sedative agent currently in Phase III trials. Metabolism via ester hydrolysis offers the advantage of quick offset between 10 and 20 min at a sedative dose of 0.10–0.20 mg/kg [56].

Endoscopic Retrograde Cholangiopancreatography (ERCP)

The decision to intubate versus sedate high-risk patients, for a moderate-risk procedure in a prone or semi-prone position still remains a topic of great debate within the anesthesia community. Although gastroenterologists do not require intubation and paralysis for the procedure, concerns about emergently needing to flip from prone to supine in order to secure the airway in an obese patient is worrisome. The morbidity with ERCP has been reported at 6.85 % with a mortality of 0.33 %[57]. Current data suggests that the preoperative ASA status, a high Malampatti score, nor elevated BMI correlate with the risk of desaturation during an ERCP [58]. The emphasis remains on optimizing ventilation, titrating drugs to effect and vigilant patient monitoring by an anesthesia provider. The art of sedation is one that is mastered with repetition. A study examined the difference amongst 1167 cases supervised by anesthesiologist who were routinely in the GI suite, versus anesthesiologists who cared for patients in GI on an ad hoc basis. It was found that the overall mean anesthesia time was 24.82 ± 12.96 versus 48.63 ± 21.53 min in each group respectively. The rates of intubation were significantly lower in the regular anesthesiologist group 0.76 % vs. 12.8 % in the ad hoc. It was further deduced that a potential

$758,536 USD would have been saved on GI suite time alone, in just this one institution, had there been an anesthesiologists from the first group doing all the cases [59]. Although an experienced provider can safely sedate patients that are morbidly obese, the decision to intubate should still be done on a case-by-case basis exercising good clinical judgment. Should the patient be left prone with an unsecured airway, the use of a Mapleson C circuit delivering higher inspired fraction of oxygen may limit hypoxemia [60] (Figs. 27.1 and 27.2).

Bronchoscopy

Bronchoscopy is increasingly used as both a diagnostic and therapeutic intervention for various conditions and has a favorable safety profile [61]. Constant bronchoscopic stimulation of the airway in conjunction with the need for akinesia are two important considerations during this anesthetic. While neuromuscular blocking agents may be utilized in combination with endotracheal intubation for certain procedures, it is less than ideal given the short duration. When targeting disease in the tracheo-broncheal tree with rigid bronchoscopy, either deep sedation or general anesthesia is warranted. Performing deep sedation on a morbidly obese patient with airway instrumentation puts that patient at high risk of hypoventilation, hypoxemia, and subsequent acidosis. Various maintenance techniques have been described to achieve an adequate depth mitigating the risk of laryngospasm and optimizing procedural conditions. Total intravenous anesthesia (TIVA) with combinations of medications such as Propofol-Remifentanil, Propofol- Dexmedetomidine, and Propofol-Midazolam are commonly used. Ventilation may be controlled, spontaneous-assisted, apneic oxygenation, manual jet, or high frequency jet [62]. Studies examining the differences between various anesthetics take into consideration oxygen saturation, level of sedation, effect on mean arterial pressure, suppression of gag reflex and cough, patient and provider satisfaction, and recovery time. Finding the perfect balance of all said factors is hard to achieve. While Dexmedetomidine is associated with less respiratory depression, it has a longer recovery time when compared to Remifentanil [63]. Unfortunately, there isn't strong data comparing anesthetic efficacy during this procedure specifically in morbidly obese patients. Our recommendation is to take into consideration the physiological changes in these high-risk patients and use agents that have minimal or short-lived effects on respiratory drive. Remifentanil is a mu receptor antagonist that is degraded by plasma cholinesterase, with a half-life of 4 min that is ideal for bronchoscopy in conjunction with Propofol [64]. The optimal dosages of Remifentanil are yet to be determined, however we suggests high dose 0.26–0.5 µg/kg/min to minimize coughing and laryngospasm [65]. The airway may be managed using a supraglottic airway device like an laryngeal mask airway, which can also serves as a conduit for bronchoscope insertion.

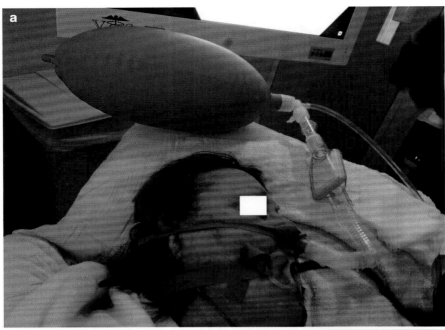

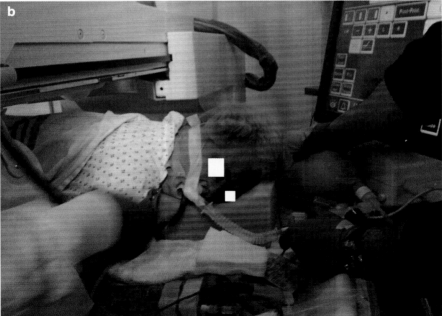

Fig. 27.1 (**a**) A nasal trumpet placed in the nose and connected to a Mapelson C breathing system with an elective endotracheal intubation (ETT) adapter. (**b**) A nasal trumpet placed in the nose and connected to a Mapelson C breathing system, bag squeezed to assist. Goudra, B. ERCP: The Unresolved question of Endotracheal Intubation

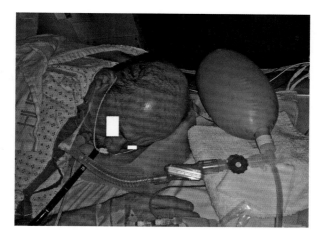

Fig. 27.2 A nasal trumpet placed in the mouth and connected to a Mapelon C breathing system with an ETT adapter

Table 27.5 Table showing cardiac procedures performed under sedation

Diagnostic angiography
Percutaneous trans-luminal coronary angioplasty (PTCA) and stenting
Valvuloplasty
Percutaneous trans-luminal rotational atherectomy (PTRA)
Trans-esophageal echocardiogram
Catheter ablation
Permanent pacemaker, lead extractions
Internal cardioverter defibrillator

Cardiac Procedures

A multitude of procedures are performed in modern cardiac catheterization laboratories that warrant assistance from an anesthesia provider. Monitored Anesthesia Care (MAC) or general anesthesia is required when there is concern for patient intolerance due to length of procedure, painful stimuli, or concern for airway compromise such as trans-esophageal echocardiogram (TEE). Common procedures are highlighted in Table 27.5. Patient specific factors of the morbidly obese all remain the same, and the anesthetic must be tailored to the procedural conditions that are required, and associated cardiovascular disease. For example a short TEE might be performed with Propofol bolus and nasal CPAP for assistance with ventilation. High-risk procedures such as lead extractions of infected pacemaker leads that were placed many years ago have the potential of becoming 'open' cases. Given the potential of becoming a cardiopulmonary bypass case, the airway is secured at the start of the case in a controlled setting and inhalational vs. TIVA is used for maintenance.

Radiology

The decision to involve an Anesthesia provider during Radiology procedures is based on numerous factors including procedure, patient compliance, and patient tolerance. It is common for nurses to administer minimal procedural sedation under the supervision of the Radiologist for interventional procedures. When preparing for an anesthetic in Radiology, the concerns of morbid obesity remain the same as highlighted in sections prior. However, unique factors in this setting stem from patient accessibility and procedure specific emergency preparedness. Monitoring from a distance via tele-monitors has become the mainstay for MRI. In order to avoid securing a difficult airway with multiple challenges including positioning an induction room is often utilized.

If general anesthesia is being induced for MRI, safety recommendations from the ASA as detailed in the Practice Advisory on Anesthetic Care for Magnetic Resonance Imaging [66] should be diligently followed. Most institutions have MRI Zones I–IV, where zone one delineates free accessibility to the general public and zones three and four are secure zones with risk of injury from ferromagnetic objects. An induction room that allows for ease of access to the patients airway and emergency equipment readily available is often used to induce general anesthesia after which the patient is transferred to Zones III–IV. Risk of injury is mitigated with the use of MRI safe equipment, and well-planned anesthetics. Although the procedure may not mandate a general anesthetic, it is important to factor in the potential for airway compromise as it relates to patient accessibility, interruption of the scan, and safety concerns with personnel emergently entering zones III–IV. For these reasons, a general anesthetic with an LMA or ETT may be warranted in morbidly obese patients in this setting.

References

1. Ogden CL, et al. Prevalence of obesity among adults: United States, 2011–2012. NCHS Data Brief. 2013;(131):1–8.
2. Ogden CL, et al. Prevalence of childhood and adult obesity in the United States, 2011–2012. JAMA. 2014;311(8):806–14.
3. Marshall NS, et al. Sleep apnea as an independent risk factor for all-cause mortality: the Busselton Health Study. Sleep. 2008;31(8):1079–85.
4. Adams KF, et al. Overweight, obesity, and mortality in a large prospective cohort of persons 50 to 71 years old. N Engl J Med. 2006;355(8):763–78.
5. Hensrud DD, Klein S. Extreme obesity: a new medical crisis in the United States. Mayo Clin Proc. 2006;81(10 Suppl):S5–10.
6. Sturm R. Increases in clinically severe obesity in the United States, 1986–2000. Arch Intern Med. 2003;163(18):2146–8.
7. Sturm R, Hattori A. Morbid obesity rates continue to rise rapidly in the United States. Int J Obes (Lond). 2013;37(6):889–91.
8. Finkelstein EA, et al. Annual medical spending attributable to obesity: payer-and service-specific estimates. Health Aff (Millwood). 2009;28(5):w822–31.

9. Metzner J, Posner KL, Domino KB. The risk and safety of anesthesia at remote locations: the US closed claims analysis. Curr Opin Anaesthesiol. 2009;22(4):502–8.
10. Joshi GP, et al. Society for Ambulatory Anesthesia consensus statement on preoperative selection of adult patients with obstructive sleep apnea scheduled for ambulatory surgery. Anesth Analg. 2012;115(5):1060–8.
11. Anesthesiologists ASo. Statement on non-operating room anesthetizing locations. Available from: http://www.asahq.org/quality-and-practice-management/standards-and-guidelines.
12. Lau DC, et al. Adipokines: molecular links between obesity and atheroslcerosis. Am J Physiol Heart Circ Physiol. 2005;288(5):H2031–41.
13. Lundgren CH, et al. Elaboration of type-1 plasminogen activator inhibitor from adipocytes. A potential pathogenetic link between obesity and cardiovascular disease. Circulation. 1996;93(1):106–10.
14. Neligan PJ. Metabolic syndrome: anesthesia for morbid obesity. Curr Opin Anaesthesiol. 2010;23(3):375–83.
15. Wajchenberg BL. Subcutaneous and visceral adipose tissue: their relation to the metabolic syndrome. Endocr Rev. 2000;21(6):697–738.
16. Kopelman P. Health risks associated with overweight and obesity. Obes Rev. 2007;8 Suppl 1:13–7.
17. Lakka HM, et al. The metabolic syndrome and total and cardiovascular disease mortality in middle-aged men. JAMA. 2002;288(21):2709–16.
18. Liese AD, Mayer-Davis EJ, Haffner SM. Development of the multiple metabolic syndrome: an epidemiologic perspective. Epidemiol Rev. 1998;20(2):157–72.
19. Bouchard C. Genetics and the metabolic syndrome. Int J Obes Relat Metab Disord. 1995;19 Suppl 1:S52–9.
20. Poirier P, et al. Obesity and cardiovascular disease: pathophysiology, evaluation, and effect of weight loss: an update of the 1997 American Heart Association Scientific Statement on Obesity and Heart Disease from the Obesity Committee of the Council on Nutrition, Physical Activity, and Metabolism. Circulation. 2006;113(6):898–918.
21. Kong AP, Chan NN, Chan JC. The role of adipocytokines and neurohormonal dysregulation in metabolic syndrome. Curr Diabetes Rev. 2006;2(4):397–407.
22. Steppan CM, et al. The hormone resistin links obesity to diabetes. Nature. 2001; 409(6818):307–12.
23. Hotamisligil GS, et al. Increased adipose tissue expression of tumor necrosis factor-alpha in human obesity and insulin resistance. J Clin Invest. 1995;95(5):2409–15.
24. Kern PA, et al. The expression of tumor necrosis factor in human adipose tissue. Regulation by obesity, weight loss, and relationship to lipoprotein lipase. J Clin Invest. 1995;95(5):2111–9.
25. Yudkin JS, et al. C-reactive protein in healthy subjects: associations with obesity, insulin resistance, and endothelial dysfunction: a potential role for cytokines originating from adipose tissue? Arterioscler Thromb Vasc Biol. 1999;19(4):972–8.
26. Wearing SC, et al. Musculoskeletal disorders associated with obesity: a biomechanical perspective. Obes Rev. 2006;7(3):239–50.
27. Grunstein R, et al. Snoring and sleep apnoea in men: association with central obesity and hypertension. Int J Obes Relat Metab Disord. 1993;17(9):533–40.
28. Alam I, et al. Obesity, metabolic syndrome and sleep apnoea: all pro-inflammatory states. Obes Rev. 2007;8(2):119–27.
29. Kaw R, et al. Unrecognized sleep apnea in the surgical patient: implications for the perioperative setting. Chest. 2006;129(1):198–205.
30. Young T, et al. Sleep disordered breathing and mortality: eighteen-year follow-up of the Wisconsin sleep cohort. Sleep. 2008;31(8):1071–8.
31. Chung F, et al. High STOP-Bang score indicates a high probability of obstructive sleep apnoea. Br J Anaesth. 2012;108(5):768–75.
32. Chung F, et al. Validation of the Berlin questionnaire and American Society of Anesthesiologists checklist as screening tools for obstructive sleep apnea in surgical patients. Anesthesiology. 2008;108(5):822–30.

33. Balk EM, et al. AHRQ comparative effectiveness reviews, in diagnosis and treatment of obstructive sleep apnea in adults. Rockville: Agency for Healthcare Research and Quality (US); 2011.
34. Kaw R, et al. Incremental risk of obstructive sleep apnea on cardiac surgical outcomes. J Cardiovasc Surg (Torino). 2006;47(6):683–9.
35. Gupta RM, et al. Postoperative complications in patients with obstructive sleep apnea syndrome undergoing hip or knee replacement: a case–control study. Mayo Clin Proc. 2001;76(9):897–905.
36. Gaddam S, Gunukula SK, Mador MJ. Post-gastrointestinal endoscopy complications in patients with obstructive sleep apnea or at high risk for sleep apnea: a systematic review and meta-analysis. Sleep Breath. 2015;20:155–66.
37. Stundner O, et al. Sleep apnoea adversely affects the outcome in patients who undergo posterior lumbar fusion. Bone Joint J. 2014;96-B(2):242–8.
38. Gaddam S, Gunukula SK, Mador MJ. Post-operative outcomes in adult obstructive sleep apnea patients undergoing non-upper airway surgery: a systematic review and meta-analysis. Sleep Breath. 2014;18(3):615–33.
39. American Society of Anesthesiologists Task Force on Perioperative Management of patients with obstructive sleep apnea. Practice guidelines for the perioperative management of patients with obstructive sleep apnea: an updated report by the American Society of Anesthesiologists Task Force on Perioperative Management of patients with obstructive sleep apnea. Anesthesiology. 2014;120(2):268–86.
40. Gross JB, et al. Practice guidelines for the perioperative management of patients with obstructive sleep apnea: a report by the American Society of Anesthesiologists Task Force on Perioperative Management of patients with obstructive sleep apnea. Anesthesiology. 2006;104(5):1081–93; quiz 1117–8.
41. Adesanya AO, et al. Perioperative management of obstructive sleep apnea. Chest. 2010; 138(6):1489–98.
42. Aldenkortt M, et al. Ventilation strategies in obese patients undergoing surgery: a quantitative systematic review and meta-analysis. Br J Anaesth. 2012;109(4):493–502.
43. Langeron O, et al. Prediction of difficult mask ventilation. Anesthesiology. 2000;92(5): 1229–36.
44. Mallampati SR, et al. A clinical sign to predict difficult tracheal intubation: a prospective study. Can Anaesth Soc J. 1985;32(4):429–34.
45. De Jong A, et al. Difficult intubation in obese patients: incidence, risk factors, and complications in the operating theatre and in intensive care units. Br J Anaesth. 2015;114(2):297–306.
46. Murphy C, Wong DT. Airway management and oxygenation in obese patients. Can J Anaesth. 2013;60(9):929–45.
47. Harbut P, et al. Continuous positive airway pressure/pressure support pre-oxygenation of morbidly obese patients. Acta Anaesthesiol Scand. 2014;58(6):675–80.
48. Chalhoub V, et al. Effect of vital capacity manoeuvres on arterial oxygenation in morbidly obese patients undergoing open bariatric surgery. Eur J Anaesthesiol. 2007;24(3):283–8.
49. Bayman EO, et al. National incidence of use of monitored anesthesia care. Anesth Analg. 2011;113(1):165–9.
50. Robbertze R, Posner KL, Domino KB. Closed claims review of anesthesia for procedures outside the operating room. Curr Opin Anaesthesiol. 2006;19(4):436–42.
51. Bhananker SM, et al. Injury and liability associated with monitored anesthesia care: a closed claims analysis. Anesthesiology. 2006;104(2):228–34.
52. Lamperti M. Adult procedural sedation: an update. Curr Opin Anaesthesiol. 2015;28:662–7.
53. Prathanvanich P, Chand B. The role of capnography during upper endoscopy in morbidly obese patients: a prospective study. Surg Obes Relat Dis. 2015;11(1):193–8.
54. Goudra BG, et al. Significantly reduced hypoxemic events in morbidly obese patients undergoing gastrointestinal endoscopy: predictors and practice effect. J Anaesthesiol Clin Pharmacol. 2014;30(1):71–7.

55. Nordt SP, Clark RF. Midazolam: a review of therapeutic uses and toxicity. J Emerg Med. 1997;15(3):357–65.
56. Pambianco DJ, et al. A phase IIb study comparing the safety and efficacy of remimazolam and midazolam in patients undergoing colonoscopy. Gastrointest Endosc. 2016;83(5):984–92.
57. Andriulli A, et al. Incidence rates of post-ERCP complications: a systematic survey of prospective studies. Am J Gastroenterol. 2007;102(8):1781–8.
58. Goudra BG, Singh PM, Sinha AC. Outpatient endoscopic retrograde cholangiopancreatography: safety and efficacy of anesthetic management with a natural airway in 653 consecutive procedures. Saudi J Anaesth. 2013;7(3):259–65.
59. Goudra BG, Singh PM, Sinha AC. Anesthesia for ERCP: impact of anesthesiologist's experience on outcome and cost. Anesthesiol Res Pract. 2013;2013:570518.
60. Goudra B, Singh PM. ERCP: the unresolved question of endotracheal intubation. Dig Dis Sci. 2014;59(3):513–9.
61. Facciolongo N, et al. Incidence of complications in bronchoscopy. Multicentre prospective study of 20,986 bronchoscopies. Monaldi Arch Chest Dis. 2009;71(1):8–14.
62. Pathak V, et al. Ventilation and anesthetic approaches for rigid bronchoscopy. Ann Am Thorac Soc. 2014;11(4):628–34.
63. Ryu JH, et al. Randomized double-blind study of remifentanil and dexmedetomidine for flexible bronchoscopy. Br J Anaesth. 2012;108(3):503–11.
64. Natalini G, et al. Remifentanil vs. fentanyl during interventional rigid bronchoscopy under general anaesthesia and spontaneous assisted ventilation. Eur J Anaesthesiol. 1999; 16(9):605–9.
65. Goudra BG, et al. Effectiveness of high dose remifentanil in preventing coughing and laryngospasm in non-paralyzed patients for advanced bronchoscopic procedures. Ann Thorac Med. 2014;9(1):23–8.
66. Practice advisory on anesthetic care for magnetic resonance imaging: an updated report by the American Society of Anesthesiologists Task Force on anesthetic care for magnetic resonance imaging. Anesthesiology. 2015;122(3):495–520.
67. American Society of Anesthesiologists Task Force on Sedation and Analgesia by Non-Anesthesiologists. Practice guidelines for sedation and analgesia by non-anesthesiologists. Anesthesiology. 2002;96(4):1004–17.

Part VIII
Future and Controversies

Chapter 28
Sedation for Gastrointestinal Endoscopy: Gastroenterologists Perspective

Andrea Riphaus and Till Wehrmann

Abstract Over the past decade the interest in sedation for gastrointestinal endoscopy has increased worldwide.

A logical consequence was the subsequent development of national guidelines to increase patients safety [1–3]. Comparing the current survey results for sedation from different countries [4–8] with older surveys, shows a significant increase in sedation frequency and the use of ultra – short-acting propofol However, sedation for endoscopy is still the subject of many discussions, which are in part controversial.

One major aspect is the exact indication for sedation, as is not necessary for all gastroenterological endoscopic interventions. Whether sedation is required, depends on the type of examination, duration, complexity, invasiveness, as well as the individual patient's characteristics. However, sedation can make the examination more comfortable for the patient as well as the examining physician. Often it is sedation that makes a successful and low risk examination possible. This is true especially for complex therapeutic interventions [1]. Patients safety as the main goal was the primary concern of the development latest published and updated international guidelines [1, 2]. While in some countries sedation might only be performed by anesthesiologists, sedation by non-anesthesiologist physicians (i.e., gastroenterologists) or a well-trained nursing staff became the standard procedure in low risk patients undergoing gastrointestinal endoscopy [1, 2]. This article provides an overview on patients best preparation, including individual risk stratification, currently most common used sedatives (especially under consideration of the increasingly employed short-acting propofol). In addition, personal and personnel-requirements, as well as technical requirements needed for sedation in gastrointestinal endoscopy are summarized.

A. Riphaus, MD, PhD (✉)
Department of Medicine, KRH Klinikum Agnes Karll Laatzen,
Hildesheimer Strasse 158, Hannover 30880, Germany
e-mail: ariphaus@web.de

T. Wehrmann, MD, PhD
Department of Gastroenterology, DKD Helios Klinik Wiesbaden,
Aukammallee 33, Wiesbaden 65191, Germany
e-mail: till.wehrmann@helios-kliniken.de

© Springer International Publishing Switzerland 2017   389
B.G. Goudra, P.M. Singh (eds.), *Out of Operating Room Anesthesia*,
DOI 10.1007/978-3-319-39150-2_28

Keywords Endoscopy • Sedation • Propofol • Benzodiazepines • Non-anesthesiologist-administered – propofol sedation (NAAP) • Nurse-administered propofol sedation (NAPS) • Monitoring • Discharge

Preparation and Pre-endoscopic Risk Assessment

Sedatives and analgesics might induce overlapping sedation states, ranging from minimal sedation (so called anxiolysis) to general anesthesia [9] (Table 28.1). Therefore, the individual cardio-respiratory risk assessment needs to be carried for any patient [1, 2]. It should include a detailed history asking for the following aspects [1, 2]:

1. Diseases of the cardiovascular and respiratory system,
2. Stridor, snoring, sleep apnea syndrome
3. Complications on previous occasions when sedatives/analgesics, regional and/or general anesthesia were administered
4. Drug allergies, current medication, and possible drug interactions
5. Most recent meal: when and what was eaten
6. Tobacco, alcohol, drug consumption

Table 28.1 Stages of sedation

	Minimal (anxiolysis)	Moderate	Deep	Anesthesia
Reaction to being addressed	Patient reacts appropriately to verbal commands	Somnolence, reaction to louder commands with additional tactile stimulation if necessary	Somnolence, hard to wake, purposeful response after repeated or painful stimulation	Patient cannot be woken, not even in response to pain stimuli
Spontaneous breathing	Not influenced	Adequate	The ability to independently maintain ventilatory function may be impaired. Patients may require assistance in maintaining a patent airway. Spontaneous ventilation may be inadequate.	Inadequate, ITN or larynx mask necessary

Modified from the American Society of Anesthesiologists [9]

Also a physical examination should be performed including vital signs and auscultation of heart and lung to indent potential cardio-respiratory problems that might occur during the procedure. A generally related classification is represented by the so-called ASA classification [9] (Table 28.2). Patients in ASA-class III or higher are known to have an increase risk due to sedation for gastrointestinal procedures. In addition, anatomical features are taken into account. A restricted mouth opening (classified according to the Mallampati score) might complicate the management of respiratory complications [1–3]. Such high risk patients are not suitable for sedation by trained nurses. In this situation one should consider to consult an anesthesiologist [1–3]. It is obligatory to provide appropriate emergency medicines and equipment such as defibrillator, equipment for airway management (bag-mask ventilation, endotracheal intubation) etc. [1–3]. Of course, should the endoscopy team also be familiar with the technique of cardiopulmonary resuscitation, refreshing it regularly as part of structured simulator courses [1–3].

Latest guidelines [1, 2] recommend a routine oxygen administration via a nasal cannula (for example with 2–3 l/min). This is based on the knowledge of the increased occurrence of hypoxemia, particularly at interventional or longer lasting procedures or in patients with high co-morbidity, pulmonary impairment or with circulatory depression (e.g., emergency cases). The administration of oxygen starting at least 2 min before the examination can significantly reduce the frequency of severe hypoxia during the endoscopic procedure [1]. If there is a pronounced hypercapnia, such as COPD, the oxygen supply must also be individually adjusted in order not to reduce the respiratory drive (by excessive O2 supplementation) [1]. The guideline of the American gastroenterologists [3] does not recommend routine prophylactic administration of oxygen. Reason is the feared delay the detection of hypoxia. However, the majority of anesthesiologists believe that the benefits of pre-oxygenation outweigh this disadvantage [1, 2].

Intra-endoscopic Monitoring

Since the transitions between the various stages of sedation (Table 28.3) are fluid, an appropriate patient monitoring is required for all patients by an independent appropriately trained person not involved in the endoscopic procedure [1–3]. The person in charge of monitoring *clinically* checks breathing by observation, palpation of thorax and abdominal wall movement, and possibly palpation of expiratory airstream.

Grade I	Healthy individual
Grade II	Mild disease, not limiting daily activities
Grade III	Severe disease, limiting daily activities
Grade IV	Severe disease, life-threatening

Table 28.2 ASA classification

Table 28.3 Guideline recommendations for sedation with propofol

Guideline, year	NAPS allowed	Limitations for NAPS	Indication for MAC
SAGES, 2009	n.a.	n.a.	ASA > III
ASGE, 2008	Yes (monitored by the doctor)	n.a.	ASA ≥ III, Emergency and complex procedures, in cases of airway difficulties
AGA, 2007	Yes	n.a.	ASA > III, high-risk patients, complex procedures
GSDMD, 2009	Yes	ASA > II, complex procedures, in cases of airway difficulties	ASA ≥ III **and** complex procedures **or** cases of airway difficulties
CAG, 2008	Yes	None	ASA ≥ III, complex procedures, in cases of airway difficulties
ASGH, 2007	Yes	None	n.a
SSGE, 2006	Yes	Complex procedures	ASA ≥ III and deep sedation. Expected difficult airway management

SAGES Society of American Gastrointestinal and Endoscopic Surgeons, *ASGE* American Society of Gastrointestinal Endoscopy, *AGA* American Gastroenterological Association, *GSDMD* German Society for Digestive and Metabolic Diseases, *CAG* Canadian Association of Gastroenterology, *ASGH* Austrian Society of Gastroenterology and Hepatology, *SSGE* Spanish Society of Gastrointestinal Endoscopy, *NAPS* Nurse administered propofol sedation, *ASA* American Society of Anesthesiologists, *MAC* Monitored anesthesia care

Standard-Monitoring recommended by different international societies includes continuous pulse oximetry and automated noninvasive blood pressure measurement (at baseline and then at 3–5-min intervals) during both NAAP and the recovery period; continuous electrocardiography is recommended in selected patients with a history of cardiac and/or pulmonary disease. Baseline, minimum and maximum heart rate/blood pressure, as well as baseline and minimum oxygen blood saturation should be recorded [1–3].

Principal Options for Sedation

Benzodiazepines

Diazepam is nowadays used very rarely because of its long half-life of 25–30 h, according to a first survey in Germany its application was stated only by around 8 % of respondents [5]. In contrast, about 80 % of respondents use midazolam [5]. Its pharmacological advantages are a shorter half-life (1,5–3 h), a better retrograde amnesia and a higher water solubility. Compared to diazepam patient tolerance and sedation efficiency are consistently well [1]. A combination of benzodiazepines and opioids (predominantly midazolam plus meperidine) was used in about one third of all gastroenterologist for colonoscopy [5]. The use in diagnostic endoscopy of the upper digestive tract (e.g., diagnostic EUS), however, is considered obsolete [5]. The advantage of a combination of benzodiazepines and opioids at endoscopy is highly controversial and can be seen rather negatively according to recent data [1, 2].

Propofol: The New Standard

Prerequisites

With respect to the introduction of the short-acting propofol (plasma half-life of 7–8 min) legal and personnel requirements are still the center of discussion. Numerous guidelines for sedation in endoscopy [1–3, 9–16], were counted in the last years worldwide, their recommendations for the use of propofol are summarized in Table 28.3. All guidelines are uniform on the assumption that the endoscopist themselves can not perform the endoscopic procedure, patient monitoring and propofol administration at the same time. Demanded is therefore a further, independent assistant person not involved in the endoscopic procedure. This can be a qualified caregiver (so called NAPS, "nurse administered propofol sedation") a second specialist in internal medicine or a gastroenterologist (usually called " gastroenterologist -directed propofol sedation, G-DPS ") or an anesthesia team ("monitored anesthesia care, MAC"). While in principle all guidelines advocate "MAC", they differed with respect to the recommendation when the gastroenterologist should consider the use of anesthesia mandatory (Table 28.3). Provided however, is that the patient is monitored according to the rules of science and that for any incident the necessary personal and instrumental equipment is given [1–3]. The qualification of medical and non-medical personnel should be maintained by regular participation in structured training curricula as developed on national [17] or European basis [18] ensuring to comply with this legal requirement in different countries and again to meet the personal requirements postulated. This is of course not only in addition to the use of propofol, but also for the use of other substances for sedation or analgesia. While currently only isolated special training guidelines exist on premedication and management of emergency situations, it could have shown that specific training courses, such as those based on simulators, might improve physicians' confidence in handling emergency situations [19].

Diagnostic Endoscopy

Propofol has the distinct advantage of sedation compared to benzodiazepines, that the effect occurs much faster [20] and patients recover more rapidly [21–30]. This also applies to the regeneration of psychomotor functions, when propofol was compared with gastroscopy or colonoscopy with a combination of midazolam and meperidine by using a driving simulator [23]. Similar results were published by a study from Japan comparing propofol with midazolam for EGG [31]. The possible improvement of diagnostic accuracy in the EGD appears an additional advantage of propofol compared to midazolam in a randomized controlled trial by Meining et al. [32].

Interventional Endoscopy

Regarding sedation with propofol the investigators evaluated the patients acceptability and tolerance for both the gastroscopy and colonoscopy, as well as for the ERCP in comparison to benzodiazepines as better [24, 25] or equally well [21, 33, 34]. In particular, for interventional examinations such as ERCP also a significantly better patient cooperation could have been shown [26, 27, 35]. Especially with the use of propofol for interventional studies one has to consider that this is not entirely without risk, as shown by data on a risk factor analysis [36]. Of 9547 patients who received propofol sedation, during the interventional upper endoscopy (EGD, ERCP, EUS) over a period of 6 years, 3151 patients received propofol as monosedation and the remaining 6396 a combination of propofol and midazolam. There were a total of 135 serious complications, premature termination of the procedure had to be made in 1.4 %. In 40 patients (0.4 %) a short-term mask ventilation and in nine patients (0.09 %) endotracheal intubation was necessary, another eight patients (0.08 %) had to be monitored on the ICU. Four patients died (mortality rate 0.03 %), in three cases potentially sedation associated side effects must be considered. As independent risk factors for the occurrence of cardiorespiratory complications emergency examinations and a higher dose of propofol were identified [36].

Risk Patients: Propofol or Midazolam?

Both during the investigation and in the post-intervention phase under midazolam elderly patients are at increased risk of documented hypoxemia [37, 38]. In the elderly, it is therefore appropriate to reduce the dose of midazolam [39]. This also suggests the modification of the recommendations of the American Society of Gastroenterology for older patients undergoing gastrointestinal endoscopy [40]. In addition, substances with low cumulative dose [40, 41] should be preferred. The careful use of propofol due to its pharmacokinetic is even safe for high-risk patients aged over 85 years, as we could have shown in a randomized trial comparing propofol with a combination of midazolam and meperidine for ERCP [37]. Similar findings were obtained in a study by Heuss et al. [42]. Since cardio-respiratory events tend to occurred more frequently, there need to be increased care in these patients. Patients with liver cirrhosis are another risk group, where a hepatic encephalopathy may increase under midazolam [43–46]. This can lead to an unforeseen anesthetic stage during sedation, a prolonged wake up period with reduced psychomotor skills.

In randomized controlled trial comparing midazolam with propofol for sedation in patients with liver cirrhosis undergoing interventional EGD the mentioned side effects did not occur when using the ultra-short acting propofol [46].

Propofol and Midazolam (So-Called Balanced Sedation)

The propofol dose required can significantly be reduced "co-induction" with small amounts of midazolam (usually 2–3 mg) [30, 47], what particularly in often prolonged interventional endoscopic procedures is possible and valid only for this. For short duration procedures, most of which are diagnostic, should be dispensed with a co-induction with midazolam, because the savings effect is only insignificantly. In addition, the advantage of rapid psychomotor recovery when using propofol as a single agent [23] and the associated possibility of faster release should not be forgiven (discharge from the recovery room to the ward or outpatient examinations) in these cases.

Propofol Plus Midazolam or Opiates

Cordruwisch et al. [48] performed sedation in 64 patients, who underwent two successive, prolonged (>30 min) endoscopic examinations following up each other. In the first procedure sedation was performed with propofol and in the subsequent examination with a combination of midazolam and propofol. The combination had the advantage of a considerable saving effect of 59 % propofol. However post-interventional wake up was twice as long as in the propofol mono-sedation group (8 min versus 4 min). Van Natta et al. [49] examined in another randomized study 200 patients who received sedation with propofol either alone, propofol plus fentanyl, propofol plus midazolam or midazolam plus fentanyl. By combining process thereby moderate sedation with a shorter recovery time was reached. On the other hand correspondingly higher doses were required with sole administration of propofol, which induced a higher sedation depth leading to a substantially longer recovery time.

Propofol and/or Opiates

Akcaboy et al. [50] studied in a randomized trial in 100 patients during a colonoscopy, the sole administration of the short-acting analgesic drug remifentanil compared to mono-sedation with propofol. It was shown that remifentanil achieved an adequate sedation, amnesia and compared to propofol better analgesia. An increased incidence of nausea and vomiting during the recovery reduced this advantage, however, significantly. Moermann et al. [51] investigated the additive dose of remifentanil for sedation with propofol in a randomized double-blind trail in 50 relatively healthy patients (ASA I and II) undergoing colonoscopy. The combination of remifentanil and propofol showed significantly more often a decrease in blood pressure and oxygen saturation. By administering remifentanil the dose of propofol required could have been reduced, however, the recovery time under propofol mono-sedation was significantly shorter (p <0.01) and patients significantly more satisfied (p <0.01).

Propofol by Non-medical Assistants

The first major studies of propofol bolus sedation by assistants in colonoscopy from the United States and Switzerland respectively included more than 2000 patients [52, 53]. No patient need to be intubated endotracheal and only in 0.2 % of cases a temporary mask ventilation was required. According to these studies, such an approach has also been discussed in other countries (e.g., Germany, Austria, Switzerland) increasingly as an alternative method. An important role was played certainly the increasing cost pressure in the health care system and the associated cost reduction for individual examination [54]. The doctor who initially introduces and delegates to the assistant staff must be informed necessarily in each individual case on the patient, i.e., for example, history and premedication, physical status etc. He/she must also regularly check on the qualifications of the assistant staff personally and assume the sedation and the resulting complications full responsibility. Appropriate training curricula e.g., on the basis of the German or European curriculum [17, 18] should be developed under consideration of different legal aspects for other countries. However, these courses are just a basic course which initially only provides a technical qualification. The practical skills should then be drawn up, for example as part of a study visit.

In some countries (e.g., France and in most states of the US) the administration of propofol is restricted by law to anesthesiologists, therefore, rendering the use of NAPS or even G-DPS impossible.

Alternative Methods

Rudin et al. were able to show in a meta-analysis [55] that the use of music in endoscopy (p=0.001) and the sedatives by 15 % (p=0.055) could contribute to a reduction of the dose of analgesics used to 29.7 %. Also sedation induced cardio-respiratory complications could be minimized by minimal sedation or through the use of ultrathin endoscopes as well as the complete renunciation of sedation [56, 57].

A simple analysis of brain wave activity within the neuromonitoring during sedation for endoscopy can now be performed by using the bispectral index (BIS monitoring) or by using the Narcotrend® process. Numerous studies in the past decade have proven that such EEG monitoring during endoscopy by 3–5 placed on the front side of the head of the patient electrodes is possible. The majority of studies, however, showed no clear advantage over the standard monitoring. Meanwhile occupy several randomized controlled trials for ERCP or performing an ESD on stomach a significant reduction in the required dose of propofol [35, 58–60]. Besides a shorter recovery time, however, these trials did not demonstrate a decisive safety advantage

Post-procedure Care

When a patient can be discharged after sedation, is already regulated since the 90s by the minimum criteria that apply regardless of the substance used [9]. These demands include stable vital signs and a complete or substantial pain relief. The patient should also drink liquids without difficulty, walk unaided and be able to control urination and are modified for more practical application [1, 2]. If necessary, the doctor should inform the patient again to the typical signs of complications. In any case it is recommended that the patient must be accompanied by another person with and to make sure of the possibilities for adequate follow-up at home. However, these discharge criteria, mainly focusing on vital signs of patients immediately after sedation, while cognitive functions and psychomotor skills are in this case not be evaluated. Even discharge criteria such as the Aldrete score [61] mainly focused on cardiovascular and respiratory functions, but may not ultimately reflect the psychomotor skills of the patient at discharge. Even though a maximum discharge score is achieved with 60–70 % of the initial value, the psychomotor skills are often significantly limited, as Willey et al. [62] were able to demonstrate in a study using midazolam in combination with pethidine for EGD. A good option is therefore the currently recommended use the use of ultra-short-acting substances as a single agent [1, 2]., because the limitation period of psychomotor functions and the half-life of the substances used are closely related. These skills recover faster after propofol compared to midazolam (possibly plus pethidine) as we [23] demonstrated in 96 patients after routine gastroscopy and colonoscopy in a driving simulator study. Under Midazolam, optionally in combination with pethidine, psychomotor skills were significantly limited 2 h after the sedation, while patients after propofol sedation showed skills comparable to their baseline performance. Finally, to clearly define the period after which patients might lead a motor vehicle safe again, would require large-scale "on-the-road" studies under well defined primary outcome parameters. Current results from simulator tests are only surrogate parameters here. Furthermore, our results refer exclusively to a mono-sedation with propofol. The effects of the combination of commonly used midazolam and propofol on the mileage, however, are not yet been investigated. The half-life of the substance used and the used sedation regimen (propofol as mono-sedation or combined with benzodiazepines or analgesics) is the decisive criterion for both the first passive on the road, and for the period of incapacity. Patients co-morbidity as well as and further individual patients factors (e.g., employment as a traffic pilot) should also be considered

[63, 64]. Usually, the patient will be able to drive, to work and to engage in legally binding decisions the next day (current European guidelines recommend a 6–12 h interval for propofol use only) [1, 2]. Strictly not recommended is the routine antagonize midazolam, for example by flumazenil to allow an earlier discharge from hospital or medical practice. The risk in this case is a relative safety for the patient, because it is first well monitored. However, the half-life of flumazenil is substantially shorter than that of midazolam and its metabolites. Thus there is a clear risk that delayed respiratory depression or an impairment of cognitive or psychomotor skills occur. Should the use of flumazenil for clinical reasons are required, the patient must be monitored for longer [1].

Conclusion for Practice

Before planning the use of sedation the cardio-respiratory risk needs to be estimated individually. A complete and fully functional emergency equipment and a team trained in airway management and resuscitation must be available. The routine prophylactic administration of 2 l of oxygen via a nasal cannula is recommended to avoid hypoxemia after any contraindications have been excluded. For purely diagnostic examinations the benefit of sedation is not clearly documented, however standard at therapeutic intention. Numerous studies have now confirming superiority of propofol compared to benzodiazepines in endoscopic interventions with an increased use in many countries. Although guidelines support the use of propofol by non-anesthesiologists, it remains not permitted in some countries. A significant advantage of propofol in purely diagnostic examinations is the rapid recovery time, also improved diagnostic accuracy seems possible. In most cases of prolonged interventional endoscopies, the advantage lies in improved patient cooperation. Propofol is safe in patients liver with cirrhosis, as well as in older high-risk patients when used carefully. A co-induction with midazolam can significantly reduce the dose of propofol, which might be required in selected patients undergoing long lasting procedures. In short procedures the disadvantage of impaired psychomotor function outweighs. The sole administration of short acting opiates instead of propofol has no advantage and is limited by their side effects such as nausea and vomiting. Sedation with propofol can safely be performed by non-anesthesiologists and might be delegated to well trained nursing staff under well defined conditions (in low-risk patients and simple procedures) in some countries. Monitoring procedures as capnography and neuro-monitoring is currently not among the standard methods and have been able to show no relevant influence or even advantage in terms of patient safety. At discharge minimum criteria should be met. In particular, patients should leave due to the current legal situation and the medical duty of care the endoscopy unit after sedation in accompaniment. It is advisable to address the organization of an accompanying person in the first explanatory meeting. The passive and active use on the road, as well as the duration of incapacity depend on the half-life of the substance used.

References

1. Riphaus A, Wehrmann T, Hausmann J, et al. Update S3-guideline: "sedation for gastrointestinal endoscopy" 2014 (AWMF-register-no. 021/014). Z Gastroenterol. 2016;54:58–95.
2. Dumonceau J-M, Riphaus A, Schreiber F, et al. Non-anesthesiologist administration of propofol for gastrointestinal endoscopy: European Society of Gastrointestinal Endoscopy, European Society of Gastroenterology and Endoscopy Nurses and Associates Guideline – updated June 2015. Endoscopy. 2015;47:1175–89.
3. Vargo JJ, Delegge MH, Feld AD, et al. Multisociety sedation curriculum for gastrointestinal endoscopy. Gastroenterology. doi:10.1053/j.gastro.2012.05.
4. Cohen LB, Wecsler JS, Gaetano JN, et al. Endoscopic sedation in the United Staters: results from an nationwide survey. Am J Gastroenterol. 2006;101:967–74.
5. Riphaus A, Rabofski M, Wehrmann T. Endoscopic sedation and monitoring practice in Germany: results from the first nationwide survey. Z Gastroenterol. 2010;48:392.
6. Paspatis GA, Manolaraki MM, Tribonias G, et al. Endoscopic sedation in Greece: results from the first nationwide survey for the Hellenic Foundation of gastroenterology and nutrition. Dig Liver Dis. 2009;41:807–11.
7. Baudet JS, Borque P, Alarcon-Fernandez O, Sanchez del Rio A, Campo R, Aviles J. Use of sedation in gastrointestinal endoscopy: a nationwide survey in Spain. Eur J Gastroenterol Hepatol. 2009;21:882–8.
8. Heuss LT, Froehlich F, Beglinger C. Changing patterns of sedation and monitoring practice during endoscopy: results of a nationwide survey in Switzerland. Endoscopy. 2005;37:161–6.
9. American Society of Anesthesiology; Gross JB, Farmington CT, Bailey PL, et al. Practice guidelines for sedation and analgesia by non-anesthsiologists. Anesthesiology. 2002;96:1004–17.
10. American Gastroenterological Association; Cohen LB, Delegge MH, Aisenberg G, et al. AGA institute review of endoscopic sedation. Gastroenterology. 2007;133:675–701.
11. Society of American Gastrointestinal and Endoscopic Surgeons; Myers J, Fanelli R, Earle D, et al. SAGES guidelines for office endoscopic services. Surg Endosc. 2009;23:1125–9.
12. German Society of Digestive and Metabolic Diseases; Riphaus A, Wehrmann T, Weber B, et al. S3-Guidelines – sedation for gastrointestinal endoscopy. Endoscopy. 2009;41:787–815.
13. Canadian Association of Gastroenterology; Byrne MF, Chiba N, Singh H, Sadowski DC. Propofol use for sedation during endoscopy in adults: a Canadian Association of Gastroenterology position statement. Can J Gastroenterol. 2008;22:457–9.
14. Austrian Society of Gastroenterology and Hepatology, Schreiber F. ÖGGH guidelines on sedation and monitoring in gastrointestinal endoscopy. Endoscopy. 2007;39:259–62.
15. Spanish Society of Gastrointestinal Endoscopy, Lopez-Roses L. Sedation/analgesia guidelines for endoscopy. Rev Esp Enferm Dig. 2006;98:685–92.
16. Section and Board of Anaesthesiology, European Union of Medical Specialists; Knape JTA, Adriaensen H, van Aken H, et al. Guidelines for sedation and/or analgesia by non-anaesthisiology doctors. Eur J Anaesthesiol. 2007;24:563–7.
17. Beilenhoff U, Engelke M, Kern-Wächter E, et al. DEGEA-Curriculum (Curriculum of the German Society of Endoscopy Nurses and Associates): sedation and emergency management in endoscopy for endoscopy nurses and associates, endopraxis. 2009;1:32–5. www.degea.de.
18. Dumonceau J, Riphaus A, Beilenhoff U, et al. European curriculum for sedation training in gastrointestinal endoscopy: position statement of the European Society of Gastrointestinal. Endoscopy. 2013;45:496–504.
19. Kiesslich R, Moenk S, Reinhardt K, et al. Combined simulation training: a new concept and workshop is useful for crisis management in gastrointestinal endoscopy. Z Gastroenterol. 2005;43:1031–9.
20. Sipe BW, Rex DK, Latinovich D, Overley C, Kinser K, Bratcher L, Kareken D. Propofol versus midazolam/meperidine for outpatient colonoscopy: administration by nurses supervised by endoscopists. Gastrointest Endosc. 2002;55:815–25.

21. Carlsson U, Grattidge P. Sedation for upper gastrointestinal endoscopy: a comparative study of propofol and midazolam. Endoscopy. 1995;27:240–3.
22. Patterson KW, Casey PB, Murray JP, O'Boyle CA, Cunningham AJ. Propofol sedation for outpatient upper gastrointestinal endoscopy: comparison with midazolam. Br J Anaesth. 1991;67:108–11.
23. Riphaus A, Gstettenbauer T, Frenz MB, Wehrmann T. Quality of psychomotor recovery after propofol sedation for routine endoscopy: a randomized and controlled study. Endoscopy. 2006;38:677–83.
24. Vargo JJ, Zuccaro Jr G, Dumot JA, Shermock KM, Morrow JB, Conwell DL, Trolli PA, Maurer WG. Gastroenterologist-administered propofol versus meperidine and midazolam for advanced upper endoscopy: a prospective, randomized trial. Gastroenterology. 2002;123: 373–5.
25. Weston BR, Chadalawada V, Chalasani N, Kwo P, Overley CA, Symms M, Strahl E, Rex DK. Nurse-administered propofol versus midazolam and meperidine for upper endoscopy in cirrhotic patients. Am J Gastroenterol. 2003;98:2440–7.
26. Jung M, Hofmann C, Kiesslich R, Brackertz A. Improved sedation in diagnostic and therapeutic ERCP: propofol is an alternative to midazolam. Endoscopy. 2000;32:233–8.
27. Wehrmann T, Kokabpick H, Jacobi V, Seifert H, Lembcke B, Caspary WF. Long-term results of endoscopic injection of botulinum toxin in elderly achalasic patients with tortuous megaesophagus or epiphrenic diverticulum. Endoscopy. 1999;31:352–8.
28. Hofmann C, Kiesslich R, Brackertz A, Jung M. Propofol for sedation in gastroscopy--a randomized comparison with midazolam. Z Gastroenterol. 1999;37:589–95.
29. Koshy G, Nair S, Norkus EP, Hertan HI, Pitchumoni CS. Propofol versus midazolam and meperidine for conscious sedation in GI endoscopy. Am J Gastroenterol. 2000;95:1476–9.
30. Reimann FM, Samson U, Derad I, Fuchs M, Schiefer B, Stange EF. Synergistic sedation with low-dose midazolam and propofol for colonoscopies. Endoscopy. 2000;32:239–44.
31. Horiuchi A, Nakayama Y, Katsuyama Y. Safety and driving ability following low-dose propofol sedation. Digestion. 2008;78:190–4.
32. Meining A, Semmler V, Kassem AM, et al. The effect of sedation on the quality of upper gastrointestinal endoscopy: an investigator-blinded, randomized study comparing propofol with midazolam. Endoscopy. 2007;39:345–9.
33. Roseveare C, Seavell C, Patel P, Criswell J, Kimble J, Jones C, Shepherd H. Patient-controlled sedation and analgesia, using propofol and alfentanil, during colonoscopy: a prospective randomized controlled trial. Endoscopy. 1998;30:768–73.
34. Ulmer BJ, Hansen JJ, Overley CA, Symms MR, Chadalawada V, Liangpunsakul S, Strahl E, Mendel AM, Rex DK. Propofol versus midazolam/fentanyl for outpatient colonoscopy: administration by nurses supervised by endoscopists. Clin Gastroenterol Hepatol. 2003;1: 425–32.
35. Wehrmann T, Grotkamp J, Stergiou N, et al. Electroencephalogram monitoring facilitates sedation with propofol for routine ERCP: a randomized, controlled trial. Gastrointest Endosc. 2002;56:817–24.
36. Wehrmann T, Riphaus A. Sedation with propofol for interventional endoscopic procedures: a risk factor analysis. Scand J Gastroenterol. 2007;10:1–7.
37. Riphaus A, Stergiou N, Wehrmann T. Sedation with propofol for routine ERCP in high-risk octogenarians: a randomized, controlled study. Am J Gastroenterol. 2005;100:1957–63.
38. Scholer SG, Schafer DF, Potter JF. The effect of age on the relative potency of midazolam and diazepam for sedation in upper gastrointestinal endoscopy. J Clin Gastroenterol. 1990;12: 145–7.
39. Dhariwal A, Plevris JN, Lo NT, Finlayson ND, Heading RC, Hayes PC. Age, anemia, and obesity-associated oxygen desaturation during upper gastrointestinal endoscopy. Gastrointest Endosc. 1992;38:684–8.
40. Qureshi WA, Zuckerman MJ, Adler DG, Davila RE, Egan JV, Gan SI, Lichtenstein DR, Rajan E, Shen B, Fanelli RD, Van Guilder T, Baron TH. ASGE guideline: modifications in endoscopic practice for the elderly. Gastrointest Endosc. 2006;63:566–9.

41. Darling E. Practical considerations in sedating the elderly. Crit Care Nurs Clin North Am. 1997;9:371–80.
42. Heuss LT, Schnieper P, Drewe J, Pflimlin E, Beglinger C. Safety of propofol for conscious sedation during endoscopic procedures in high-risk patients-a prospective, controlled study. Am J Gastroenterol. 2003;98:1751–7.
43. Assy N, Rosser BG, Grahame GR, Minuk GY. Risk of sedation for upper GI endoscopy exacerbating subclinical hepatic encephalopathy in patients with cirrhosis. Gastrointest Endosc. 1999;49:690–4.
44. Vasudevan AE, Goh KL, Bulgiba AM. Impairment of psychomotor responses after conscious sedation in cirrhotic patients undergoing therapeutic upper GI endoscopy. Am J Gastroenterol. 2002;97:1717–21.
45. Hamdy NA, Kennedy HJ, Nicholl J, Triger DR. Sedation for gastroscopy: a comparative study of midazolam and Diazemuls in patients with and without cirrhosis. Br J Clin Pharmacol. 1986;22:643–7.
46. Riphaus A, Lechowicz I, Frenz MB, Wehrmann T. Propofol sedation for upper gastrointestinal endoscopy in patients with liver cirrhosis as an alternative to midazolam to avoid acute deterioration of minimal encephalopathy: a randomized, controlled study. Scand J Gastroenterol. 2009;44:1244–51.
47. Seifert H, Schmitt TH, Gultekin T, Caspary WF, Wehrmann T. Sedation with propofol plus midazolam versus propofol alone for interventional endoscopic procedures: a prospective, randomized study. Aliment Pharmacol Ther. 2000;14:1207–14.
48. Cordruwisch W, Doroschko M, Wurbs D. Deep sedation in gastrointestinal endoscopic interventions: safety and reliability of a combination of midazolam and propofol. Dtsch Med Wochenschr. 2000;125:619–62.
49. Van Natta ME, Rex DK. Propofol alone titrated to deep sedation versus propofol in combination with opioids and/or benzodiazepines and titrated to moderate sedation for colonoscopy. Am J Gastroenterol. 2006;101:2209–17.
50. Akcaboy ZN, Akcaboy EY, Albayrak D, et al. Can remifentanil be a better choice than propofol for colonoscopy during monitored anesthesia care? Acta Anaesthesiol Scand. 2006;50: 736–41.
51. Moerman AT, Struys MM, Vereecke HE, Herregods LL, De Vos MM, Mortier EP. Remifentanil used to supplement propofol does not improve quality of sedation during spontaneous respiration. J Clin Anesth. 2004;16:237–43.
52. Sipe BW, Rex DK, Latinovich D. Propofol versus midazolam/meperidine for outpatient colonoscopy: administration by nurses supervised by endoscopists. Gastrointest Endosc. 2002;55:815–25. Erratum in: Gastrointest Endosc 2002; 56: 324.
53. Heuss LT, Schnieper P, Drewe J, Pflimlin E, Beglinger C. Risk stratification and safe administration of propofol by registered nurses supervised by the gastroenterologist: a prospective observational study of more than 2000 cases. Gastrointest Endosc. 2003;57:664–71.
54. Hassan C, Rex DK, Cooper GS, Benamouzig R. Endoscopist-directed propofol administration versus anesthesiologist assistance for colorectal cancer screening: a cost-effectiveness analysis. Endoscopy. 2012;44:456–64.
55. Rudin D, Kiss A, Wetz RV, Sottile VM. Music in the endoscopy suite: a meta-analysis of randomized controlled studies. Endoscopy. 2007;39:507–10.
56. Liebermann DA, Wuerker CK, Katon RM. Cardiopulmonary risk of esopagogastroduodenoscopy. Role of endoscope diameter and systemic sedation. Gastroenterology. 1985;88:468–72.
57. Cooper MW, Davison CM, Uastin CA. Arterial oxygen saturation during upper gastrointestinal endoscopy in elderly patients: the role of endoscope diameter. Age Ageing. 1995;24:254–6.
58. Paspatis GA, Chainaki I, Manolaraki M, et al. Efficacy of bispectral monitoring as an adjunct to propofol deep sedation for ERCP: a randomized controlled trial. Endoscopy. 2009;41: 1046–51.
59. Imagawa A, Fujiki S, Kawahara Y, et al. Satisfaction with bispectral index monitoring of propofol-mediated sedation during endoscopic submucosal dissection: a prospective, randomized study. Endoscopy. 2008;40:905–9.

60. Aldrete JA. Modifications to the postanesthesia score for use in ambu- latory surgery. J Perianesth Nurs. 1998;13:148–55.
61. Al-Sammak Z, Al-Falaki MM, Gamal HM. Predictor of sedation during endoscopic retrograde cholangiopancreatography – bispectral index vs. clinical assessment. Middle East J Anaesthesiol. 2005;18:141–8.
62. Willey J, Vargo JJ, Connor JT, et al. Quantitative assessment of psychomotor recovery after sedation and analgesia for outpatient EGD. Gastrointest Endosc. 2002;56:810–6.
63. Mueller M, Wehrmann T. How best to approach endoscopic sedation? Nat Rev Gastroenterol Hepatol. 2011;8:481–90.
64. Vargo JJ. Doc, can I drive home? Am J Gastroenterol. 2009;104:1656–7.

Chapter 29
Propofol Infusion Platforms

Preet Mohinder Singh and Basavana Goudra

Abstract Propofol is the most popular drug used for sedation assisted procedures. Many drug delivery systems taking advantage of propofol pharmacokinetics are available in the market. Target controlled infusion systems have strong evidence in support of their use in the operating room. TCIs help to maintain a constant sedation level via computer generated propofol dosing regimens. Many new studies have shown that propofol based TCI guided sedation has the potential to alter patient outcomes, decrease sedation provider's workload and allow rapid patient turnovers in a busy sedation suite. Going one step further, new personalized sedation concept has emerged. Sedasys is a recently approved semi-automatic propofol based sedation delivery system. Sedasys can be used for mild to moderate sedation in adults undergoing gastroenterological endoscopic procedures. It uses a computer based dosing protocol based upon patient's demographic parameters. Sedasys continuously monitors the sedation depth using patient's responsiveness to automated verbal stimulus and can lower the propofol doses if needed.

Keywords Propofol delivery systems • Target controlled infusions • Sedasys

Newer Propofol Sedation Delivery Systems

Introduction

Propofol has come a long way since its discovery in 1977. Once its unique properties of short duration of action and clear headed recovery were identified, it became a popular target for drug development companies. Multiple modifications have been

P.M. Singh, MD, DNB, MNAMS (✉)
Department of Anesthesiology, Critical Care and Pain Medicine,
All India Institute of Medical Sciences, Ansari Nagar, New Delhi 110029, India
e-mail: preetrajpal@gmail.com

B. Goudra, MD, FRCA, FCARCSI
Department of Anesthesiology and Critical Care Medicine, Hospital of the University of Pennsylvania, 3400 Spruce Street, 5042 Silverstein Building, Philadelphia, PA 19104, USA
e-mail: goudrab@uphs.upenn.edu

© Springer International Publishing Switzerland 2017
B.G. Goudra, P.M. Singh (eds.), *Out of Operating Room Anesthesia*,
DOI 10.1007/978-3-319-39150-2_29

made in its commercial preparations, improving its pharmacological profile over the years. Unparalleled by any drug, a lot of research has also been directed towards improving the technology used to deliver propofol to the patients. Although, no changes in the actual structure of propofol have been made, the delivery systems have seen drastic transformation. From manual boluses it has emerged into a drug being delivered by automated systems like- Sedasys.

Principles of Drug Delivery Systems

The number of clinical uses of propofol probably surpass any other drug. Other than an established use as an induction agent its utility for procedural sedation is unmatched. The pharmacological profile that is typically targeted by drug delivery system are

- Propofol is capable of providing dose dependent depth of sedation. The sedation spectrum for propofol varies from general anesthesia → Deep sedation → conscious sedation → light sedation.
  The drug delivery systems thus can incorporate protocols to decrease the dose delivered and thus alter the sedation depth. This can allow propofol being effectively used for procedures ranging from rigid bronchoscopy (deeper sedation) to wound dressing change (light sedation).
- No residual effect- Propofol being a highly lipid soluble drug undergoes extensive redistribution. Additionally, it undergoes significant extrahepatic metabolism (up to 30%). Due to these properties the context sensitive half-life after long infusions is also not much prolonged. As a result, the delivery systems can actually calculate estimated does without needing alterations accounting for minor organ system ailments.
- Availability- This is often an understated factor that has played a vital role in development of wide range of propofol delivery systems. With generic drug available since almost early nineties, the opportunities for development of delivery systems were overtaken by many manufacturers. A classic example of limitation that could have been posed by exclusive patent is remifentanil. Despite having most of the properties of an ideal drug its delivery systems still lag behind that of propofol. Generic propofol preparations are easily available across the globe allowing more opportunity for researchers to further develop its delivery systems.
- Validated sedation depth measurement- this is one of the most recent developments. Electroencephalographic monitors can estimate objectively the sedation "level" achieved with the propofol infusion. In our own study we were able to demonstrate the effectiveness of one such monitoring "Sedline" for the use in patients undergoing clolonoscopy under propofol based sedation [1].
- Compatibility with other drugs- Another unique feature that has been exploited by the newer delivery systems is the lack of significant drug interaction with opioids. Both opioids and propofol can lower each other's dose requirements.

Rather than the possibility of increasing the depth of sedation disproportionately, sedation systems use this property to their advantage. Lowering individual doses decreases the associated individual side effects.

These unique features specific to propofol form the basis of drug development systems. Going beyond the manual boluses and simple infusion pumps, propfol delivery in now venturing into the "computer assisted sedation" systems.

Several propofol infusion platforms have been devised to address the inherent safety problems associated with propofol administration. These platforms include

Target Controlled Infusion Systems

One of the most desired property of a drug administered intravenously would be the ability to measure its actual blood concentration at a given point of time. This would allow the sedation provider to titrate the drug to the required clinical sedation level. Target controlled infusion (TCIs) simulate this principle but rather than being able to measure the blood concentrations they estimate the same using computer based models. Interestingly, these calculated values show a high degree of accuracy with only 5 % patients being the outliers [2]. Extensive experience exists for the use of propofol based TCI during procedures under general anesthesia.

How Do TCIs Work?

TCIs use population based normograms to estimate poropfol concentration in either the plasma or even at the site where poropfol acts (brain- effect site). TCIs thus can work in two modes. The user can set to deliver a particular concentration in the blood (Plasma site mode) or the choose a concentration in the brain (effect site mode). The development of these models is analogous to the anesthesia models used during the inhalational anesthetics. By convention, during the gas based anesthesia it is assumed that the partial pressure of gas being exhaled from the lung is the concentration/ partial pressure of gas in the brain. Under inhalation anesthesia it is believed that the venous blood (inflowing into the lung from the brain) has fully equilibrated with the tissue in the brain. The concentration of expired gas- thus expresses the concentration in the brain and is the MAC value determined for the agent. This is analogous to the effect site mode. Unlike, the inhalation anesthetics the TCI system gives the user the luxury to choose desired brain site concentration directly.

The plasma site mode allows the user to choose the desired drug concentration in the plasma. It is analogous to the concentration of inhalation anesthetics being delivered into the lung by the fresh gas flow. As the clinical effects actually depend upon the brain concentration- effect site modes have become more popular and are more reliable [3].

Propofol Sedation and TCI

TCIs derive their evidence from population based studies. Propofol is the drug that has undergone extensive testing and use with TCI models. Many researchers have performed studies on propofol distribution after intravenous use. It is believed that once propofol is injected its distribution/metabolism follows a three compartment model. These three compartments as described initially by Gept's et al. include-Central drug compartment and two peripheral compartments (high perfusion and low perfusion compartments). For the development of TCI, once the propofol is administered the volume of distribution is calculated by computer generated model. Based upon different research protocols, different models of propofol TCI exist. The most well developed models for adults include the Marsh and the Schnider's model. The specific implications of these models pertaining to sedation procedures is given in the Table 29.1.

Many studies have evaluated the benefits of TCI based propofol delivery systems and the well-known benefits include

(a) Hemodynamic stability- Studies have shown that with the use of TCI based propofol delivery the total amount of propofol consumed is lower than that administered via manual boluses or fixed rate continuous infusions. This decreased amount of propofol delivered translates into better preserved hemodynamic stability. Patients sedated in intensive care units have shown to need fewer vasopressors with the use of propofol TCI [4].

(b) Decreased airway intervention- Evidence suggests that with the use of TCI based sedation the overshoot and undershoot of propofol concentration is less likely. The overshoot of concentration (when given as bolus) has the propensity to cause apnea or airway obstruction. Hsu et al. demonstrated that these episodes in patients undergoing endoscopy were significantly lower with the use of propofol TCI in comparison to fixed infusion of propofol.

(c) Faster recovery- one of the aim of developing technology is to improve the safety and also lower the associated costs. As already stated, the total amount of propofol injected can be decreased with TCI use the patient wakeup times are actually smaller. Lin et al. showed that patients sedated with propofol TCI for bronchoscopic procedures had smaller discharge times with lower complication rates [5]. These rapid turn overs can reflect in terms of saving vital operating room time that can have long term economic impact [6].

(d) Better patient and endoscopist satisfaction towards the procedure- Propofol based TCIs maintains a steady state of concentration and prevents changes in patient's depth of sedation. This helps to avoid procedural interruptions and thus improves the endoscopist satisfaction. On the other hand, frequent episodes of light sedation can lead to patient awareness and thus cause poor patient satisfaction. TCI being able to maintain a steady state of sedation helps in both the above goals. These aspects of propofol TCI used were demonstrated by Fanti et al. during gastroenterological sedation procedures [7].

Table 29.1 TCI- Propofol models and their implications for sedation procedures

Propofol TCI modelling for procedures under sedation			
	Marsh model	Schnider model	Implication for sedation
Concentration target/ recommended mode	Plasma concentration Sedation- 1.5–5 µgm/ml	Effect site concentration- brain	
Central compartment volume for initial dose	15.9 l (for 70 kg male)	4.27 l (independent of age and weight)	Initial doses smaller for Schndier model – Less hemodynamic instability Fixed initial dose in Schnider model irrespective higher weight or age- poorer predictability
Infusion rates estimated immediately after bolus	Generally higher for all patients	Lower	Lesser dose may reflect into better hemodynamic stability (especially in moribund patients)
Over pressure technique (higher initial bolus)	Can be performed manually	Inherent part of protocol- gradual higher dose	Faster onset with Schnider model Rapid increase in depth available- e.g., bronchoscopies etc.
Initial infusion rate estimation based on	Total body weight	Total body weight and Lean body mass (calculated value)	Studies show poor predictability with increasing BMI in Schnider model Marsh model may overestimate total dose
Effect site equilibration constant (KeO)	0.26	0.456	Predicted time to peak effect (TTPE) is smaller with Schnider- Rapid onset More hemodynamic instability in elderly – as drug overshoots higher
Estimated rate of drop of concentration	Independent for age	Age accounted	Elderly would have smaller level fall- maintenance may be overestimated
Evidence based overall total dose	Higher	Lower	No Direct comparison available- wake up times may be better in Schnider model

(e) Improved efficiency of the sedation provider- This is an indirect benefit. Manual titration of propofol dose requires constant vigilance. Frequent adjustments in infusion doses can divert the attention from monitoring. TCI after initial bolus automatically adjusts its dose to maintain a steady state of sedation. This can allow the sedation provider to focus on patient monitoring more effectively.

Presently, "Open TCI Pumps" are available in the market. They allow the operator to not only choose what modelling for a particular drug to use but also allow to alter the drug. Thus in a single TCI system in addition to propofol an additional drug can be used as well (in a separate syringe). This would cut down hospital costs allowing to buy single device to run TCI for drugs like propofol and remifentanil. A few of these open TCI systems include -CATIA, IVA-SIM (University of Bonn, Germany), STANPUMP (Stanford University, USA), STELPUMP (University of Stellenbosch, South Africa) etc.

The Future of TCI

Newer TCI system where patient can control to TCI-based propofol sedation has been developed. This system allows the patient to step up the propofol infusion dose as per his/her depth. As the patient becomes light, he can increase the dose using a hand held switch. The TCI system is programmed to only to allow slight increase on patient's demand. As a safety feature, these devices allow only small step up in propofol dose avoiding over sedation with larger rise in propofol dose. Many studies have evaluated these devices and have reported their favorable profile in indications such as ERCP, colonoscopy, dental and oral surgery [8]. The safety of these delivery systems has been demonstrated even in patients undergoing complex procedures such as ERCP [9]. Another emerging concept is electroencephalography (EEG)-based sedation depth control. Preclinical trials have shown the utility of this method for short-acting opioids (remifentanil) and propofol among patients undergoing endoscopic procedures [10].

Personalized of Sedation

One of the major limitation of propofol use has been its pharmacodynamic variation. Although, the TCI systems can predict what concentration reaches the brain but they fail to predict how the brain responds to a particular concentration. Thus patient responses despite knowing the drug concentrations are largely unpredictable. A new concept that has emerged is to access the patient's sedation level using automated monitoring system and allowing this monitoring system to alter the propofol dose. This idea forms the basis of introduction of "computer assisted personalized sedation system". The FDA recently approved one such propofol drug delivery system- The Sedasys

Sedasys

Sedays has often been introduced as a sedation delivering robot. It is as system approved for delivering propofol based moderate to light sedation for procedures outside the operating room. It is approved for use in ASA I and II adults (>18 years) for gastroenterological endoscopic procedures. Although Sedasys is licensed to be used by non-anesthesiologist for sedation but one of the prerequisites is the presence of a formally trained anesthesiologist in the vicinity.

Sedasys introduces a new monitoring technology called the automated responsiveness monitoring (ARM). ARM measures patient's depth of sedation by his/her ability to squeeze a hand held switch in response to an auditory or vibrational stimulus. This forms a unique feature of the Sedays system. Unlike all previous technologies that attempted to measure non-specific parameters like hemodynamics, respiratory rate- Sedasys by measuring actual patient responsiveness tires to solve the problem of pharmacodynamic variations.

Sedasys: What Can It Do and Cant?

Sedasys is a semi-automatic propofol infusion system. Being semi-automatic means that is does need operator inputs for dose adjustments. Sedasys, is programmed to decrease the propofol dose but not to increase it. This feature although seems like a limitation but adds a safety check. For increasing the propofol dose in the Sedasys system, manual intervention is required. Once the Sedasys system detects that the patient's response to ARM is blunted and possibility of deeper level of sedation exists. It cuts down the propofol infusion dose. On the other hand even if it measures the patient to be light- it is incapable of stepping up the propofol dose by itself.

Once the Sedasys is set up for a procedure it is programmed to account for only first single fentanyl bolus (25–100 μgms). Any further boluses of fentanyl (or any other opioid) cannot lead to automated propofol dose adjustments. Thus warranting operator intervention for dose adjustment.

Sedasys Technical Aspects

The Sedasys system consists of two main units. These are-

(a) Bedside monitoring unit (BMU)- This incorporates all the conventional monitors including pulse oximeter, blood pressure, electrocardiogram and ARM monitor. The BMU is designed to follow the patient through pre-procedure, procedure, and postprocedure.
(b) Procedure Room Unit (PRU)- PRU is the main propofol delivery unit of the Sedasys system. It incorporates all the above monitoring in addition to capnography during the procedure.

PRU uses a drug delivery algorithm and intravenous infusion pump to deliver propofol with a variable infusion rate to achieve and maintain a desired sedation level. It enables the physician team to adjust the patient's level of sedation by entering a dose rate that they by experience believe will maintain the desired sedation level. The System calculates an appropriate loading dose based on the patient's demographic parameters. The loading dose is delivered over 3 min; immediately after, the System automatically starts delivering the entered dose rate. Another feature incorporated in to the Sedasys is a PRN button (*pro re nata*) that allows the sedation provider to provide a propofol bolus of 0.25 mg/Kg.

Propofol Drug Delivery Safety Concerns

No matter what delivery system is used for propofol, concerns about the device safety will always cloud its use. It is not unusual for propofol based sedation to accidently develop into deep sedation even with most experience hands. Concerns for "Who should be allowed to use propofol?" have been a matter for constant debate. ASA has expressed concerns about patient safety due to compromised airway and has been against the use of Non-anesthesiologist administrated propofol (NAAP). A recent meta-analysis showed that propofol administration by experienced endoscopist may be equally safe as that by an anesthesiologist [11]. The newer delivery systems in the pipeline aim towards further operator independent drug delivery techniques. They aim for development of feedback systems to objectify assess the patient sedation state and readjust the propofol dose. Thus in such systems the role of anesthesiologist may actually be limited and safety of NAAP may actually further improve.

References

1. Goudra B, Singh PM, Gouda G, Borle A, Carlin A, Yadwad A. Propofol and non-propofol based sedation for outpatient colonoscopy-prospective comparison of depth of sedation using an EEG based SEDLine monitor. J Clin Monit Comput. 2015. [Epub ahead of print].
2. Schnider TW, Minto CF, Struys MMRF, Absalom AR. The safety of target-controlled infusions. Anesth Analg. 2016;122(1):79–85.
3. Enlund M. TCI : target controlled infusion, or totally confused infusion? Call for an optimised population based pharmacokinetic model for propofol. Ups J Med Sci. 2008;113(2):161–70.
4. Le Guen M, Liu N, Bourgeois E, Chazot T, Sessler DI, Rouby J-J, et al. Automated sedation outperforms manual administration of propofol and remifentanil in critically ill patients with deep sedation: a randomized phase II trial. Intensive Care Med. 2013;39(3):454–62.
5. Lin T-Y, Lo Y-L, Hsieh C-H, Ni Y-L, Wang T-Y, Lin H-C, et al. The potential regimen of target-controlled infusion of propofol in flexible bronchoscopy sedation: a randomized controlled trial. PLoS One. 2013;8(4):e62744.
6. Goudra BG, Singh PM, Sinha AC. Anesthesia for ERCP: impact of anesthesiologist's experience on outcome and cost. Anesthesiol Res Pract. 2013;2013:570518.

7. Fanti L, Gemma M, Agostoni M, Rossi G, Ruggeri L, Azzolini ML, et al. Target controlled infusion for non-anaesthesiologist propofol sedation during gastrointestinal endoscopy: the first double blind randomized controlled trial. Dig Liver Dis. 2015;47(7):566–71.
8. Sheahan CG, Mathews DM. Monitoring and delivery of sedation. Br J Anaesth. 2014;113 Suppl 2:ii37–47.
9. Gillham MJ, Hutchinson RC, Carter R, Kenny GN. Patient-maintained sedation for ERCP with a target-controlled infusion of propofol: a pilot study. Gastrointest Endosc. 2001;54(1): 14–7.
10. Gambús PL, Jensen EW, Jospin M, Borrat X, Martínez Pallí G, Fernández-Candil J, et al. Modeling the effect of propofol and remifentanil combinations for sedation-analgesia in endoscopic procedures using an Adaptive Neuro Fuzzy Inference System (ANFIS). Anesth Analg. 2011;112(2):331–9.
11. Goudra BG, Singh PM, Gouda G, Borle A, Gouda D, Dravida A, et al. Safety of non-anesthesia Provider-Administered Propofol (NAAP) sedation in advanced gastrointestinal endoscopic procedures: comparative meta-analysis of pooled results. Dig Dis Sci. 2015;60(9):2612–27.

Chapter 30
Regional Techniques: Role and Pitfalls

Shelley Joseph George and Maimouna Bah

Abstract Employing regional anesthesia outside of the operating room equips the clinician with another set of tools to optimally treat pain and allow for and improved patient recovery. Although regional anesthesia may not be appropriate in all situations, it is very effective in the right situation. When doing nerve blocks outside of the operating room setting, it is helpful to set up a portable block cart that can carry all equipment and medication necessary. The chapter outlines the instances when regional anesthesia may truly be beneficial to patient care, which nerve blocks should be employed, how to do the nerve blocks, and special considerations that should be thought of prior to placing a nerve block. The local anesthetic systemic toxicity algorithm is also placed in the chapter.

Keywords Interscalene Block • Supraclavicular Block • Infraclavicular Block • Axillary nerve block • Median nerve block • Radial nerve block • Ulnar Nerve block • Musculocutaneous Nerve block • IV regional block • Femoral Nerve block • Fascia Iliaca Block • Intercostal Nerve Block • Paravertebral Block • Neuraxial Anesthesia • Rib Fracture • Hip Fracture • Interstitial brachytherapy • Uterine Artery embolization

Upper Extremity Blocks

Brachial Plexus

Anatomy

The brachial plexus is formed from union of the anterior rami of C5-T1, with variable contributions of C4 and T2. Once the nerves leaves their intervertebral foramina, they course anterolaterally and inferiorly between the anterior and middle scalene muscles where the nerve roots unite to form three trunks, which lie posterior to the subclavian artery as it courses along the upper surface of the first rib [1–3]. The

S.J. George, MD (✉) • M. Bah, MS, MD
Department of Anesthesiology, Hahnemann University Hospital,
245 N. 15th St, Mailstop 310, Philadelphia, PA 19102, USA
e-mail: shelley.george@drexelmed.edu; maimouna.bah@drexelmed.edu

© Springer International Publishing Switzerland 2017
B.G. Goudra, P.M. Singh (eds.), *Out of Operating Room Anesthesia*,
DOI 10.1007/978-3-319-39150-2_30

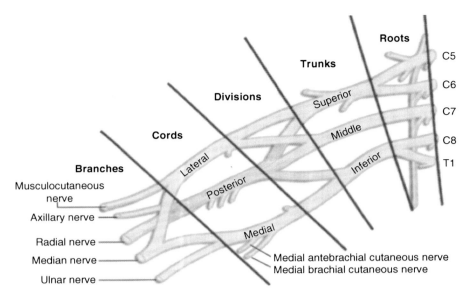

Fig. 30.1 Roots, trunks, divisions, cords, and branches of the brachial plexus (Reproduced from Elsevier, Miller's Anesthesia , Ronald D. Miller MD, MS , 2015, Ch 57, pp 1724–1724, Figure 57-3)

superior (C5 and C6), middle (C7), and inferior (C8 and T1) trunks are arranged accordingly and each trunk forms anterior and posterior divisions that pass posterior to the mid-portion of the clavicle to enter the axilla. Within the axilla, these divisions form the lateral, posterior, and medial cords, named according to their relationship with the second part of the axillary artery. At the border of the pectoralis minor muscle each cord gives off a large branch before ending as a major terminal nerve. The lateral cord gives rise to the lateral branch of the median nerve and terminate as the musculocutaneous nerve; the medial cord gives rise to the median nerve, and terminate as the ulnar nerve; and the posterior cord divides into the axillary and radial nerves (Fig. 30.1) [1]. Aside from the main terminal nerves several other branches arise from the roots of the brachial plexus including the suprascapular nerve, which arises from C5-C6 and supplies the muscles of the dorsal aspect of the scapula, and sensory supply of the shoulder joint. Local anesthetic may be applied along any point of the brachial plexus to provide a desired nerve block. Branches derived directly from cervical roots are usually blocked with the interscalene block approach.

Interscalene Block

Clinical Applications

An interscalene block is recommended for shoulder and proximal humerus surgical procedure therefore ideal for reduction of dislocated shoulder. When performed the roots of the brachial plexus (C5- C7) are most commonly blocked with this technique. Due to location, blockage of the ulnar nerve, which originates from C8-T1, usually does not occur; and for complete surgical anesthesia of the shoulder, the C3-C4 cutaneous branches may need to be block with local infiltration or use of superficial cervical block. Interscalene blocks are appropriate in nearly all patients, even the obese due to ease of identifiable necessary landmarks [2–4]. However, Interscalene blocks should be avoided in patients with significant impaired pulmonary function due to blockage of the phrenic nerve and in patients with contralateral vocal cord paralysis [1]. Contraindication includes local infection, severe coagulopathy, local anesthetic allergy, and patient refusal.

Technique

Surface anatomy of importance includes the larynx, sternocleidomastoid muscle, and external jugular vein. This block can be performed with the arm in any position. The patient should be in the supine position, with the head turned away from the side to be blocked. The block is often performed at the level of the C6 vertebral body, which is at the level of the cricoid cartilage. The plexus courses between the anterior and middle scalene muscles, superior and posterior to the second and third parts of the subclavian artery. The interscalene groove can be palpated by rolling the fingers posterolaterally over the anterior scalene muscle into the groove. A line is extended laterally from the cricoid cartilage to intersect the interscalene groove, indicating the level of the transverse process of C6 [2]. Although the external jugular vein often overlies this point of intersection, it is not a constant or reliable landmark [2].

This block is well suited with ultrasound guidance as it is easy to obtain a supraclavicular view of the subclavian artery and brachial plexus; then trace the plexus up the neck with the ultrasound probe until the plexus are visualized as hypoechoic structures between the anterior and medial scalene muscles [4, 5]. A 22–25-gauge with 4-cm needle should be used. The needle is inserted perpendicular to the skin with a 45° caudad and slightly posterior angle [2, 5]. The needle is then advanced in an out-of-plane or an in-plane approach until a paresthesia or nerve stimulator response is elicited. After desired response is obtained and there is negative aspiration, local anesthetic solution is injected incrementally depending on the desired extent of blockade. This is one of the brachial plexus block in which large volume of local anesthetic allows effective anesthesia therefore large volumes up to 40 ml are typically used [1–4, 6].

Side Effects and Complications

Blockage of the ipsilateral phrenic nerve block is almost guaranteed with the interscalene block, which result in diaphragmatic paresis in majority of patients, even with dilute solutions of local anesthetics, and is associated with significant reduction in pulmonary function [2, 6]. Hemidiaphragmatic paresis may result in dyspnea, hypercapnia, and hypoxemia. Techniques to decrease blockade of the phrenic nerve include using very small volumes of local anesthetic and localizing the brachial plexus at a lower level in the neck. Horner's syndrome may also result from blockage of sympathetic fibers to the cervicothoracic ganglion. The risk of pneumothorax is small when the needle is correctly placed at the C5 or C6 level because of the distance from the dome of the pleura. The proximity of significant neurovascular structures can increase the risk of serious neurologic complications when an interscalene block is performed in heavily sedated or anesthetized patients [4]. Therefore, an interscalene block should be placed with the patient awake or under light sedation.

Supraclavicular Block

Clinical Applications

The supraclavicular block is recommended for procedures of the upper arm, elbow, forearm, wrist, and hand. This technique blocks the divisions of the brachial plexus, at this level the distal trunk-proximal division of the brachial plexus is compact therefore the supraclavicular block result in faster onset and effective blockage of almost the entire upper extremity below the shoulder compared to other upper extremity blocks [5]. Studies have shown small volume of local anesthetic produces rapid onset of reliable blockade of the brachial plexus [4, 5, 7].

The neurovascular bundle of the brachial plexus lies midpoint inferior to the clavicle and the nerve bundles are located vertically over the first rib posterior to the subclavian artery, which can be palpated in some patients. The first rib which is short, broad, and flat, with an anteroposterior orientation at the site of the plexus typically prevents the needle's reaching the pleural. Contraindication includes local infection, severe coagulopathy, and patient refusal. This block is cautioned in patients who are uncooperative or cannot tolerate any degree of respiratory compromise.

Technique

The patient is positioned supine with the head turned away from the side to be blocked with then arm adducted and the hand extended along the side. The midpoint of the clavicle is typically identified and the posterior border of the sternocleido-mastoid palpated over the anterior scalene muscle into the interscalene groove, identification of the subclavian artery at this point confirms the landmark. With the use of the ultrasound one can visualize the brachial plexus structures, as well as the subclavian artery and pleura, just below the first rib [8]. A 22-gauge, 4-cm needle is directed in a caudad, slightly medial to posterior direction until a paresthesia or motor response is elicited or the first rib is encountered. If the first rib is encountered without elicitation of a paresthesia, the needle can be systematically moved anteriorly or posteriorly along the rib with continuous visualization of the needle tip with the ultrasound until the other landmarks are located such as the subclavian artery/vein and pleura. After localization of the brachial plexus, aspiration for blood should be performed before incremental injections of local anesthetic.

Side Effects and Complications

The supraclavicular block is more difficult to perform on obese patients, however there is no increased risk of complications documented [2]. The prevalence of pneumothorax after supraclavicular block is 0.5–6% and diminishes with increased experience and use of ultrasound [1]. If pneumothorax occurs the onset of symptoms is usually delayed and it can take up to 24 h therefore a routine chest radiography post procedure is not recommended [4]. Other complications include phrenic nerve block, at a lesser degree than the interscalene block, Horner's syndrome, and neuropathy, which usually is self-limited.

Infraclavicular Block

Clinical Applications

The infraclavicular block is recommend for procedures at or distal to the elbow, arm, and hand. It provides blockage of the brachial plexus at the level of the cords. An ultrasound and nerve stimulator is required with this block because there are no palpable vascular landmarks to aid in directing the needle. This technique is distal from the neuraxial structures and the lungs, thus minimizing the complication of an interscalene or supraclavicular block.

Technique

The Patient is typically positioned supine but no special arm positioning is required. The ultrasound is placed below the midpoint of the inferior border of the clavicle near the palpable coracoid process and used to visualize the neurovascular bundle. The needle is inserted and advanced laterally until, the brachial plexus identified and confirmed by the nerve stimulator. An incremental local anesthetic is injected around the axillary artery.

Side Effects and Complications

Due to the proximity of the axillary artery there is risk of vascular puncture and systemic local anesthetic toxicity. It is recommended to avoid this approach on patient with catheters or pacemakers at this region [2].

Axillary Block

Clinical Applications

Among the brachial plexus blocks, the axillary approach is by far the most popular due to its ease, reliability, and safety [3, 4]. Blockade occurs at the level of the terminal nerves therefore it is suitable for procedure of the forearm and hand. The musculocutaneous nerve however is usually spared, at this level as it has already left the sheath and lies with the coracobrachialis muscle. This block is suited for outpatients and is easily adapted to the pediatric population [4, 7]. Arm position is very important therefore axillary blockade is unsuitable for patients who are unable to abduct the arm to perform the block.

Technique

The patient should be placed in supine position with the arm to be blocked placed at a right angle to the body, elbow flexed to 90°. The dorsum of the hand rests on a bed or pillow. The axillary artery can then be palpated and traced from the lower axilla to as proximal as possible. The artery is then fixed against the patient's humerus and the ultrasound is placed to visualize neurovascular bundle. Although anatomic variations exist the median nerve is typically found superior to the artery, the ulnar nerve is inferior, and the radial nerve is posterior to lateral. A short 22-gauge needle is then inserted and advanced until the axillary sheath is entered and desire (including muscular cutones) nerve stimulation is obtained. Local anesthetic is injected after negative aspiration. The ultrasound aids visualization of local anesthetic spread around the nerves. Proximal needle placement and maintenance of distal pressure facilitate proximal spread of the solution.

Side Effects and Complications

Nerve injury and systemic toxicity are the most significant complications associated with the axillary block [5, 9]. Hematoma and infection are rare complications.

Terminal Nerve Blocks

Clinical Applications

Peripheral nerve blocks are useful for procedures at the wrist and elbow requiring limited anesthesia or has contraindications to brachial plexus block such as infection, bilateral procedure, coagulopathy, or difficult anatomy [2, 8]. Peripheral blocks performed at the level of the elbow and wrist are typically performed as "field" blocks without requiring the use of nerve stimulator or ultrasound. Benefits include ease of blocks and reduce complications.

Median Nerve Block

The median nerve originates from the lateral and medial cords of the brachial plexus. It travels medial to the brachial artery. In the antecubital space, it is medial to the insertion of the biceps tendon. It gives off multiple motor branches before it enters the carpal tunnel. Then it is located between the flexor carpi radialis and palmaris longus tendon in the carpal tunnel.

Blocking the median nerve provides anesthesia to the palmar surface of the first, second, third, and lateral half of the fourth digit, motor blockade causing Loss of pronation of forearm, weakness in flexion of the hand at the wrist, loss of flexion of radial half of digits and thumb, and loss of abduction and opposition of thumb. The median nerve block requires the patient's arm supine, the medial and lateral epicondyles of the humerus identified. The major landmark for this technique is the brachial artery, which is found medial to the biceps tendon at the intercondylar line.

To block the median nerve at the elbow, one identifies the brachial artery in the antecubital crease just medial to the biceps insertion and inserts a short 22-gauge needle just medial to the artery, and directed toward the medial epicondyle until desired wrist flexion and/or thumb opposition is obtained. A small amount of local anesthetic is then injected.

The median nerve is blocked at the wrist by identifying the palmaris longus tendon which can be discentered when the patient is instructed to flex at the way. A short 22-gauge needle is inserted just medial to the palmaris longus tendon at the carpal tunnel and small amount of local is injected.

Radial Nerve Block

The radial nerve originates from the terminal branch of the posterior cord of the brachial plexus and travels posterior to the humerus innervating the triceps and entering the spiral groove of the humerus. It then moves laterally at the elbow and travel thru the posterior lateral of the forearm.

Blockage of the radial nerve provides anesthesia to the lateral aspect of the dorsum of the hand and the proximal portion of the first, second, third and lateral half of the fourth digit. The Radial nerve can be block at the elbow or the wrist.

The radial nerve is blocked at the elbow by locating the biceps tendon and tracing it until it contacts the epicondyle. A small 22 gauge needle is inserted lateral to the biceps tendon near the epicondyle, a small local anesthetic is inject around the radial nerve as it passes over the anterior aspect of the lateral epicondyle.

The radial nerve is blocked at the wrist by identifying the palmaris longus and flexor carpi radialis tendon. A small needle is inserted over this tendon at the base of the first metacarpal; a small local anesthetic is injected proximally along the tendon and a right angle across the anatomic snuffbox. This injection tends to be very superficial.

Ulnar Nerve Block

The ulnar nerve originated from the medial cords of the brachial plexus and travel alongside the axillary and brachial arteries. It is easily located in the ulnar groove, which is bony space between the medial epicondyle of the humerus and olecranon process. In the forearm the nerve travel between the flexor digitorum profundus and the flexor carpi ulnaris.

Blockade of the ulnar nerve provides anesthesia of the ulnar side of the hand, the fifth digit, the medial part of fourth digit, and all the small muscles of the hand, except the thenar eminence and the first and second lumbrical muscles.

At the elbow, the ulnar nerve is blocked by inserting a small needle proximal to the arcuate ligament and posterior to the medial epicondyle until desire the nerve stimulation is obtained. Due to the superficial location of this nerve at this site there is a high incidence of nerve injury.

At the wrist, the ulnar nerve is located beneath the flexor carpi ulnaris tendon between the ulnar artery and the pisiform bone. The nerve is blocked by placing the needle alongside the tendon until desire nerve stimulation is obtained. A small anesthetic is injected alongside the area.

Musculocutaneous Nerve Block

The musculocutaneous nerve originates as the terminal branch of the lateral cord. It innervates the biceps, brachialis muscles, and terminates as the lateral cutaneous nerve of the forearm providing sensory to the radial side of the forearm up to the radiocarpal joint.

The musculocutaneous nerve block is usually performed as a supplement block to the axillary block of the brachial plexus. The nerve is usually located superior and proximal to the brachial artery thru the coracobrachialis muscle. An ultrasound is helpful to visualize the nerve between the muscle tissues. A small amount of local anesthetic is then injected along the nerve.

Side Effects and Complications

In general, terminal peripheral nerve blocks have a less frequent risk of complications. However there is a higher risk of nerve injury due to the nerves being superficially placed between ligamentous and bony structures [8]. Intravascular injection can occur therefore injection after aspiration is recommended.

Intravenous Regional Blocks

Clinical Applications

Intravenous regional blocks also known as Bier block were first described in 1908 by a German surgeon, August Bier [1–3, 6]. The technique involves the patient resting supine an intravenous cannula placed. Proximal and distal tourniquets are then applied on the desired limb. The goal of the tourniquet is to contain the anesthetic injected locally therefore cuffs should have secure closures and reliable pressure gauges. The Bier block has multiple advantages, including ease of administration, and rapid onset and recovery; therefore it is excellent for short procedures.

Technique

Prior to the intravenous administration of local anesthetic the desired limb is first exsanguinated by either tightly wrapping the extremity with an Esmark elastic bandage from distal to proximal direction or elevating it for 3–4 min to allow gravity to exsanguinate it [2]. The proximal cuff is then inflated greater than the systolic pressure until the absence of a distal pulse. The local anesthetic is then injected slowly; the total dose is based on the patient's weight [6]. The onset of anesthesia is usually within 5 min. When the patient complains of tourniquet pain, the distal tourniquet, which overlies anesthetized skin, is inflated, and the proximal tourniquet is released. The tourniquet can be safely release slowly after 25 minutes and the patient monitored closely for local anesthetic toxicity. For very short duration procedure the tourniquet must be left inflated for at least 15–20 min to avoid rapid intravenous systemic bolus of local anesthetic resulting into toxicity.

Side Effects and Complications

Most common problems associated with bier blocks include tourniquet discomfort, painful exsanguination, and rapid recovery leading to postoperative pain [2, 6]. Early deflation of the tourniquet or excessive doses of local anesthetics can result in systemic anesthetic toxicity. Rare complications including development of compartment syndrome and limb loss have also been noted [2, 8].

Lower Extremity Blocks

The most common indication for regional anesthesia outside of the OR is hip fracture. Pain from hip fracture, both intracapsular and extracapsular, can be treated with a lower extremity nerve block [10]. These blocks include femoral nerve block, fascia iliaca block, and lumbar plexus block. The femoral nerve block, sometimes called a 3-in-1 block, is an excellent block to treat pain from hip fracture and other injuries to the leg [11, 12]. A fascia iliaca block can also be used to treat hip and lower extremity pain, however, the efficacy of the femoral nerve block is greater than the fascia iliaca block [13]. A lumbar plexus block can also provide pain relief for hip fracture, however, the block is technically challenging, has a higher complication rate than the femoral block, and should only be performed by those with advanced training in nerve blocks [1, 14]. In addition, the femoral block is as effective as the lumbar plexus block in controlling pain after surgical repair of hip fractures [15].

Femoral Nerve Block [1, 16]

Anatomy

The femoral nerve innervates the leg- including the anterior and medial thigh distally to the knee and the medial aspect of the lower leg and foot. The femoral nerve also provides branches to the hip.

Indications

Hip fracture, injury to the anterior or medial thigh, femur, or knee

Procedure

The femoral nerve block is done adjacent to the femoral artery, in the inguinal crease. The block is usually done in the supine position, although some practitioners prefer Trendelenburg positioning of the table if the goal is analgesia to the hip [11]. The area should be prepped and draped in a sterile fashion. In the obese patient, tape can be used to secure the pannus out of the procedure field. The pulsation of the femoral artery can be used as a landmark in correct placement of the ultrasound transducer, although this can be difficult in the obese patient, and it is not necessary for the procedure. The ultrasound transducer should be placed in the inguinal crease in a transverse plane and adjusted until the femoral artery is identified. The femoral nerve can then be located lateral to the femoral artery, deep to the fascia illaca, superficial to the iliopsoas muscle. The femoral nerve is hyperechoic and can be oval or triangular in shape.

Once the femoral nerve is identified, the skin is anesthetized with a superficial infiltration of local anesthetic or skin wheal, 1 cm laterally to the ultrasound transducer. A 22-guage insulated stimulating needle is then inserted in-plane to the femoral nerve. A "pop" can often be felt as the needle moves deep to the fascia iliaca. A nerve stimulator is not necessary for a successful block, however, it can aid in optimal positioning. To verify appropriate position of the needle, a patellar twitch should be present between 0.3 and 0.5 mA. After negative aspiration, 10–20 mL of local anesthetic is injected in divided doses adjacent to the femoral nerve, checking for negative aspiration between each dose. A finger can be used to apply pressure just distal to the point of injection to encourage proximal spread of the local anesthetic to improve analgesia to the hip. The Injection should be stopped if high injection pressures are noted or if the patient experiences pain during injection.

Complications

The complication rate for femoral blocks is low. Complications include failed block, nerve injury, intravascular injection of local anesthetic, local anesthetic systemic toxicity, bleeding, and infection [1].

Fascia Iliaca Block [17]

Anatomy

The fascia iliaca block relies on the location of the femoral nerve and the lateral femoral cutaneous nerve, coursing beneath the fascia iliacus and above the iliacus muscle. Spread of local anesthestic along this plane provides the block of the nerves.

Indications

Hip fracture, injury to the anterior, anterolateral, or medial thigh, femur, or knee

Procedure

As with the femoral block, the fascia iliaca block is done in the supine position, at the inguinal crease. After sterile prep and drape of the field, the transducer is placed in a transverse plane in the inguinal crease to identify the femoral artery. The hyperechoic femoral nerve is then located lateral to the femoral artery, deep to the fascia iliaca, superficial to the iliopsoas muscle. Once these structures are identified, the transducer is moved laterally to identify the sartorius muscle. Local anesthetic can be used to anesthetize the skin and subcutaneous tissue at the needle insertion point. Insert the needle in plane until the fascia iliaca is pierced. A "pop" may be felt as the needle moves deep to the fascia iliaca. After negative aspiration, 30–40 mL of local anesthetic is injected in divided doses. The transducer can be moved medically to confirm spread to the femoral nerve and laterally to confirm spread beneath the sartorius muscle.

Complications

The complications of the fascia iliaca block are similar to the femoral block, although the chance of intravascular injection is less as the block is not perivascular [1].

Thoracic Blocks

Regional anesthesia can be superior to systemic analgesia when a patient suffers from multiple rib fractures. There is often a possibility of coinciding lung injury. Regional analgesia will relieve the patient's pain and allow for improved breathing. The pain, otherwise, can impair ventilation and ability to clear secretions, which may progress. Up to 1/3 of patients with rib fractures develop nosocomial pneumonia [18]. Not only will epidural anesthesia decrease pain but it will double vital capacity and reduce flail chest [18]. While opioids may relieve the patient's pain, side effects such as sedation are common and may lead to further respiratory compromise. The pain management guidelines for blunt thoracic trauma recommend epidural analgesia as the preferred mode of pain relief unless contraindicated [18]. Reasons for inability to provide epidural anesthesia may include infection, coagulopathy, spinal fractures, hemodynamic instability [19, 20].

Intercostal Nerve Blocks

Indications

Pain relief from rib fractures, herpes zoster or cancer pain. Blockade of two dermatomes above and below the cause of pain is necessary.

Contraindications

Local Infection, Coagulatopathy, and if inadvertent pneumothorax would cause serious consequences.

Anatomy

The intercostal nerve runs with the intercostal artery and vein on the underside of corresponding rib. The nerve is formed from the dorsal and ventral rami of the thoracic spinal nerves. The nerve usually runs below both the vein and artery. The nerve block will anesthetize the sensory and motor fibers of that specific side.

Technique

Position: Put the patient in a supine or lateral decubitus position. Palpate and mark each rib at the mid and posterior axillary line to help visualize the length of the rib. Most commonly the block is placed 6–8 cm from (lateral to) the spinous process. Place a skin wheal at the inferior border of the rib and then place a 20–25 g needle needle at the inferior portion of the rib. Hit the rib and then walk off the rib inferiorly. Advance the needle 5 mm underneath the rib and aspirate. If aspiration for blood and air is negative inject 3–5 ml of local anesthetic. If a catheter is desired an 18–20 g Tuohy needle should be placed and a catheter can then be threaded through the Tuohy.

Complications

Intercostal nerve blocks have the highest levels of local anesthetic in the blood. Doses must be carefully titrated to avoid LAST.
Pneumothorax
Intravascular injection.
Spinal anesthesia
hematoma

Thoracic Paravertebral Nerve Block

Indications

The thoracic paravertebral block is an alternative to a thoracic epidural which is less complicated and has minimal hemodynamic changes.

Indications

Malignant and benign neuralgias
Post herpetic neuralgia
Multiple rib Fractures

Contraindications

Infection at the site
Empyema
Neoplasm
Coagulopathy
Deformed spine

Anatomy

The TPNB will anesthetize the spinal nerve as it emerges from the from the intervertebral foramina and divides into two rami. A larger anterior ramus, which innervates the muscles and the skin of the anterolateral body and limbs and a smaller posterior ramus which innervates the skin and muscles of the back and neck. This will create a unilateral, somatic and sympathetic block. The thoracic paravertebral space is defined as the parietal pleura as the anterolateral border, the base as the vertebral body. The posterior boundary is the transverse process and superior costotransverse ligament

Technique

Place the patient in the sitting or lateral decubitus position. Identify the midline. The C7 spinous process is the most prominent process when the neck is flexed. After identifying C7 continue to mark the thoracic spinous processes. T7 corresponds to the lower tip of the scapulae. Place a 22 g block needle 2.5 cm lateral to the midline (spinous process) of the side desired to be anesthetized. A 22 gauge block needle should enter perpendicular to the skin and contact the transverse process, approximately 3–4 cm. Because the thoracic spinous processes have an acute angle the middle of one spinous process correlates to the transverse process one level below. Eg. T5 spinous process and T6 transverse process. If the transverse process is not contacted at 4 cm, withdraw the needle and reinsert it caudad or cephalad. Once bone is contacted the needle should be withdrawn and redirected cauded 1 cm further. At this point a pop may be felt correlating with the costrotransverse ligament. This may correlate with a loss or resistance technique. After negative aspiration for air and blood 4 ml of local anesthetic may be administered. The nerve block must be redone at each level desired to be anesthetized. If placing for rib fractures a catheter may be placed at the halfway mark between the lowest and highest fracture. If placing a catheter it is common to feel resistance which can be overcome by creating a pocket with 5–10 ml of saline.

Dosing

If proceeding with multiple injections of 3–4 cc then 0.5–0.75 % ropivicaine may be bolused.

If placing a catheter an 18 g tuohy needle may be used to intraduce the gather then 0.2 % ropivicaine may be infused.

Complications

Pneumothorax
Intervascular injection
Inadvertant epidural injection and contralateral anesthetic spread

Intrathecal injection
Inadvertant intraplural catheter placemnt

Intrapleural Blocks

Intrapleural blocks are another option to give local anesthetic, but it runs a high risk of local anesthetic toxicity secondary to high absorption [21].

Neuraxial

Neuraxial anesthesia may be administered to the appropriate patient population. Thoracic epidural anesthesia may be appropriate for rib injury while lumbar neuraxial anesthesia may benefit the patient undergoing a gynecologic procedure in IR OR in offsite locate.

Anatomy

The epidural space is a potential space that is located between the ligamentum flavum and the dura mater. Its range is from the foramen magnum to the sacral hiatus and contains emerging nerve roots of the spinal cord, fat and veins. The spinal cord ends at L2L3.

An epidural can be placed in the sitting or lateral decubitus position. Landmarks used include the posterior superior iliac crests which coincide with L4L5. Then the midline is found by palpating the spine and feeling the finger come off of the spinous process into the interspace.

Once the location has been determined, administer a local anesthetic skin wheal and create a track.

Place the Tuohy needle through the skin wheal. The Tuohy needle will pass through the skin, superspinous, and interspinous ligaments before it reaches the ligamentum flavum. Engage the Tuohy needle at the ligamentum flavum.

Attach a fluid or air filled plastic or glass syringe. Advance the Tuohy needle in tiny increments and feel for a loss of resistance after each time the Tuohy is advanced.

If there is a positive loss of resistance without blood or csf, than an epidural catheter may be advanced

The catheter may be advanced 4–6 cm into the space.

Aspirate the catheter for blood or csf. If negative give a test dose of local anesthetic with epinephrine to verify once more that the catheter is not sitting in the csf or an epidural vessel.

Secure the epidural.

Thoracic Epidural Analgesia

Epidurals have been shown to reduce mechanical ventilation times and the incidence of pneumonia in patients with rib injury when the epidural corresponds with the level of the injury

Contraindications

Hypotension and hypovolemia, uncooperative patient, head or spinal injuries, systemic infection and hemostatic possibilities.

Anatomy

The thoracic spinous process are angled downward. This will affect the angle at which the Tuohy needle is introduced.

Technique

The needle will be inserted one fingerbreadth lateral to the desired interspace. The needle is inserted perpendicular to the skin until the lamina is met. Then the needle is angled 45° medially and 45° cephalad and walked to the ligamentum flavum
    The loss of resistance technique is then employed to enter the epidural space

Gynecologic

Combined spinal epidural anesthesia or patient controlled epidural analgesia is a technique that allows for an anesthetic to be continued for post operative pain control after uterine artery embolizations. Uterine artery embolizations are an option for patients who do not wish to undergo hysterectomy for symptomatic uterine fibroids.

Combined Spinal Epidural: CSE

A CSE may be perfomed by finding the epidural space with a Tuohy needle and then advancing a spinal needle through the Tuohy needle, past the dura. Once CSF is confirmed, local anesthetic may be injected through the spinal needle to quickly achieve a spinal dose. Once the patient is dosed, the spinal needle is removed and an epidural catheter is threaded through the Tuohy to leave an epidural for the rest of the case if needed or postoperative pain.

Interstitial Brachytherapy

Interstitial brachytherapy is associated with significant postoperative pain and PCEA is an effective method for post-operative pain

Sedation and Regional Anesthesia

Peripheral nerve blocks have been established since the early stages of anesthesia. It been performed since the 1880s, when Halsted and Hall described the injection of cocaine into peripheral nerves for minor surgical procedures [1]. To this day, regional anesthesia has grown significant popularity as it decreases the need for postoperative analgesics, incidence of nausea, shortens post-anesthesia care unit time, and increases patient satisfaction [1, 6]. Most importantly, peripheral nerve block can be performed in non-operative room settings.

The regional techniques are chosen depending on the surgical site, ambulation requirements, and the desired postoperative pain control. Anesthesia providers should have a detailed anatomic knowledge to choose the appropriate technique for the intended surgical procedure and avoid complications. Nerve blocks should be administered in areas with standard hemodynamic monitors, supplemental oxygen, and resuscitation medications including lipid emulsion readily available [1–3, 6]. Patients should be monitored with pulse-oximetry, Noninvasive blood pressure and electrocardiogram. Sedation for regional anesthesia is not a requirement. However sedation is readily used to reduce anxiety and minimize discomfort.

Goal, of sedation will depend on the technique being employed. Paresthesia seeking techniques are reliant on patient cooperation and participation to guide the local anesthetic injection accurately; therefore, only small doses of sedation medication are recommended [1]. Paresthesia techniques have been criticized for causing patient discomfort, although clinical studies have not shown a significant increase in neurologic complications with this technique [1, 2]. However the use of peripheral nerve stimulators allows for localization of a specific peripheral nerve without requiring the elicitation of a paresthesia, thus allowing patients to be more heavily sedated during block placement.

Short-acting benzodiazepine and opioids such as Midazolam and fentanyl respectively are widely used. Other well-documented drugs are Propofol, ketamine, or Etomidate. Regardless of drugs or techniques employed the most important goals are to titrate for comfort while ensuring the patient respond to verbal clues as well as patients' comorbidities [2].

The Benefits of Regional Anesthesia

One of the greatest benefits of regional anesthesia is the improved pain control and decreased need for opioids and sedation. Trauma patients are commonly under-treated for pain Reasons, include ongoing resuscitation, as well as concerns for the side-effects of systemic medications like NSAIDS and opioids [3]. Elderly patients with hip fractures are at high risk of delirium after injury. Practitioners are reluctant to prescribe opioid medications to elderly patients, and elderly patients receive less opioid medication when compared to younger patients with the same injuries [22]. Unfortunately, elderly patients who do not receive systemic pain medication are not protected from delirium. In fact, both inadequately treated pain and use of IV opioid medication increase the risk for delirium [23, 24]. Femoral nerve blocks provide better pain control when compared to opioid only pain control strategies [11]. In addition, regional anesthesia has been shown to decrease delirium in patients at intermediate-risk of developing delirium after hip fracture [25].

Peripheral nerve blocks can also replace the need for sedation for some procedures in the emergency department. This decreases complications related to sedation as well as staffing required to monitor patients after sedation, which can also reduce costs. Shoulder reductions performed under brachial plexus blocks had a decreased length of stay when compared to reductions performed under sedation, with no decrease in patient satisfaction [26].

Pain from rib fractures can lead to significant complications [12]. Pain often prevents patients from taking adequate breaths, leading to atelectasis, V/Q mismatch, hypoxemia, pneumonia, and respiratory failure. Opioid medications can worsen these symptoms. In treating rib fractures, epidural anesthesia has been shown to increase comfort, reduce incidence of pneumonia, reduce ICU length of stay, and reduce days on mechanical ventilation [19, 27]. When an epidural is contraindicated, a paravertebral nerve block catheter can also provide superior pain control and facilitated ambulation and return to normal activities [12].

Special Considerations

Compartment Syndrome

It has been debated if peripheral nerve blocks should be placed in patients at risk for acute compartment syndrome, because it could possibly mask pain. Pain is one of the most important symptoms in diagnosing the syndrome. Acute compartment syndrome occurs most often in men less than 35 years who have had a tibial or forearm fractures, and crush injuries, spare Femoral neck and ankle fractures are less susceptible to compartment syndrome [18]. The concern of using nerve blocks or continuous catheters is that the onset of ischemic pain may not be appreciated if the nerve block has anesthetized the area of injury. Failure to diagnose and treat compartment syndrome early can lead to sequelae such as amputation, rhabdo-myolyis, and cardiac arrhythmias [18]. Only a handful of case reports have been published describing nerve blocks with acute compartment syndrome. They describe either break through pain or a nerve block that was unable to resolve the pain. Thus new breakthrough pain or a failed nerve block may be a sign of early acute compartment syndrome. The risks and benefits of placing a peripheral nerve block on susceptible patients should be thoroughly discussed with the patient as well as the patient's perioperative care team. If choosing to do a regional nerve block one must keep a high index of suspicion, frequently assess the patient and monitor for compartmental pressures [21].

Elderly

The elderly pose several challenges to adequately treating pain. Opioids may have negative neurologic effects in a population that may already have diagnosed cognitive or vascular disorders [28]. Narcotics may also cause severe constipation and lead to nausea and vomiting in a population that may not be able to adequately protect their airway leading to aspiration pneumonia. Treating these patients with non-steroidal anti- inflammatory drugs (NSAIDS), poses issues of its own. NSAIDS can lead to gastrointestinal bleeds which may need further intervention, make the patient anemic and require transfusion. Yet inadequately treating these patients' pain especially after hip fracture, yields to delayed recovery.

Nerve blocks after hip surgery can decrease the need for systemic pain medications. While the femoral block and the fascia-iliaca block are helpful to control post operative pain, they may be also be considered in the ED setting for pre-operative analgesia. The fascia iliaca block has been found to be nearly as effective as parenteral NSAIDS after hip fracture. It has also been found to control patient pain without the need for additional narcotics [28].

Coagulation

The coagulation status of the patient must be taken into consideration when deciding if a peripheral nerve block would be appropriate. Spontaneous hematomas have been reported in patients who were on anticoagulants. A hematoma within the nerve sheath may increase the risk of ischemic nerve injury [6]. Of the cases that have been reported all patients with neuro deficits had neurologic recovery within 6–12 months [1]. Symptoms of bleeding that patients may present with include pain in the region of the peripheral nerve block, a drop in the hemoglobin, hypotension, and neurologic deficits. Diagnosis of a hematoma may be made via CT. Treatment includes surgical consultation and necessary supportive treatments.

ASRA guidelines recommend using the same neuraxial injection guidelines for peripheral nerve blocks. Patients who are to receive a peripheral nerve block while anticoagulated must be aware of the risks as well as be closely monitored after. An INR of ≤1.4 is considered acceptable for both neuraxial and peripheral nerve blocks [1].

Peripheral Nerve Injury PNI

There is conflicting information regarding whether the incidence of nerve injury has decreased with the use of ultrasound. The reported rate of long term injury is 2–4/10,000 blocks [28, 29]. There is usually resolution of sensory deficits that occur within the territory of the peripheral block within days to weeks [30] .

There is some evidence that suggests that proximal nerves may be at higher risk to injury than more distal [31, 32].

Get a neurologic consult to begin managing all treatable causes [33]. In the case that all treatable causes have been excluded a pain consultation can be useful to coordinate the patient's care and monitor the patient for chronic pain from the injury

Because of the various reporting mechanisms delineating the risk factors for PNI is difficult.

Infection

Infection in the blood is a relative contraindication for peripheral nerve blocks, but placing catheters may add another source of infection.

Local Anesthetic Toxicity

LAST is a known serious but rare complication of peripheral nerve blocks, The practitioner should be aware of signs and be prepared to treat the patient if necessary. This should be given even more careful consideration since these Religional blocks will be done outside of the operating room and necessary equipment may not be as readily available. It will be helpful to create a mobile cart with all equipment necessary to treat LAST, so there is no delay in treatment.

Absorption of Local Anesthetics (Most to Least)

Intravenous > Intercostal > Caudal epidural > Lumbar epidural > Brachial plexus > Subcutaneous

Checklist by ASRA [34] : Treatment:

Ventilate with 100% FiO$_2$

Seizure suppression with benzodiazapenes (e.g., Midazolam IV), avoid Propofol if hemodynamically unstable.

Alert OR for possible need for Cardiopulmonary bypass

Management of Cardiac Dysrythmias

AVOID vasopressin, calcium channel blockers, beta blockers, or local anesthetic

Begin Lipid Emulsion Therapy (Intralipid)

Record LAST events at www.lipidrescue.org and report use of lipid to www.lipidregistry.org

Intralipid: 1.5 mL/kg IV bolus; Repeat 1–2 times for asystole

Start infusion 0.25–0.5 mL/kg/min for 30–60 mins for hypotension

Epinephrine: total dose: <1 mcg/kg

References

1. Horlocker Terese T, KSL, Wedel Denise J. Peripheral nerve blocks. In: D. MR, editors. Miller's anesthesia. Elsevier; 2015. p. 1721–51.
2. Brown DL. Atlas of regional anesthesia. 3rd ed. Philadelphia: Elsevier Saunders; 2006.
3. Choi JJ, Lin E, Gadsden J. Regional anesthesia for trauma outside the operating theatre. Curr Opin Anaesthesiol. 2013;26(4):495–500.
4. Neal JM, Gerancher JC, Hebl JR, Ilfeld BM, McCartney CJ, Franco CD, et al. Upper extremity regional anesthesia: essentials of our current understanding, 2008. Reg Anesth Pain Med. 2009;34(2):134–70.
5. Ryu T, Kil BT, Kim JH. Comparison between ultrasound-guided supraclavicular and interscalene brachial plexus blocks in patients undergoing arthroscopic shoulder surgery: a prospective, randomized, parallel study. Medicine. 2015;94(40):e1726.
6. Madison SJ, Ilfeld BM. Peripheral nerve blocks. In: Butterworth JFI, Mackey DC, Wasnick JD, editors. Morgan & Mikhail's clinical anesthesiology. 5eth ed. New York: McGraw-Hill; 2013.
7. De Jose Maria B, Banus E, Navarro Egea M, Serrano S, Perello M, Mabrok M. Ultrasound-guided supraclavicular vs infraclavicular brachial plexus blocks in children. Paediatr Anaesth. 2008;18(9):838–44.
8. Liebmann O, Price D, Mills C, Gardner R, Wang R, Wilson S, et al. Feasibility of forearm ultrasonography-guided nerve blocks of the radial, ulnar, and median nerves for hand procedures in the emergency department. Ann Emerg Med. 2006;48(5):558–62.
9. Maga JM, Cooper L, Gebhard RE. Outpatient regional anesthesia for upper extremity surgery update (2005 to present) distal to shoulder. Int Anesthesiol Clin. 2012;50(1):47–55.
10. Dickman E, Pushkar I, Likourezos A, Todd K, Hwang U, Akhter S, et al. Ultrasound-guided nerve blocks for intracapsular and extracapsular hip fractures. Am J Emerg Med. 2016;34(3): 586–9.
11. Beaudoin FL, Haran JP, Liebmann O. A comparison of ultrasound-guided three-in-one femoral nerve block versus parenteral opioids alone for analgesia in emergency department patients with hip fractures: a randomized controlled trial. Acad Emerg Med. 2013;20(6):584–91.

12. Gadsden J, Warlick A. Regional anesthesia for the trauma patient: improving patient outcomes. Local Reg Anesth. 2015;8:45–55.
13. Newman B, McCarthy L, Thomas PW, May P, Layzell M, Horn K. A comparison of preoperative nerve stimulator-guided femoral nerve block and fascia iliaca compartment block in patients with a femoral neck fracture. Anaesthesia. 2013;68(9):899–903.
14. Lumbar Plexus Block. 2013. Available from: http://www.nysora.com/techniques/neuraxial-and-perineuraxial-techniques/ultrasound-guided/3279-lumbar-plexus-block.html.
15. Amiri HR, Safari S, Makarem J, Rahimi M, Jahanshahi B. Comparison of combined femoral nerve block and spinal anesthesia with lumbar plexus block for postoperative analgesia in intertrochanteric fracture surgery. Anesth Pain Med. 2012;2(1):32–5.
16. Ultrasound Guided Femoral Nerve Block. 2013. Available from: http://www.nysora.com/techniques/ultrasound-guided-techniques/lower-extremity/3056-ultrasound-guided-femoral-nerve-block.html.
17. Ultrasound guided fascia iliaca block. 2013. Available from: http://www.nysora.com/techniques/ultrasound-guided-techniques/lower-extremity/3057-ultrasound-guided-fascia-iliaca-block.html.
18. Wu JJ, Lollo L, Grabinsky A. Regional anesthesia in trauma medicine. Anesthesiol Res Pract. 2011;2011:713281.
19. Bulger EM, Edwards T, Klotz P, Jurkovich GJ. Epidural analgesia improves outcome after multiple rib fractures. Surgery. 2004;136(2):426–30.
20. Available from: http://www.pitt.edu/~regional/Epidural/epidural.htm.
21. De Buck F, Devroe S, Missant C, Van de Velde M. Regional anesthesia outside the operating room: indications and techniques. Curr Opin Anaesthesiol. 2012;25(4):501–7.
22. Jones JS, Johnson K, McNinch M. Age as a risk factor for inadequate emergency department analgesia. Am J Emerg Med. 1996;14(2):157–60.
23. Vaurio LE, Sands LP, Wang Y, Mullen EA, Leung JM. Postoperative delirium: the importance of pain and pain management. Anesth Analg. 2006;102(4):1267–73.
24. Morrison RS, Magaziner J, Gilbert M, Koval KJ, McLaughlin MA, Orosz G, et al. Relationship between pain and opioid analgesics on the development of delirium following hip fracture. J Gerontol A Biol Sci Med Sci. 2003;58(1):76–81.
25. Mouzopoulos G, Vasiliadis G, Lasanianos N, Nikolaras G, Morakis E, Kaminaris M. Fascia iliaca block prophylaxis for hip fracture patients at risk for delirium: a randomized placebo-controlled study. J Orthop Traumatol Off J Ital Soc Orthop Traumatol. 2009;10(3):127–33.
26. Blaivas M, Adhikari S, Lander L. A prospective comparison of procedural sedation and ultrasound-guided interscalene nerve block for shoulder reduction in the emergency department. Acad Emerg Med. 2011;18(9):922–7.
27. Ullman DA, Fortune JB, Greenhouse BB, Wimpy RE, Kennedy TM. The treatment of patients with multiple rib fractures using continuous thoracic epidural narcotic infusion. Reg Anesth. 1989;14(1):43–7.
28. Godoy Monzon D, Iserson KV, Vazquez JA. Single fascia iliaca compartment block for post-hip fracture pain relief. J Emerg Med. 2007;32(3):257–62.
29. Orebaugh SL, Williams BA, Vallejo M, Kentor ML. Adverse outcomes associated with stimulator-based peripheral nerve blocks with versus without ultrasound visualization. Reg Anesth Pain Med. 2009;34(3):251–5.
30. Borgeat A, Ekatodramis G, Kalberer F, Benz C. Acute and nonacute complications associated with interscalene block and shoulder surgery: a prospective study. Anesthesiology. 2001;95(4):875–80.
31. Moayeri N, Bigeleisen PE, Groen GJ. Quantitative architecture of the brachial plexus and surrounding compartments, and their possible significance for plexus blocks. Anesthesiology. 2008;108(2):299–304.
32. Neal JM, Barrington MJ, Brull R, Hadzic A, Hebl JR, Horlocker TT, Huntoon MA, Kopp SL, Rathmell JP, Watson JC. The second ASRA practice advisory on neurologic complications

associated with regional anesthesia and pain medicine: executive summary 2015. Reg Anesth Pain Med. 2015;40(5):401–30.

33. Neal JM, Kopp SL, Pasternak JJ, Lanier WL, Rathmell JP. Anatomy and pathophysiology of spinal cord injury associated with regional anesthesia and pain medicine: 2015 update. Reg Anesth Pain Med. 2015;40(5):506–25.

34. Neal JM, Mulroy MF, Weinberg GL, American Society of Regional Anesthesia and Pain Medicine. American Society of Regional Anesthesia and Pain Medicine checklist for managing local anesthetic systemic toxicity: 2012 version. Reg Anesth Pain Med. 2012;37(1):16–8.

Chapter 31
Newer Drugs for Sedation: Soft Pharmacology

Janette Brohan and Peter John Lee

Abstract Drugs traditionally used for sedation and anaesthesia, such as benzodiazepines, clonidine, etomidate and propofol have each some of the features of the ideal sedative for the out-of-operating room (OR) environment. However the search for the ideal sedative in this environment continues and has resulted in the development of newer agents for sedation. There is a growing interest in 'soft pharmacology'. 'Soft drugs' is a term used to describe agents, often analogs of a parent compound, with a chemical configuration designed to allow rapid metabolism into inactive metabolites after exerting their desired therapeutic effect (s). 'Soft' sedative drugs, such as remimazolam, dexmedetomidine, etomidate analogs and fospropofol may approach the ideal out-of-OR sedative, as they can potentially offer well-controlled titratable activity and ultrashort action. The salient features of these drugs are discussed in this chapter (Table 31.1)

Keywords Soft pharmacology • Soft drugs • Remimazolam • Dexmedetomidine • Etomidate analogs • MOC-etomidate • Carboetomidate • Fospropofol

Introduction

The out-of-operating room (out-of-OR) environment presents unique challenges to the anesthesiologist. Such challenges can include remote locations, lack of immediate assistance from colleagues and potentially less experienced assistance. An area of interest and potential improvement is the drugs used for sedation.

J. Brohan, MB, BCh, BAO (✉)
Department of Anaesthesia, Cork University Hospital, Wilton, Cork, Cork, Ireland
e-mail: janettebrohan@gmail.com

P.J. Lee, MB, BCh, BAO, FCARCSI, MD
Department of Anaesthesia, Intensive Care and Pain Medicine,
Cork University Hospital, Wilton, Cork, Ireland
e-mail: peter.lee@hse.ie

© Springer International Publishing Switzerland 2017
B.G. Goudra, P.M. Singh (eds.), *Out of Operating Room Anesthesia*,
DOI 10.1007/978-3-319-39150-2_31

An ideal out-of-OR sedative agent would have the following properties:

1. Ease of use, helpful where suboptimal staffing and monitoring facilities might occur in an out-of-OR anaesthesia setting
2. Rapid onset of effect, given the time and resource limitations inherent to some out-of-OR anaesthesia environments
3. Quick recovery on discontinuation of sedation, important due to the ambulatory nature of out-of-OR anesthesia, and the potentially remote locations and poor recovery facilities that may be involved
4. Minimal residual sedation to allow for neurological evaluation

The search for this ideal drug for sedation has intensified in recent years [1, 2] and several new agents are presented here. 'Soft drugs' is a term sometimes used to describe agents, often analogs of a parent compound, with a chemical configuration designed to allow rapid metabolism into inactive metabolites after exerting their desired therapeutic effect(s) [3]. The following 'soft' sedative drugs may approach the ideal out-of-OR sedative, as they can offer well controlled titratable activity and ultrashort action.

Table 31.1 Summary of salient features and pharmacokinetics of newer sedative agents

	Remimazolam	Dexmedetomidine	Etomidate analogs[a]	Fospropofol
Class	Benzodiazepine	α2 adrenoceptor agonist	Imidazole	Propofol prodrug
Receptor	$GABA_A$	α2 adrenoceptors	$GABA_A$	$GABA_A$
Sedative dose	0.1–0.2 mg/kg	1 mcg/kg over 10 min, then 0.2–0.7 mcg/kg/h infusion	To be determined	6.5 mg/kg followed by 1.6 mg/kg at 4 min intervals
Dose reduction for elderly	No	Yes	To be determined	Yes
Dose reduction for hepatic impairment	No	Yes	To be determined	Limited data but dose reduction advised
Dose reduction for renal impairment	No	No	To be determined- carboxylic acid metabolite may accumulate in renal impairment	No dose reduction with creatinine clearance > 30 ml/ min. Limited data for patients with creatinine clearance < 30 ml/ min
Onset	1.5–2.5 min	5–8 min	To be determined- rapid in animal models	4–8 min

(continued)

Table 31.1 (continued)

	Remimazolam	Dexmedetomidine	Etomidate analogs[a]	Fospropofol
Metabolism	Ester hydrolysis	Hepatic metabolism via cytochrome p450 and glucuronidation	Ester hydrolysis	Fospropofol metabolized to propofol by endothelial and hepatic alkaline phosphatases Propofol metabolized by hepatic and erythrocyte dehydrogenases
Offset	6.8–9.9 min	6 min	To be determined- rapid in animal models	5–18 min
Active metabolite	No	No	Carboxylic acid metabolite	No

[a]Etomidate analogues such as MOC-etomidate and carboetomidate are currently under development and data available at time of publication comes from animal models

Remimazolam

Remimazolam is an ester-based benzodiazepine derivative with, as the name might suggest, certain properties of both remifentanil and midazolam [4]. It is derived from its parent compound midazolam, but with the incorporation of the pharmacokinetic properties of remifentanil. The design of remimazolam with the inclusion of a carboxylic ester linkage results in rapid hydrolysis in the body by ubiquitous tissue esterases to an inactive carboxylic acid metabolite (CNS 7054) (Table 31.1).

Benzodiazepine use for procedural sedation has two main limitations: the absence of analgesic properties, and persistence of sedative effects beyond the duration of the procedure. This latter feature relates to both diffuse drug distribution and prolonged elimination. The use of midazolam, which has the shortest half-life of any of the benzodiazepines, can lead to prolonged sedation and unpredictable recovery due to a half-life of 1.8–6.4 h and accumulation of an active metabolite, α-hydroxy-midazolam, which has a sedative effect [4, 5].

Remimazolam, in contrast, may bypass these limitations of benzodiazepines, and may indeed have many of the properties of the ideal sedative agent for use in the out-of-OR setting [6, 7]. In addition to producing dose-dependant sedation, remimazolam has a rapid offset when compared to midazolam. This is due to metabolism and clearance by tissue esterases, in addition to an inactive metabolite [8]. Another important feature of remimazolam for the out-of-OR setting is the lack of accumulation, with the context-sensitive half-time similar to that of remifentanil [9].

Uses

Pre-operative   Pre-procedural premedication
Intra-operative   Initiation and maintenance of procedural sedation
                   Rapid onset and offset sedation for procedural sedation [10]
                   Co-induction of anaesthesia
                   Benzodiazepine anaesthesia
Post-operative   Shorter duration of recovery from anesthetic/sedation,
                   owing to reduction in intraoperative anesthetic and
                   opioid requirements

Structure

The structures of midazolam and remimazolam are presented in Fig. 31.1. The significant difference between the two molecules is the introduction of a carboxylic ester linkage to remimazolam, which allows metabolism by non-specific tissue esterases in the blood- in a similar way to remifentanil.

Dosing

– Sedative dose 0.1–0.2 mg/kg [10]
– Due to organ-independent elimination, no dosage adjustments are required for patients with hepatic or renal impairment.
– Age-related deterioration of hepato-renal drug handling is unlikely to have impact on remimazolam's metabolism

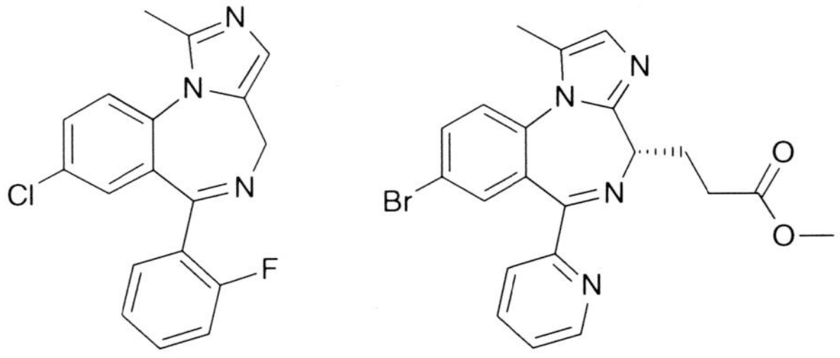

Fig. 31.1 Structures of midazolam and remimazolam [11]

Midazolam   Remimazolam

Kinetics

- Like other benzodiazepines, remimazolam acts on GABA receptors, specifically GABA$_A$ [8], modulating the effects of GABA at the GABA receptors
- Onset 1.5–2.5 min [10]
- Metabolized by dose-independent ester hydrolysis into inactive metabolite CNS 7054
- Rapid clearance 70.3 ± 13.9 L/h (midazolam clearance 23 ± 4.5 L/h) [8]
- Volume of distribution 23 ± 4.5 L/h (midazolam volume of distribution 81.8 ± 27.1 L/h) [8]
- Half life 0.75 ± 0.15 h [8]
- Mean offset time 6.8–9.9 min [10]
- Minimal accumulation- context sensitive halftime 7–8 min after a 2-h infusion [9]
- Slow clearance of inactive metabolite (4.22 ± 1.25 L/h) with terminal half-life of 2.89 ± 0.65 h
- Reversed by flumazenil

Adverse Effects

At the time of publication, there was ongoing recruitment for a phase III trial investigating efficacy and adverse effects of remimazolam in patients undergoing colonoscopy [12]. From the results of the phase I and II trials of remimazolam, the adverse effects of remimazolam appear to be similar to those of other benzodiazepines, including hypotension, respiratory depression, and desaturation [9, 10].

Dexmedetomidine

Clonidine was the first α2-adrenoceptor agonist, and was formulated in the 1960s. It was initially marketed as a nasal decongestant but was subsequently recognized as an effective antihypertensive and sedative drug. Dexmedetomidine, which is also an α2-agonist, was approved by the Food and Drug Administration at the end of 1999 for short-term (<24 h) analgesia and sedation in the intensive care unit. Its use has since expanded to include the perioperative period.

Dexmedetomidine has greater specificity for the α2-adrenoceptor compared to clonidine (ratios of α2:α1 activity, 1620:1 for dexmedetomidine, 220:1 for clonidine) [13]. Presynaptic α2- adrenoceptors regulate the release of norepinephrine and adenosine trisphosphate through a negative feedback mechanism, which results in

Fig. 31.2 The action of dexmedetomidine at a synapse

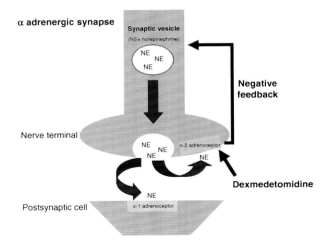

the analgesic effects of dexmedetomidine (Fig. 31.2). The sedative effects of dexmedetomidine result from agonism of central α2 receptors in the presynaptic neurons and subsequent inhibition of neuronal firing in the brain, particularly the locus coeruleus, and in the spinal cord [14].

The analgesic effects of dexmedetomidine are a result of:

1. direct α2-adrenoceptor agonism and inhibition of norepinephrine release
2. α2-adrenoceptor modulation of G-protein-gated potassium channels, resulting in membrane hyperpolarization and decreased firing rate in excitable cells in the CNS
3. G protein coupled reduction in calcium conductance through cell membranes and inhibition of neurotransmitter release [15]

There are many advantages to dexmedetomidine as an out-of-OR sedative. Because its actions are not mediated by the GABA-mimetic system, it has sedative, analgesia, and antishivering properties, but does not cause respiratory depression [16]. 'Cooperative sedation' is a term used to describe the sedative effect of dexmedetomidine, whereby the patient can be deeply sedated yet rousable and able to interact with healthcare providers [17].

Uses

Pre-operative	Pre-procedural premedication [18]
Intra-operative	Initiation and maintenance of procedural sedation
	Reduction of anaesthetic requirements [19, 20]
	Dose-dependant sedation without respiratory depression [21]
	Arousability maintained at deep levels of sedation [22]
	Attenuation of sympathoadrenal effects of surgical stimulation and endotracheal intubation [23]
	Analgesia, in addition to reduction of opioid requirements [23, 24]

Post-operative	Reduced duration of recovery from anesthetic/sedation, owing to reduction in intraoperative anesthetic and opioid requirements
	Reduction in analgesic requirements [24]
Other	Initiation and maintenance of intensive care sedation [25, 26]

Structure

Dexmedetomidine is an imidazole compound and is the pharmacologically active dextroisomer of medetomidine, which displays selective α2-agonism.

Presentation

Dexmedetomidine is presented in 200 mcg/2 mL (100 mcg/mL) glass vial to be used after dilution. Dexmedetomidine must be diluted with 48 ml 0.9 % sodium chloride injection to achieve a concentration of 4 mcg/ml.

Dosing

- Initial loading dose 1 mcg/kg over 10 min, followed by continuous IV infusion of 0.2–0.7 mcg/kg/h [27]
- For patients >65 years a loading infusion of 0.5 mcg/kg over 10 min and a reduction in the maintenance infusion should be considered [27]
- Hepatic impairment- dose reduction recommended [27]
- Renal impairment- no dose reduction required [28]

Kinetics

- Time to onset of action 5–8 min [27]
- Peak effect 10–20 min [27]
- Peak plasma concentrations achieved within 1 h after continuous infusion [27]
- Distribution half-life (t1/2) of approximately 6 min; a terminal elimination half-life (t1/2) of approximately 2 h [27]
- Highly bound to plasma proteins (94 %) [27]
- Lipophilic- Steady-state volume of distribution (Vss) of approximately 118 l
- Metabolism by the liver via cytochrome P450 & glucuronidation [13]
- Clearance is approximately 39 L/h [27]
- Mean offset time after single dose 6 min [27]

- Context sensitive halftime increases, depending on duration of infusion- ranging from 4 min after a 10 min infusion to 250 min after an 8 h infusion [29]
- No active metabolites
- Inactive metabolites excreted in urine (~95 %) and faeces (4 %) [27]

Adverse Effects [27]

Cardiovascular

- Hypotension incidence (56 %) and bradycardia incidence (42 %), both of which are due to inhibition of central sympathetic outflow [30, 31]
- Hypertension on initial bolusing, owing to peripheral α2B-adrenoceptor stimulation of vascular smooth muscle incidence (16 %) [30, 31]
- Arrhythmias including atrial fibrillation (4 %), extrasystoles, supraventricular tachycardia, ventricular arrhythmia and heart block

Respiratory

- Respiratory depression incidence (37 %)
- Respiratory failure incidence (6 %)
- Acute respiratory distress syndrome incidence (3 %)
- Pleural effusion incidence (2 %)

CNS

- Agitation incidence (8 %)
- Anxiety incidence (5 %)

GI

- Nausea incidence (11 %)
- Constipation incidence (6 %)
- Dry mouth incidence (4 %)

Others

- Hypokalaemia incidence (9 %)
- Pyrexia incidence (7 %)
- Hyperglycaemia incidence (7 %)
- Anemia incidence (3 %)
- Oliguria incidence (2 %)

Etomidate Analogs- MOC-Etomidate & Carboetomidate

Etomidate is a rapidly acting imidazole-based intravenous sedative-hypnotic agent that is used to induce general anesthesia through potentiation of GABA$_A$ receptor activation. As is the case with other intravenous anaesthetic agents, etomidate's hypnotic action ceases following bolus delivery when it is redistributed from the brain to other tissues. Etomidate undergoes elimination by the liver with a half-life of several hours [32]. One of the main advantages of etomidate over other induction agents is its ability to maintain hemodynamic stability even in the setting of cardio-vascular compromise [33]. The predominant issue surrounding the use of etomidate however, is adrenocortical suppression [34]. Etomidate potently inhibits 11β-hydroxylase, an enzyme in the biosynthetic pathway leading to adrenocortical steroid synthesis [35, 36]. Alternative etomidate analogs are currently under inves-tigation in the hopes of developing a rapidly metabolized hypnotic agent with the haemodynamic stability of etomidate but without the adrenocortical suppression characteristic of the parent compound. At the time of publication, these agents were under development and had not yet undergone human testing.

Methoxycarbonyl etomidate (MOC-etomidate), is a rapidly metabolized and ultra-short acting soft analog of etomidate that does not produce prolonged adreno-cortical suppression in rats after bolus administration [37]. MOC-etomidate has been found to potently enhance GABA$_A$ receptor function and produce a loss of righting reflex in rats that was extremely brief [37, 38]. In common with remifent-anil and remimazolam, it contains a metabolically-labile ester moiety that is rapidly hydrolyzed by esterases to form a carboxylic acid metabolite [37]. This metabolite is 300-fold less potent than MOC-etomidate but may accumulate in patients with renal failure [39], the clinical significance of which is yet to be determined. The structures of etomidate, MOC-etomidate and MOC-etomidate carboxylic acid are shown in Fig. 31.3.

Carboetomidate has a pyrrole ring in place of the imidazole ring of etomidate responsible for binding with 11β-hydroxylase [40]. Thus carboetomidate was devel-

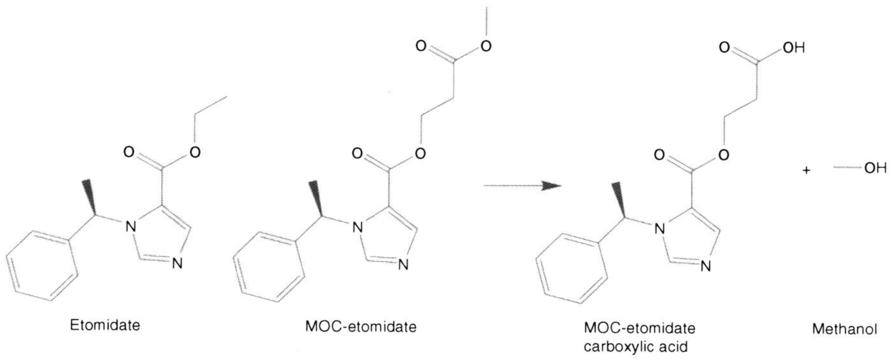

Fig. 31.3 Structures of etomidate, MOC-etomidate and MOC-etomidate carboxylic acid [48] (With permission from Oxford University Press, Sneyd and Rigby-Jones [48])

oped to have a low affinity for 11β-hydroxylase. Carboetomidate retains the GABA$_A$ receptor modulatory function, hypnotic activity and cardiovascular effects of etomidate [40]. It is three orders of magnitude less potent an inhibitor of in vitro cortisol synthesis compared to its parent compound and does not suppress steroid synthesis in rats [41]. Similar to MOC-etomidate, carboetomidate also contains a metabolically-labile ester moiety that is rapidly hydrolyzed by esterases to form the same carboxylic acid metabolite. There may also be the same issues with metabolite accumulation in patients with renal failure.

Water Soluble Propofol Analogues- Fospropofol

Since propofol was introduced in 1977 it has established itself as the most popular agent for induction of anaesthesia, in addition to a popular intravenous sedative agent; with many characteristics of the conceptually ideal drug [42, 43]. There are some disadvantages with propofol use, however. Close to 30 % of patients experience pain on intravenous injection of propofol [44]. In addition, propofol as a sedative agent can have a 'narrow therapeutic window' resulting in a sudden transition from moderate sedation to general anaesthesia which can be difficult to control [42, 44, 45].

Several water soluble analogues of propofol have been developed that avoid these disadvantages. Fospropofol is a water soluble prodrug of propofol with pharmacokinetic attributes different from those of propofol. Within the fospropofol molecule the propofol moiety is linked with a methylphosphate group at C-1 (a noncharged hydroxyl group is replaced with a charged phosphate group), resulting in electronegativity and polarity within the molecule, thus leading to water solubility of fospropofol [46]. It is metabolized to propofol, phosphate, and formaldehyde by endothelial alkaline phosphatases (Fig. 31.4). The metabolism of 1 mg of fospropofol in vivo releases 0.54 mg of propofol [47]. The sedative and anaesthetic properties of fospropofol result from the released propofol subsequently potentiating GABA-inhibitory pathways.

Fospropofol has a number of potential advantages over propofol. The water soluble nature of the compound may result in less severe pain on injection when compared to that of the propofol lipid emulsion [48]. When compared with propofol emulsion, fospropofol may be more suitable for use in the out-of-OR setting [49]. Following fospropofol administration, the active propofol metabolite is released following time-dependent enzymatic conversion. As a result, sedation following fospropofol administration has a slower onset of action than that following propofol administration. The relatively slow breakdown process of fospropofol subsequently results in sustained levels of propofol, with fewer peaks and troughs, and a longer duration of action compared to that with propofol administration [47]. This might be an advantage for very brief outpatient procedures where a single loading dose may be enough for an entire procedure. It is important that those administering fospropofol have an awareness of this delayed onset of clinical effect however, as additional boluses could lead to deeper level of sedation that intended.

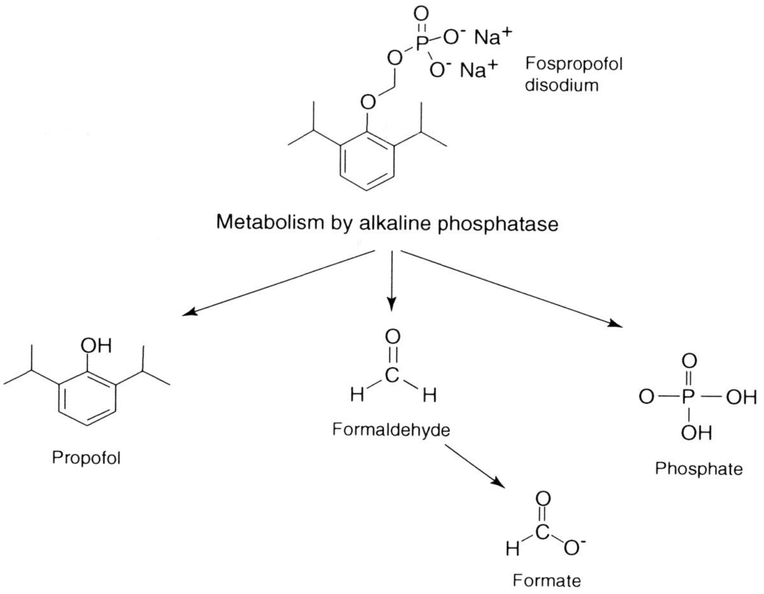

Fig. 31.4 Metabolism of fospropofol to propofol, phosphate, and formaldehyde by endothelial alkaline phosphatases

The metabolism of fospropofol results in the release of propofol, phosphate and formaldehyde. Alkaline dehydrogenase and formaldehyde dehydrogenase break down the formaldehyde to formate, which liberates carbon dioxide and water. This latter reaction involves the co-enzyme tetrahydrofolate. Formate is an end-metabolite of fospropofol. Accumulation of formate can have toxic effects, including metabolic acidosis and retinal toxicity leading to blindness. These toxic concentrations far exceed those that are reached with usual metabolism during standard fospropofol dosing regimens. Provided tetrahydrofolate concentrations are normal and maximum dosing rates are not exceeded, there is a negligible chance of toxicity related to formaldehyde liberation via fospropofol [50].

Uses

MAC sedation for diagnostic procedures (bronchoscopy, endoscopy) or therapeutic procedures (minor surgical procedures) [51, 52]

Structure

Fospropofol is a N-phosphono-O-methyl prodrug of propofol. The comparative structures of fospropofol and propofol and illustrated in Fig. 31.4.

Presentation

Fospropofol is formulated as a clear aqueous solution. The commercially available formulation contains 3.5 % of fospropofol per milliliter in water. Each 30 ml single use vial contains 35 mg of fospropofol disodium per ml (a total of 1050 mg of fospropofol disodium in a 30 ml vial) [51].

Dose

- Initial intravenous bolus of 6.5 mg/kg followed by supplemental doses of 1.6 mg/kg intravenously, at 4 min intervals as required [47]
- Patients >65 years- initial intravenous bolus of 4.9 mg/kg followed by supplemental doses of 1.2 mg/kg intravenously at 4 min intervals as required [47]
- Patients with renal impairment [47]:

  • No dosage reduction required with creatinine clearance >30 ml/min
  • Limited safety and efficacy data are available for use in patients with creatinine clearance < 30 ml/min.

- Limited studies involving patients with hepatic impairment. Caution advised when using fospropofol in patients with hepatic impairment [47]

Kinetics

- Time to onset of action 4–8 min [49]
- Mean offset time after single dose 5–18 min
- Volume of distribution of fospropofol 0.33 ± 0.069 L/kg, volume of distribution of propofol metabolite 5.8 L/kg
- Half-life (t1/2) of fospropofol 48–52 min. Half-life of liberated propofol 2.06 ± 0.77 h but this does not reflect the duration of sedation due to rapid redistribution [51]
- 98 % protein bound
- Fospropofol metabolized to propofol, formaldehyde and phosphate by alkaline phosphatases present in endothelium and liver (Fig. 31.4) [46, 52, 53]
- Propofol metabolite further metabolized to propofol glucuronide and other metabolites, catalyzed by glutathione dependent and independent dehydrogenases in the liver and erythrocytes
- Formaldehyde metabolite further metabolized to formate by enzyme systems, including formaldehyde dehydrogenase, present in various tissues, particularly the red blood cells. The formate produced is rapidly eliminated by oxidation to carbon dioxide
- Clearance of fospropofol 0.280 ± 0.053 L/h/kg, with clearance of propofol metabolite approximately 39 L/h/kg
- Elimination- 0.02 % excreted unchanged in urine

Adverse Effects

- Paresthesia, including perineal discomfort or burning sensation (incidence ~50–70%) [47, 54, 55]
- Pruritus (incidence 16–20%) [47, 54, 55]
- Both paresthesia and pruritis side effects are mild and self-limiting, lasting 1–2 min [55]
- Hypoxemia (incidence 4%)- The risk of which is reduced by appropriate positioning of the patient and the use of supplemental oxygen [56]
- Hypotension (incidence 4%)- Patients with compromised myocardial function, reduced vascular tone, or who have reduced intravascular volume may be at an increased risk for hypotension [46]
- Respiratory depression (incidence 1%) [46]

References

1. Johnson KB. New horizons in sedative hypnotic drug development: fast, clean, and soft. Anesth Analg. 2012;115(2):220–2.
2. Sear JW, Brown WE. Research into new drugs in anesthesia: then and now. Anesth Analg. 2012;115(2):233–4.
3. Buchwald P, Bodor N. Recent advances in the design and development of soft drugs. Pharmazie. 2014;69:403–13.
4. Midazolam hydrochloride injective FDA approved labeling by Baxter Healthcare Corporation dated April 2010. Available at: http://dailymed.nlm.nih.gov/dailymed/lookup.cfm?setid=373fc1d0-9bd2-414b-8798-7bf04526a12e. Accessed 16 Sept 2015.
5. Nordt SP, Clark RF. Midazolam: a review of therapeutic uses and toxicity. J Emerg Med. 1997;15:357–65.
6. Kilpatrick GJ, McIntyre MS, et al. CNS 7056: a novel ultra-short-acting Benzodiazepine. Anesthesiology. 2007;107:60–6.
7. Sneyd R. Remimazolam: new beginnings or just a me-too? Anesth Analg. 2012;115(2):217–9.
8. Wiltshire HR, Kilpatrick GJ, et al. A placebo and midazolam-controlled phase I single ascending dose study evaluating the safety, pharmacokinetics, and pharmacodynamics of remimazolam (CNS 7056). Part II: populating pharmacokinetic and pharmacodynamic modeling and simulation. Anesth Analg. 2012;115:284–96.
9. Antonik LJ, Goldwater R, et al. A placebo and midazolam-controlled phase I single ascending-dose study evaluating the safety, pharmacokinetics, and pharmacodynamics of remimazolam (CNS 7056): part I. Safety, efficacy and basic pharmacokinetics. Anesth Analg. 2012;115:274–83.
10. Borkett KM, Riff DS, et al. A phase II, randomized, double-blind study of remimazolam (CNS 7056) versus midazolam for sedation in upper gastrointestinal endoscopy. Anesth Analg. 2015;120(4):771–80.
11. Goudra BG, Singh PM. Remimazolam: the future of its sedative potential. Saudi J Anaesth. 2014;8(3):388–91.
12. A phase III of remimazolam in patients undergoing colonoscopy
13. Gertler R, Brown HC, et al. Dexmedetomidine: a novel sedative-analgesic agent. Proc (Bayl Univ Med Cent). 2001;14(1):13–21.

14. Hunter JC, Fontana DJ, et al. Assessment of the role of alpha 2-adrenoceptor subtypes in the antinociceptive, sedative andhypothermic action of dexmedetomidine in transgenic mice. Br J Pharmacol. 1997;122:1339–44.

15. Birnbaumer L, Abramowitz J, et al. Receptor-effect or coupling by G proteins. Biochim Biophys Acta. 1990;1031:163–224.

16. Bhana N, Goa KL, et al. Dexmedetomidine. Drugs. 2000;59:263–8.

17. Pandharipande P, Ely EW, et al. Dexmedetomidine for sedation and perioperative management of critically ill patients. Semin Anesth Perioper Med Pain. 2006;25:43–50.

18. Taittonen MT, Kirvela OA, et al. Effect of clonidine and dexmedetomidine premedication on perioperative oxygen consumption and haemodynamic state. Br J Anaesth. 1997;78:400–6.

19. Aho M, Lehtinen AM, et al. The effect of intravenously administered dexmedetomidine on perioperative hemodynamics and isoflurane requirements in patients undergoing abdominal hysterectomy. Anesthesiology. 1991;74:997–1002.

20. Fragen RJ, Fitzgerald PC. Effect of dexmedetomidine on the minimum alveolar concentration (MAC) of sevoflurane in adults age 55 to 70 years. J Clin Anesth. 1999;11:466–70.

21. Belleville JP, Ward DS, et al. Effects of intravenous dexmedetomidine in humans. I. Sedation, ventilation, and metabolic rate. Anesthesiology. 1992;77:1125–33.

22. Turkmen A, Alten A, et al. The correlation between the Richmond agitation-sedation scale and bispectral index during dexmedetomidine sedation. Eur J Anaesthesiol. 2006;23:300–4.

23. Scheinin B, Lindgren L, et al. Dexmedetomidine attenuates sympathoadrenal responses to tracheal intubation and reduces the need for thiopentone and perioperative fentanyl. Br J Anaesth. 1992;68:126–31.

24. Aho MS, Erkola OA, et al. Effect of intravenously administered dexmedetomidine on pain after laparoscopic tubal ligation. Anesth Analg. 1991;73:112–8.

25. Venn RM, Bradshaw CJ, et al. Preliminary UK experience of dexmedetomidine, a novel agent for postoperative sedation in the intensive care unit. Anaesthesia. 1999;54:1136–42.

26. Jakob SM, Ruokonen E, et al. Dexmedetomidine vs midazolam or propofol for sedation during prolonged mechanical ventilation. JAMA. 2012;307(11):1151–60.

27. Dexmedetamodine prescribing information. http://www.drugs.com/pro/precedex.html. Accessed 4 Dec 2015.

28. De Wolf AM, Fragen RJ, et al. The pharmacokinetics of dexmedetomidine in volunteers with severe renal impairment. Anesth Analg. 2001;93:1205–9.

29. Venn RM, Karol MD, et al. Pharmacokinetics of dexmedetomidine infusions for sedation of postoperative patients requiring intensive care. Br J Anaesth. 2002;88:669–75.

30. Bloor BC, Ward DS, et al. Effects of intravenous dexmedetomidine in humans. II. Hemodynamic changes. Anesthesiology. 1992;77:1134–42.

31. Xu H, Aibiki M, et al. Effects of dexmedetomidine, an alpha 2-adrenoceptor agonist, on renal sympathetic nerve activity, blood pressure, heart rate and central venous pressure in urethane-anesthetized rabbits. J Auton Nerv Syst. 1998;71:48–54.

32. de Ruiter G, Popescu DT, et al. Pharmacokinetics of etomidate in surgical patients. Arch Int Pharmacodyn Ther. 1981;249:180–8.

33. Gooding JM, Corssen G. Effect of etomidate on the cardiovascular system. Anesth Analg. 1977;56:717–9.

34. Lundy JB, Slane ML, et al. Acute adrenal insufficiency after a single dose of etomidate. J Intensive Care Med. 2007;22:111–7.

35. Wagner RL, White PF. Etomidate inhibits adrenocortical function in surgical patients. Anesthesiology. 1984;61:647–51.

36. Wagner RL, White PF, et al. Inhibition of adrenal steroidogenesis by the anesthetic etomidate. N Engl J Med. 1984;310:1415–21.

37. Cotten JF, Husain SS, et al. Methoxycarbonyl-etomidate: a novel rapidly metabolized and ultra-short-acting etomidate analogue that does not produce prolonged adrenocortical suppression. Anesthesiology. 2009;111:240–9.

38. Cotton JF, Le Ge R, et al. Closed-loop continuous infusions of etomidate and etomidate analogs in rats: a comparitive study of dosing and the impact on adrenocortical function.
Anesthesiology. 2011;115:764–73.
39. Le Ge R, Pejo E, et al. Pharmacological studies of methoxycarbonyl etomidate's carboxylic
acid metabolite. Anesth Anal. 2012;115(2):305–8.
40. Pejo E, Cotton JF, et al. In vivo and in vitro pharmacological studies of methoxycarbanyl-
carboetomidate. Anesth Analg. 2012;115:297–304.
41. Cotten JF, Forman SA, et al. Carboetomidate: a pyrrole analog of etomidate designed not to
suppress adrenocortical function. Anesthesiology. 2010;112:637–44.
42. Kay B, Rolly G. I.C.I. 35868, a new intravenous induction agent. Acta Anaesthesiol Belg.
1977;28:303–16.
43. Chen S, Rex D. Registered neurse-administered propofol sedation for endoscopy. Aliment
Pharmacol Ther. 2004;19:147–55.
44. Bachmann-Mennanga B, Ohlmer A, et al. Incidence of pain after intravenous injection of a
medium-/long-chain triglyceride emulsion of propofol. An observational study in 1375
patients. Arzneimittelforschung. 2003;53:621–6.
45. Fischer MJ, Leffler A, et al. The general anesthetic propofol excites nociceptors by activating
TRPV1 and TRPA1 rather than GABAA receptors. J Biol Chem. 2010;285:34781–92.
46. Abdelmalak B, Khanna A, et al. Fospropofol, a new sedative anesthetic, and its utility in the
perioperative period. Curr Pharm Des. 2012;18:6241–52.
47. Lusedra US Prescribing Information. http://medlibrary.org/lib/rx/meds/lusedra/. Accessed 8
Nov 2015
48. Sneyd JR, Rigby-Jones AE. New drugs and technologies, intravenous anaesthesia is on the
move (again). Br J Anaesth. 2010;105:246–54.
49. Welliver M, Rugari SM. New drug, fospropofol disodium: a propofol prodrug. AANA
J. 2009;77(4):301–8.
50. Dhareshwar SS, Stella VJ. Your prodrug releases formaldehyde: should you be concerned?
No! J Pharm Sci. 2008;97:4184–93.
51. Mueller SW, Moore GD, et al. Fospropofol disodium for procedural sedation: emerging evidence of its value? Clin Med Insights Ther. 2010;2:513–22.
52. Levitzky B, Varge J. Fospropofol disodium injection for the sedation of patients undergoing
colonoscopy. Ther Clin Risk Manag. 2008;4:733–8.
53. Schywalsky M, Ihmsen H, et al. Pharmacokinetics and pharmacodynamics of the new propofol prodrug GPI 15715 in rats. Eur J Anaesthesiol. 2003;20(3):182–90.
54. Rex DK, Cohen LB, Kline JK, et al. Fospropofol disodium for minimal-to-moderate sedation
during colonoscopy produces clear-headed recovery: results of a phase 3, randomized, double-
blind trial. Gastrointest Endosc. 2007;65:AB367.
55. Pruitt RE, Cohen LB, et al. A randomized open-label, multicenter, dose-ranging study of sedation with Aquavan injection (GPI 15715) during colonoscopy. Gastrointest Endosc.
2005;61:AB111.
56. Silvestri GA, Vincent BD, et al. A phase 3, randomized, double-blind study to assess the efficacy and safety of fospropofol disodium injection for moderate sedation in patients undergoing
flexible bronchoscopy. Chest. 2009;135:41–7.

Chapter 32
Future Research and Directions in Out of Operating Room Anesthesia

Basavana Goudra and Preet Mohinder Singh

Abstract The traditional surgeries are declining and with that the role of surgeons. The last decade has seen an unprecedented growth of "procedures" that are threatening to replace many conventional surgeries. More importantly, these procedures have moved to places away from the safe operating rooms. As a result, the role of traditional anesthesiologists will wane and anesthesia providers will be required to learn new skills to face the new challenges. This chapter has examined some of the risks associated with providing deep sedation and anesthesia in out of operating room locations. Airway related adverse events dominate along with fluctuating anesthesia needs. Every location poses unique challenges and no single anesthesia provider will be able to master all the skills necessary. Research and publications are lacking in this area. It is hoped that mainstream anesthesia journals will recognize this area of anesthesia and give its due importance.

Keywords Propofol • Sedation • Cardiac electrophysiology • Airway

Introduction

Rarely a surgical approach or an interventional procedure is developed to exploit a newly invented anesthesia technique. Traditionally, anesthesia providers have developed innovative ways to render any novel surgery/procedure pain free and acceptable to patients. Pioneering new techniques, whether in the area of drug delivery or device development, have helped the growth of surgical and non-surgical

B. Goudra, MD, FRCA, FCARCSI (✉)
Department of Anesthesiology and Critical Care Medicine,
Hospital of the University of Pennsylvania, 3400 Spruce Street,
5042 Silverstein Building, Philadelphia, PA 19104, USA
e-mail: goudrab@uphs.upenn.edu

P.M. Singh, MD, DNB, MNAMS
Department of Anesthesiology, Critical Care and Pain Medicine,
All India Institute of Medical Sciences, Ansari Nagar, New Delhi, Delhi 110029, India
e-mail: preetrajpal@gmail.com

© Springer International Publishing Switzerland 2017
B.G. Goudra, P.M. Singh (eds.), *Out of Operating Room Anesthesia*,
DOI 10.1007/978-3-319-39150-2_32

specialties. For example, extensive use of propofol in endoscopy sedation popularized screening colonoscopy. Similarly, application of jet ventilation in electrophysiological procedures has rendered the procedural conditions more favorable to interventional cardiologists. Many soft drugs are in the making and these sedative/hypnotics will be looking for an appropriate "home". Although Sedasys® is dead, the idea of computer assisted personalized sedation (CAPS) is very much alive.

In order to foresee future anesthetic challenges in the area of out of operating room anesthesia (OORA), it is essential to focus on the current developments in related fields. Additionally, the existing anesthetic challenges in out of operating room locations are far from resolved and need consideration. Some of the challenges facing OORA are related to patent safety while others are related to its practice.

Patient Safety and Outcome

Hypoxemia and associated adverse events continue to dominate OORA practice. An often mentioned study in relation to OORA practice is that of Metzner et al. She analyzed the American Society of Anesthesiologists Closed Claims database and specifically studied the pattern of injury associated with OORA practice [1]. An important finding was, that 50 % of the claims from remote locations involved monitored anesthesia care. There were more deaths in remote locations compared to those arising from operating room practice. Respiratory adverse outcomes dominated out of operating room location claims. Moreover, oxygenation/ventilation related events were the most common. Most notably, remote location claims were frequently judged as preventable by better monitoring.

The findings of our own study published in Nov 2015 were no different [2]. In this single center retrospective analysis of 73,029 gastrointestinal (GI) endoscopic procedures, the incidence of cardiac arrest and death (all causes, until discharge) was 6.07 and 4.28 per 10,000 in patients sedated with propofol. This was in comparison to non–propofol-based sedation where the incidence was 0.67 and 0.44 for cardiac arrest and death respectively. The incidence of cardiac arrest during and immediately after the procedure (in the recovery area) for all endoscopies was 3.92 per 10,000, of which 72 % were airway management related. In this study, about 90.0 % of all peri-procedural cardiac arrests occurred in patients who received propofol. Additionally, even non-cardiac arrest adverse events were more likely to occur in patients who received propofol sedation [3]. The latest addition to the reports of propofol related adverse events is the study of Wernli et al. [4, 5]. This study involving patients undergoing colonoscopy concluded, that propofol sedation is associated with a 13 % increase in all complications.

Adverse events like air embolism leading to death are reported during procedures such as endoscopic retrograde cholangiopancreatography (ERCP) and has been a subject of recent research [6–8]. Selected patients might benefit from the use of doppler ultrasound to detect any ERCP related air embolus. It was recently reported that ineffective sedation and unnecessary patient movements might contribute to poorer therapeutic outcomes in patients undergoing advanced endoscopic procedures [9, 10]. In this study, the authors investigated the impact of anesthesia and deep sedation on the efficacy of esophageal radiofrequency ablation (RFA) procedures. They found a high frequency of sedation related adverse events (SRAEs) in patients receiving both general endotracheal anesthesia (GET) and deep sedation. However, they also found an association between the occurrence of SRAE and the number of RFAs needed to achieve complete eradication of dysplasia. This study highlights the important role of anesthesia providers in OORA. Not only do our actions improve the patent comfort, they can impact the therapeutic outcome.

Newer procedures like peroral endoscopic myotomy (POEM) are getting popular. Standardization of anesthesia practice during such procedures is important. Failure of standardization might contribute to adverse events like pulmonary aspiration [11]. Organizations like American Society of anesthesiologists (ASA) and the European Society of Anesthesiologists (ESA) should take a lead role in designing evidence based guidelines for OORA practice.

In summary, respiratory and cardiovascular complications remain a significant factor in patients receiving anesthesia in out of OR locations. Tackling these issues will be a challenge for researchers. Developments of new airway devices and drugs are steps in the right direction [12–15]. Initial results with remimazolam, a new short acting benzodiazepine with a fixed context sensitive half-life are encouraging [16, 17]. It remains to be seen if the drug can keep its initial promise. In our opinion, remimazolam has kinetics that are better suited for intensive care unit (ICU) sedation or as a hypnotic component of total intravenous anesthesia (TIVA), than for GI endoscopy.

Non-anesthesia Providers and Propofol

Administration of propofol by non-anesthesia providers is a very controversial area. We published a meta-analysis reporting the safety of propofol in the hands of non-anesthesia providers [18]. In this study, we compared the safety of propofol sedation in patients who underwent advanced endoscopic procedures. Propofol was administered by either anesthesia providers (AAP) or non-anesthesia providers (NAAP). NAAP were predominantly registered nurses who worked under the supervision of gastroenterologists. After analyzing a total of 3018 and 2374 patients from twenty-six studies in each group (16 NAAP and 10 AAP, respectively), the meta-analysis found a significantly higher incidence of hypoxia (oxygen saturation less than 90%) and airway intervention rates in the AAP group. However, both patient and endoscopist satisfaction rates were lower in the NAAP group. A higher mean dose of propofol administered by the anesthesia providers was the most likely explanation. This might have contributed to both better satisfaction as well as higher sedation-related adverse event rates.

Cost and Efficiency

With the rising cost of US health care, it has become imperative to demonstrate that anesthesia providers not only provide safe sedation, but also bring value for money. Questions have been raised about the value of anesthesia providers in endoscopy suites [19–21]. The most common justification for extensive use of propofol in screening colonoscopy relates to patient acceptability. The patient satisfaction is unquestionably higher with propofol sedation. The success of any national screening program is determined by its uptake. Without public participation, such programs are likely to fail. Fear of discomfort is likely to keep away many of these patients. Considering that the incidence of colonic cancer is demonstrably less since the advent of screening colonoscopy, an argument can be made for propofol use in all the patients. In spite of added sedation risks, the overall gains might swing the balance. Even in relation to cost, the savings in terms of cancer treatment might offset any propofol administration related expenses. Additionally, the burden of dealing with cancer in the family, both financial and psychological cannot be overlooked. The increased efficiency that can be achieved with propofol is another important factor. However, there is no evidence to prove any of these assumptions. A large prospective randomized trial is might answer most of these questions.

Anesthesia Providers

Having a competent group of dedicated anesthesia providers is demonstrated to improve the outcome during the ERCP (Endoscopic Retrograde Cholangiopancreatography) anesthesia [22]. In this single center study of 1167 ERCP procedures, 653 (56%) were assisted by regular and 514 (44%) by non-regular anesthesia consultants. Across all American Society of Anesthesiologists (ASA) grades, regular anesthesiologists provided safer and more efficient care than non-regular anesthesiologists (overall mean anesthesia time of 24.82 ± 12.96 versus 48.63 ± 21.53 min). Safety was established by higher mean oxygen saturations and in the regular anesthesiologists group. This was in spite of the fact that regular anesthesiologists tended to intubate these patients more frequently. Monetarily, if all the procedures were to be performed by regular anesthesiologists, the hospital could have saved US \$758536.00 over the 2 years. This savings was from ERCP associated anesthesia costs alone. As a result, it is important to consider the use of appropriately trained and dedicated anesthesia providers in OORA practice. These findings are important for manpower planning in any large endoscopy center.

Withdrawal of Sedasys® from the US market and the death of Joan Rivers are likely to increase anesthesia provider's requirement during endoscopy sedation [23, 24]. Sedasys is unlikely to be bought by any other company due to inherent flaws in the design [25, 26]. Propofol is an inappropriate sedative for any computer administered personalized sedation. Partially this is because of its enormous pharmacokinetic and pharmacodynamic variability. In the Northeastern United

States, 53 % of all colonoscopies are performed with the use of propofol, while in the Western region only 8 % use propofol [4, 5]. This trend is likely to change.. As a result, anesthesia providers should prepare themselves for a major increase in the use of propofol in OORA. Assuring both safety and comfort to our patients is the key to success.

Documentation

As reported by metzner et al., closed claim studies have highlighted the additional risks experienced by anesthesia providers who choose to work in this OORA [1, 27, 28]. The additional risks will translate to more litigation related activity. Accurate documentation is an area that deserves special attention. Paper based documentation is used by most free standing endoscopy centers. Accurate and timely documentation of all vital events is not always possible with paper charting. However, electronic documentation has its own limitations.

A recent study observed the effect of the introduction of Epic (an electronic data documentation system) on the safety and efficacy of ERCP procedures [29]. In this study, retrospective data of 305 patients who underwent ERCP (wherein electronic charting was used – "Epic group") were compared with 288 patients who underwent the same procedure with paper documentation ("paper group"). Time of various events involved in the procedure such as anesthesia start, endoscope insertion, endoscope removal, and transfer to the post-anesthesia care unit were regularly documented. It was observed that both "anesthesia start to scope insertion" times and "scope removal to transfer" times were significantly less in the Epic group compared to the paper documentation group. Use of Epic system led to a net saving of 4 min per patient. However, the mean oxygen saturations were significantly less in the Epic group that might not be related to true oxygen desaturations. It was concluded that although the electronic documentation allows seamless flow of patients, failure to remove all artifacts can lead to errors and become a source of potential litigation hazard. As a result, it is important to have an understanding of the boundaries of any new electronic documentation system before making what might be a long time commitment.

Emerging Procedures and Opportunities in OORA

A brief mention of peroral endoscopic myotomy (POEM) was made earlier. Other endoscopic procedures may be in the offing. Endoscopic therapy of reflux might become common place. The robot aided endoscope intubation would allow the endoscopists reach intervention sites throughout the large bowel [30, 31]. Effectiveness of gastric neurostimulation in patients with gastroparesis is being actively investigated [32]. As the data on its safety and effectiveness accumulates,

FDA might approve this modality of gastroparesis management. Natural orifice transluminal endoscopic surgery (NOTES) has ushered in a new era in flexible endoscopy [33]. Endoscopic procedures such as full-thickness resection, endoscopic myotomy, direct endoscopic pancreatic necrosectomy and bariatric endoscopy are some of the benefits of this technology. With natural orifice transluminal endoscopic surgery, the scope of the gastroenterologist will expand to treat conditions that have traditionally been out of the reach of the near or foreseeable future endoscopes. As it happened with cardiac surgery in 80s, the role of gastrointestinal surgeon is likely to decrease significantly in the years to come. It is to be expected that procedures will take longer and deep sedation/general anesthesia might be needed more frequently.

Along with major advancements in the field of intracardiac electrophysiology, extracardiac electrophysiology is likely to play a major role in the future. Procedures like epicardial ablation, LAA ligation, pericardial drug and cell delivery are performed in the epicardial space [34–37]. Minimally invasive closed-chest ultrasound-guided substance delivery into the pericardial space is currently experimental. In patients with chronic atrial fibrillation, transcatheter left atrial appendage (LAA) ligation may represent a safer substitute to oral anticoagulation.

In the area of radiotherapy, anesthesiologist's involvement is likely to increase in the area of brachytherapy. As patient's immobility is necessary for placement of many targeted radiation delivery devices, the role of OORA provider will become important.

Conclusions

In the above paragraphs, we have tried to draw the attention of the readers to some of the emerging, controversial and challenging areas as they relate to OORA. Obviously, there is significant work that needs to be done. It is hoped that the chapter will motivate future generation of anesthesia providers to meet the challenges of OORA.

References

1. Metzner J, Posner KL, Domino KB. The risk and safety of anesthesia at remote locations: the US closed claims analysis. Curr Opin Anaesthesiol. 2009;22(4):502–8.
2. Goudra B, Nuzat A, Singh PM, Gouda GB, Carlin A, Manjunath AK. Cardiac arrests in patients undergoing gastrointestinal endoscopy: a retrospective analysis of 73,029 procedures. Saudi J Gastroenterol Off J Saudi Gastroenterol Assoc. 2015;21(6):400–11.
3. Goudra B, Nuzat A, Singh PM, Borle A, Carlin A, Gouda G. Association between type of sedation and the adverse events associated with gastrointestinal (GI) endoscopy-an analysis of five years' data from a tertiary center in the USA. Clin Endosc. 2016. doi: 10.5946/ce.2016.019.
4. Wernli KJ, Brenner AT, Rutter CM, Inadomi JM. Risks associated with anesthesia services during colonoscopy. Gastroenterology. 2016;150:888–94.
5. Goudra B, Singh PM. Forward progress of sedation for gastrointestinal endoscopy requires taking a step back. Gastroenterology. Accpted for publication.

6. Mathew J, Parker C, Wang J. Pulseless electrical activity arrest due to air embolism during endoscopic retrograde cholangiopancreatography: a case report and review of the literature. BMJ Open Gastroenterol. 2015;2(1):e000046.

7. Park S, Ahn JY, Ahn YE, Jeon S-B, Lee SS, Jung H-Y, et al. Two cases of cerebral air embolism that occurred during esophageal ballooning and endoscopic retrograde cholangiopancreatography. Clin Endosc. 2016;49:191–6.

8. Marchesi M, Battistini A, Pellegrinelli M, Gentile G, Zoja R. Fatal air embolism during endoscopic retrograde cholangiopancreatography (ERCP): an "impossible" diagnosis for the forensic pathologist. Med Sci Law. 2016;56(1):70–3.

9. Mizrahi M, Sengupta N, Pleskow DK, Chuttani R, Sawhney MS, Berzin TM. Minor anesthesia-related events during radiofrequency ablation for Barrett's esophagus are associated with an increased number of treatment sessions. Dig Dis Sci. 2016;61(6):1591–6.

10. Goudra B, Singh PM. Providing deep sedation for advanced endoscopic procedures-more than just pushing propofol. Dig Dis Sci. 2016;61(6):1426–8.

11. Goudra B, Singh PM, Gouda G, Sinha AC. Peroral endoscopic myotomy-initial experience with anesthetic management of 24 procedures and systematic review. Anesth Essays Res. 2016;10(2):297–300.

12. Goudra B, Chandramouli M, Singh P, Sandur V. Goudra ventilating bite block to reduce hypoxemia during endoscopic retrograde cholangiopancreatography. Saudi J Anaesth. 2014;8(2):299.

13. Goudra bite block for upper gastrointestinal endoscopy. PubMed – NCBI [Internet]. [cited 2016 Mar 21]. Available from: http://www.ncbi.nlm.nih.gov/pubmed/25657763.

14. Testing the Efficacy and Safety of the WEI Nasal Jet – Full Text View – ClinicalTrials.gov [Internet]. [cited 2016 Mar 21]. Available from: https://clinicaltrials.gov/ct2/show/NCT02005406.

15. Goudra B, Singh P. Remimazolam: the future of its sedative potential. Saudi J Anaesth. 2014;8(3):388.

16. Borkett KM, Riff DS, Schwartz HI, Winkle PJ, Pambianco DJ, Lees JP, et al. A phase IIa, randomized, double-blind study of remimazolam (CNS 7056) versus midazolam for sedation in upper gastrointestinal endoscopy. Anesth Analg. 2015;120(4):771–80.

17. Pambianco DJ, Borkett KM, Riff DS, Winkle PJ, Schwartz HI, Melson TI, et al. A phase IIb study comparing the safety and efficacy of remimazolam and midazolam in patients undergoing colonoscopy. Gastrointest Endosc. 2016;83(5):984–92.

18. Goudra BG, Singh PM, Gouda G, Borle A, Gouda D, Dravida A, et al. Safety of Non-anesthesia Provider-Administered Propofol (NAAP) sedation in advanced gastrointestinal endoscopic procedures: comparative meta-analysis of pooled results. Dig Dis Sci. 2015;60(9):2612–27.

19. Dumonceau J-M. Nonanesthesiologist administration of propofol: it's all about money. Endoscopy. 2012;44(5):453–5.

20. Kumar P. Science and politics of propofol. Am J Gastroenterol. 2005;100(5):1204–5.

21. Rex DK. The science and politics of propofol. Am J Gastroenterol. 2004;99(11):2080–3.

22. Goudra BG, Singh PM, Sinha AC. Anesthesia for ERCP: impact of anesthesiologist's experience on outcome and cost. Anesthesiol Res Pract. 2013;2013:570518.

23. Ethicon Pulling Sedasys Anesthesia System [Internet]. [cited 2016 Mar 11]. Available from: http://www.outpatientsurgery.net/news/2016/03/10/ethicon-pulling-sedasys-anesthesia-system.

24. Rice S. Joan Rivers' death highlights risks in outpatient surgery for seniors. Mod Healthc. 2014;44(37):11.

25. Goudra BG, Singh PM. SEDASYS, sedation, and the unknown. J Clin Anesth. 2014;26:334–6.

26. Goudra BG, Singh PM, Chandrasekhara V. SEDASYS(®), airway, oxygenation, and ventilation: anticipating and managing the challenges. Dig Dis Sci. 2014;59:920–7.

27. Metzner J, Domino KB. Risks of anesthesia or sedation outside the operating room: the role of the anesthesia care provider. Curr Opin Anaesthesiol. 2010;23(4):523–31.

28. Metzner J, Posner KL, Lam MS, Domino KB. Closed claims' analysis. Best Pract Res Clin Anaesthesiol. 2011;25(2):263–76.

29. Goudra B, Singh P, Borle A, Gouda G. Effect of introduction of a new electronic anesthesia record (Epic) system on the safety and efficiency of patient care in a gastrointestinal endoscopy suite-comparison with historical cohort. Saudi J Anaesth. 2016;10(2):127.

30. Rozeboom ED, Bastiaansen BA, de Vries ES, Dekker E, Fockens PA, Broeders IAMJ. Robotic-assisted flexible colonoscopy: preliminary safety and efficiency in humans. Gastrointest Endosc. 2016;83(6):1267–71.

31. Rozeboom ED, Broeders IAMJ, Fockens P. Feasibility of joystick guided colonoscopy. J Robot Surg. 2015;9(3):173–8.

32. Ross J, Masrur M, Gonzalez-Heredia R, Elli EF. Effectiveness of gastric neurostimulation in patients with gastroparesis. Journal of the Society of Laparoendoscopic Surgeons. 18(3):[e2014.00400].

33. Watson RR, Thompson CC. NOTES spin-off for the therapeutic gastroenterologist: natural orifice surgery. Minerva Gastroenterol Dietol. 2011;57(2):177–91.

34. Piers SRD, van Huls van Taxis CFB, Tao Q, van der Geest RJ, Askar SF, Siebelink H-MJ, et al. Epicardial substrate mapping for ventricular tachycardia ablation in patients with non-ischaemic cardiomyopathy: a new algorithm to differentiate between scar and viable myocardium developed by simultaneous integration of computed tomography and contrast-enhanced magnetic resonance imaging. Eur Heart J. 2013;34(8):586–96.

35. Bartus K, Han FT, Bednarek J, Myc J, Kapelak B, Sadowski J, et al. Percutaneous left atrial appendage suture ligation using the LARIAT device in patients with atrial fibrillation: initial clinical experience. J Am Coll Cardiol. 2013;62(2):108–18.

36. Price MJ, Gibson DN, Yakubov SJ, Schultz JC, Di Biase L, Natale A, et al. Early safety and efficacy of percutaneous left atrial appendage suture ligation: results from the U.S. transcatheter LAA ligation consortium. J Am Coll Cardiol. 2014;64(6):565–72.

37. Laakmann S, Fortmüller L, Piccini I, Grote-Wessels S, Schmitz W, Breves G, et al. Minimally invasive closed-chest ultrasound-guided substance delivery into the pericardial space in mice. Naunyn Schmiedebergs Arch Pharmacol. 2013;386(3):227–38.

Index

© Springer International Publishing Switzerland 2017
B.G. Goudra, P.M. Singh (eds.), *Out of Operating Room Anesthesia*,
DOI 10.1007/978-3-319-39150-2

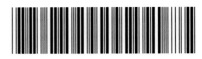